Sexualized Brains

Sexualized Brains

Scientific Modeling of Emotional Intelligence from a Cultural Perspective

edited by Nicole C. Karafyllis and Gotlind Ulshöfer

A Bradford Book
The MIT Press
Cambridge, Massachusetts
London, England

MIT Press books may be purchased at special quantity discounts for business or sales promotional use. For information, please email special_sales@mitpress.mit.edu or write to Special Sales Department, The MIT Press, 55 Hayward Street, Cambridge, MA 02142.

This book was set in Stone sans & Stone serif by SNP Best-set Typesetter Ltd., Hong Kong. Printed and bound in the United States of America.

Library of Congress Cataloging-in-Publication Data

Sexualized brains : scientific modeling of emotional intelligence from a cultural perspective / edited by Nicole C. Karafyllis and Gotlind Ulshöfer.
     p. cm.
  "A Bradford Book".
  Includes bibliographical references and index.
  ISBN 978-0-262-11317-5 (hardcover : alk. paper) 1. Sex differences (Psychology) 2. Sex role–Psychological aspects. 3. Emotional intelligence. I. Karafyllis, Nicole C., 1970– II. Ulshöfer, Gotlind, 1967–
  BF692.2.S497 2008
  155.3'3—dc22
                                    2008008736

10 9 8 7 6 5 4 3 2 1

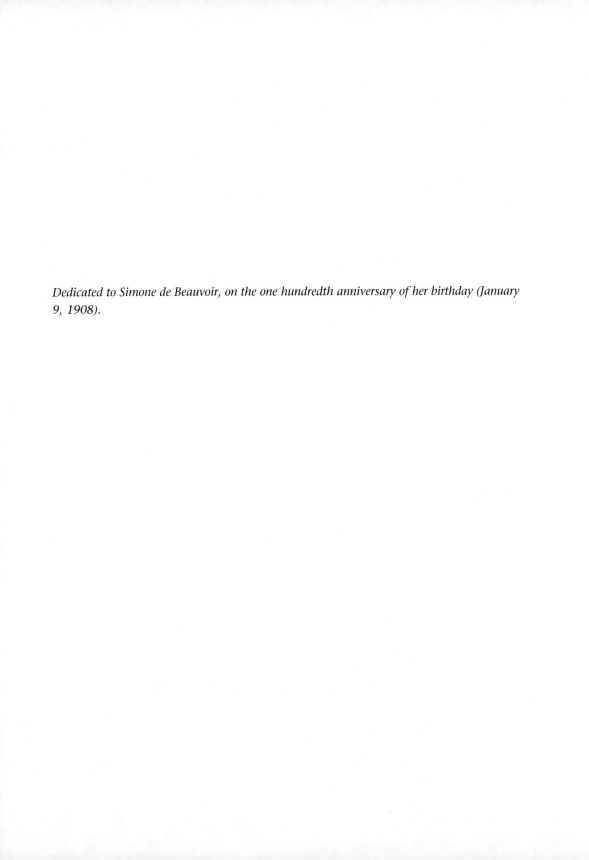

Dedicated to Simone de Beauvoir, on the one hundredth anniversary of her birthday (January 9, 1908).

Contents

Preface   ix
Acknowledgments   xiii
List of Abbreviations   xv

1   Introduction: Intelligent Emotions and Sexualized Brains—Discourses, Scientific Models, and Their Interdependencies   1
Nicole C. Karafyllis and Gotlind Ulshöfer

I   Historical Analysis: Cultural and Scientific Forces

2   Genius, Gender, and Elite in the History of the Neurosciences   53
Michael Hagner

3   The Biosexual Foundations of Our Modern Concept of Gender   69
Robert A. Nye

4   Emotional Styles and Modern Forms of Life   81
William M. Reddy

II   Emotions in the Laboratories: Methods and Impacts

5   Technology Assessment of Neuroimaging: Sex and Gender Perspectives   103
Bärbel Hüsing

6   Emotional Intelligence, Professional Qualifications, and Psychologists' Need for Gender Research   117
Myriam N. Bechtoldt

7   Emotional Intelligence as Pop Science, Misled Science, and Sound Science: A Review and Critical Synthesis of Perspectives from the Field of Psychology   131
Carolyn MacCann, Ralf Schulze, Gerald Matthews, Moshe Zeidner, and Richard D. Roberts

III   Socioeconomic Contexts: Emotional Brains at Work

8   Emotional Capital, Therapeutic Language, and the Habitus of
"The New Man"   151
Eva Illouz

9   Technologies of the Emotional Self: Affective Computing and the "Enhanced
Second Skin" for Flexible Employees   179
Carmen Baumeler

10   The Economic Brain: Neuroeconomics and "Post-Autistic Economics" through
the Lens of Gender   191
Gotlind Ulshöfer

IV   Self-Representations: The Human Person and Her Emotional Media

11   Emotional Intelligence at the Interface of Brain Function, Communication, and
Culture: The Role of Media Aesthetics in Shaping Empathy   221
Kathrin Fahlenbrach and Anne Bartsch

12   Oneself as Another? Autism and Emotional Intelligence as Pop Science, and the
Establishment of "Essential" Differences   237
Nicole C. Karafyllis

13   Social Emotions and Brain Research: From Neurophilosophy to a
Neurosociology of Law   317
Malte-Christian Gruber

References   329
About the Authors   391
Name Index   399
Subject Index   405

Preface

Our title promises an interdisciplinary inquiry into the role of scientific research on emotions and its cultural implications in a broad sense. Scientific culture has a long history of creating the brain as an epistemic object, and science has always intermingled with the life worlds beyond the laboratory's boundaries and shaped practices and ideas. But now, some new developments have prompted us to ask new questions, foremost among them those concerning gender and elite issues—because at present, we observe a fundamental (hetero)sexualization of the brain, which is based on neuroscientific research on emotions and neuroimages of emotions. Other than the rational capacities of the human (usually male) brain, a person's emotional components were long considered to be diffuse properties open to all sexes and gender roles. However, in light of cognitive science research, emotions have acquired cognitive content and thus serve certain functions—for example, in the workplace, for mating, for raising children. The central aim of this book is to elucidate the different architectures of means and ends, in which emotions are scientifically and culturally implemented and according to which they are transmuted into actions and policies.

The idea that emotions have an intelligent core (and vice versa: that intelligence has an emotional core) was triggered by both the neurosciences and psychology, but it recently became popular because of a specific cultural climate. This is also true of the new interest in "essential differences" of male and female brains and behaviors. The book offers a thorough analysis and critical reflection upon both discourse fields and the scientific models underlying these new developments.

The editors' Introduction provides transdisciplinary insight into the basic concepts (e.g., sex, gender, elite, brain, emotion) involved in the neuroscientific discourses and the ones on emotional intelligence (EI), preparing the reader for the chapters that follow and showing the cultural range of neuroscientific impact. It also explains why these fields of expertise, and their experts, were chosen to investigate the interconnected models and discourses of EI, sexualized brains, and emotions research. Outlining the goal envisioned, the development of a cultural philosophy of science that takes "brains" (strictly speaking: persons) and meanings inside and outside the laboratory into account will give readers an idea of how different discourse fields—for example, on leadership and on cognitive emotions—correlate in their basic assumptions.

In part I, historians of science and culture thus explore *historical views* of gender, sex, and elite brains, which are still present driving forces. They show how the relations between emotion and intelligence have been reconfigured. Which leading assumptions derive from which epistemic cultures (including science), with their own codes, symbols, and metaphors? Michael Hagner analyzes the outstanding idea of genius thinking in the history of brain research and shows that the brain is an object highly contaminated by symbols. To possess, to measure, and to open the skulls of prominent men like Friedrich Schiller or Albert Einstein, looking for the essence of their exceptional abilities, has always been an investigative topic for medical research. Women's brains, on the other hand, were of less scientific interest until recently. The focus of the second chapter in part I is on the categories of sex and gender. Robert A. Nye reflects on the resexualization of gender categories in modern biological research, especially on hormones and (trans)sexuality. The words "sex" and "gender," he argues, are used interchangeably to refer to men and women and to male and female. "Gender" now has a biological dimension that feminist radicals in the 1960s never meant for it to have when they popularized the term as a socially constructed category of analysis. William M. Reddy analyzes emotional styles, that is, modern forms of life that are constituted by ways of showing, naming, and hiding emotions. Since this perspective provides an occasion for cultural comparisons, his chapter gives a hint of how strange the discourse on EI must seem to other, non-Western cultures.

Following this historical approach, part II explores various methods of representing and measuring emotions and EI. The focus is on different *techniques* (including apparatuses, instruments, questionnaires employed, i.e., the techniques' media) used to make emotions *visible* and accessible. Thus, this part of the book examines how emotions are modeled as "real." Using the terms introduced to philosophy of science by Ian Hacking (1983), the relation between *representing* and *intervening* is explored. Biologist Bärbel Hüsing looks at the new visualization techniques and different types of brain experiments ("neuroimaging") from a gender point of view. She explains the normative benchmarks set within the methods of functional imaging, showing the brains of men and women "at work." While analyzing current technology from an assessment perspective, the chapter anticipates possible future applications outside the research context and critically discusses their impact. For instance: Could and should neuroimaging be used as a diagnostic tool to determine the "proper sex" of persons prior to transsexual surgery?

Research on intelligence, in the field of psychology, is confronted with the pop-science construct of EI. Psychologist Myriam N. Bechtoldt provides an overview of its history, describes the principal testing methods such as the George Washington Social Intelligence Test and the Mayer–Salovey–Caruso Emotional Intelligence Test, analyzes crucial problems in measurement, and calls for gender research in this area. Carolyn MacCann and her coauthors, Ralf Schulze, Gerald Matthews, Moshe Zeidner, and Richard D. Roberts, make a contribution to the question of whether EI is pop science, is pseudoscience, or constitutes a reputable branch of scientific study. They examine how popular discourse on EI differs from serious scientific study by psychologists, outlining a set of guidelines for distinguishing between the empty rhetoric of pseudoscience and the evidential basis of a science of EI.

Furthermore, the structures of present-day society and the media shape our perceptions and evaluations of emotions and intelligences. In part III we ask, in what socioeconomic contexts are debates on elites, EI, and gender situated? The studies gathered here analyze the cultural mentality of the present discourses on EI, particularly related to the impact on personal success in the workplace. The brain is often not explicitly referred to in these contexts, but it remains a powerful model "underneath" to legitimize social disparities. Eva Illouz contributes a detailed sociological analysis of emotion and of the interrelations of habitus and gender in "therapy-driven" societies. She depicts the image of "the new man" in the age of late capitalism, where everyone has to sell his or her "emotional capital." Elitist thinking triggers the creation of this image, showing that it is not new at all. The self-conception of the employee in flexible capitalism is also a topic in sociologist Carmen Baumeler's analysis. Not only mental training but also enhancement of efficiency by means of technical devices placed close to the body can help to rationalize emotions. Affective and wearable computing give modern employees an "enhanced second skin," signaling and amplifying the natural skin's sensitive capacities. Consequently, flexible employees do not even have to use their brains for communicating job-relevant emotions like stress any more. The brain/body divide is manifested by technological efforts, as sensor and chip detect and communicate rapid pulse rates and perspiration to "somebody" else. The concept of EI mirrors these "technologies of the self," as Michel Foucault has put it.

Gotlind Ulshöfer turns to the ideal market participant in neoclassical economics, the *Homo oeconomicus*, and shows his (!) reconfigurations in recent neuroeconomics. The topos of his "autistic behavior" is also discussed in the critical post-autistic economics (PAE) movement, which has recently developed. Emphasizing the socioeconomic element of emotions and EI from a gender perspective, Ulshöfer's chapter places neuroeconomics in relation to economic elites, emotional labor, and fair p(l)ay.

The chapters in part IV, the final section, deal with philosophical and cultural perspectives in the narrower sense of the term "culture," exploring the media of emotions and self-representations. The first chapter in part IV takes the reader to the cinema. Media scientists Kathrin Fahlenbrach and Anne Bartsch show the aesthetic shaping of emotions between neuro- and EI research. They analyze the communication of audiovisual meta-emotions and the performance of the meta-subject "brain." The second chapter in part IV focuses on the *extreme-male-brain theory* against the background of

EI and autism and starts by asking why autists recently became so popular in the movies and what the sciences have to do with it. Even if the neurosciences and the psychology of EI both regard the *brain* as a boundary object, their views on the self and the other have different implications, as philosopher and biologist Nicole C. Karafyllis points out. Where neurobiology stresses the somatic determination of the *self* and somehow apologizes for antisocial behavior (e.g., autism), organizational psychology, in contrast, emphasizes individuals' responsibility for their own social effectiveness and offers methods for increasing it. Both approaches undermine the reflexive structure of the "self," as it is known in phenomenology (Ricœur 1992), and depict a human being who leads the life of an *autist*. The wide-ranging implications of depersonalization give added importance to uncovering the unspoken assumptions about gender and social stratification which underlie, but have not yet explicitly figured within, the terms of this ongoing debate. Autists have deficiencies in affect and empathy. However, simply because four out of five diagnosed autists are men, is it legitimate to say that "the male brain" is *essentially* autistic? And if the answer is "yes," does this really legitimize saying that men are more suitable for information technology and science jobs in the future, as top brain scientist Simon Baron-Cohen (2004, 185) has suggested? And, lastly: How do you find a male brain—is it always inside a man's body?

Finally, lawyer and philosopher Malte-Christian Gruber scrutinizes the idea of neurosociology and the meta-subject of an organism-like society in light of Antonio R. Damasio's writings. In addition, he demonstrates how the distinct border between animal and human behavior affects the idea of useful and sociable emotions. The law, in general, is dependent on a clear-cut distinction between the two. Ideas of justice and, at the same time, the idea of humanity are both challenged by recent neuroscientific findings.

We tackle the problems mentioned above with experts from psychology, sociology, biology, philosophy, history, cultural anthropology, media studies, economics, and law—and try to untie at least a few of the knots, because we believe there is a common thread: the unperceived attempts to control the autonomous individual and personal growth, and the discursive strategies of persuasion to appreciate exactly that mode of control in the name of science. Reasons and emotions might not be natural antagonists, but they are cultural antagonists in knowledge societies. This may lead to a renewed recognition (Honneth 1996) of emotions, which takes individual experiences and goals seriously, instead of an appreciation of sex-specific, "intelligent" behavior that is extrinsically motivated.

Acknowledgments

We would like to thank—really emotionally!—the people who made this book possible, starting with all our inspiring authors. Working with them—across Lake Constance, the Mediterranean, the Atlantic, and the Pacific—was both a great pleasure and an honor.

We would also like to thank the following individuals, groups, and institutions: the students of Johann Wolfgang Goethe University Frankfurt (Germany), where the initiating congress on "Emotional Intelligence, Gender, and Elites" took place in Spring 2006, who challenged us with interesting discussions and inspired us to embark on a larger research project related to this topic; the Templeton Research Foundation (United States) and the Protestant Academy Arnoldshain (Germany), which cofunded the congress; and the chair of the Frankfurt lecture series on "The Human Person" (2005–2008), Thomas M. Schmidt.

Native speakers Stephen L. Starck and Staci von Boeckmann did a tremendous job fine-tuning the translated texts. Ramsay Richmond and many of the European authors' English-speaking colleagues proofread the chapters first. Other intellectual debts are acknowledged in the authors' chapters. Administrative assistants Gabriele Blumer, Yasar Damar, Sebastian Duchatsch, and Karin Weintz helped with correcting and formatting the manuscript.

Thomas E. Stone, senior editor at MIT Press, and Katherine A. Almeida, in-house editor at MIT Press, were more than helpful in supporting this project and were a pleasure to work with. We also thank the anonymous reviewers of the manuscript for recommending this work for publication. We are indebted to our colleagues, acquaintances, and friends Astrid Dinter, Moritz Epple, Hille Haker, Silvia Krömmelbein, Alan Mittleman, Barbara Murphy, Ruxandra Sireteanu, Anja Schäfers, Elke Tönges, and Elke Wagner for their advice and support. Last but not least, we would like to thank the psychologists John ("Jack") D. Mayer, Richard D. Roberts, Keith Oatley, and Jeannette Haviland-Jones for being open-minded and making many helpful suggestions.

For permission to quote copyrighted materials, we are grateful to the following: Antonio R. Damasio for the lines in *Looking for Spinoza: Joy, Sorrow, and the Feeling*

Brain (2003); Daniel Goleman, and Bantam Books, for the lines from *Emotional Intelligence: Why It Can Matter More than IQ* (1995); Anne C. Krendl, and the journal *Social Neuroscience*, for the images in Anne C. Krendl, C. Neil Macrae, William M. Kelley, Jonathan A. Fugelsang, Todd F. Heatherton, 2006, "The good, the bad, and the ugly: An fMRI investigation of the functional anatomic correlates of stigma" (*Social Neuroscience* 1, 1: 5–15); Rosalind W. Picard, and MIT Press, for the lines in *Affective Computing* (1998); Rosalind W. Picard and Charles Q. Du, for the lines in "Monitoring stress and heart health with a phone and wearable computing" (*Offspring* 1, 1 [2002]: 14–22); Tania Singer, and the journals *Science* and *Nature*, for the images in Tania Singer, Ben Seymour, John P. O'Dougherty, Klaas E. Stephan, Raymond J. Dolan, and Chris D. Frith, 2006, "Empathic neural responses are modulated by the perceived fairness of others" (*Nature* 439: 466–469), and for the images in Tania Singer, Ben Seymour, John O'Doherty, Holger Kaube, Raymond J. Dolan, and Chris D. Frith, 2004, "Empathy for pain involves the affective but not sensory components of pain" (*Science* 303, no. 5661: 1157–1162).

Some of the paragraphs of Eva Illouz' chapter come from chapter 6 in her new book *Saving the Modern Soul: Therapy, Emotions, and the Culture of Self-Help* (2008), University of California Press, The Regents of the University of California.

The historical images in Michael Hagner's chapter appeared in his book *Geniale Gehirne: Die Geschichte der Elitegehirnforschung* (2004), Wallstein Publisher, Göttingen.

List of Abbreviations

ACC	Anterior cingulate cortex
ADHD	Attention-deficit/hyperactivity disorder
AES	Assessing Emotions Scale
AI	Artificial intelligence
AQ	Autism spectrum quotient
BBC	British Broadcasting Corporation
CEO	Chief executive officer
CPI	California Psychological Inventory
CT	(Roentgen-Ray) Computed tomography
DNA	Deoxyribonucleic acid
DSM–II–R	American Psychiatric Association's Diagnostic and Statistical
DSM–III	Manual of Mental Disorders (II–R, second revised ed.; III, third
DSM–III–R	ed.; III–R, third revised ed.; IV, fourth ed.)
DSM–IV	
EEG	Electroencephalography
EI	Emotional intelligence
EQ	Emotional quotient
EQ-i	Emotional Quotient Inventory
ERP	Event-related potential
FDA	U.S. Food and Drug Administration
fMRI	functional magnetic resonance imaging
FTM	Female to male (transsexuals)
g	general intelligence

GMIF	UNESCO's Gender Mainstreaming Implementation Framework for 2002–2007
GWSIT	George Washington Social Intelligence Test
HFA	High-functional autists
HIV	Human immunodeficiency virus
IQ	Intelligence quotient
IT	Information technology
LFA	Low-functional autists
LSD	Lysergic acid diethylamide
MEG	Magnetoencephalography
MEIS	Multifactor Emotional Intelligence Scale
MLQ	Multifactor leadership questionnaire
MPD	Multiple personality disorder
MRI	Magnetic resonance imaging
MSCEIT	Mayer–Salovey–Caruso Emotional Intelligence Test
NA	Nucleus accumbens
NASA	National Aeronautics and Space Administration
NEO-FFI	NEO Five-Factor Inventory
	NEO: Neuroticism, Extraversion, Openness
NIRS	Near infrared spectroscopy
NSA	National Security Agency (U.S.)
OT	Oxytocin
PAE	Post-autistic economics
PC	Personal computer
	Political correctness
PDD	Pervasive developmental disorder
PDG	Prisoner's dilemma game
PET	Positron emission tomography
r	Pearson correlation coefficient

SII	Second somatosensory area of cerebral cortex
sMRI	structural magnetic resonance imaging
SPECT	Single photon emission computed tomography
SQ	Systemizing quotient
TEIQue	Trait emotional intelligence questionnaire
TMS	Transcranial magnetic stimulation
UNESCO	United Nations Educational, Scientific, and Cultural Organization

1   Introduction: Intelligent Emotions and Sexualized Brains—Discourses, Scientific Models, and Their Interdependencies

Nicole C. Karafyllis and Gotlind Ulshöfer

The last decade, despite its bad news, has also seen an unparalleled burst of scientific studies of emotion. Most dramatic are the glimpses of the brain at work, made possible by innovative methods such as new brain-imaging technologies. They have made visible for the first time in human history what has always been a source of deep mystery: exactly how this intricate mass of cells operates while we think and feel, imagine and dream. This flood of neurobiological data lets us understand more clearly than ever how the brain's centers for emotion move us to rage or tears, and how more ancient parts of the brain, which stir us to make war as well as love, are channeled for better or worse. This unprecedented clarity on the workings of emotions and their failings brings into focus some fresh remedies for our collective emotional crisis.

—Daniel Goleman, *Emotional Intelligence: Why It Can Matter More than IQ,* 1995, xi.

1.1   The Starting Point

In this book, leading scholars from both sides of the Atlantic focus on the new neurodisciplines, their sexual stereotyping and use of gender role clichés, and their underlying relations to the "hype" around Emotional Intelligence (EI). The latter was kicked off by Daniel Goleman's best-sellers on EI, which have appeared since the mid-1990s[1] and include his most recent publication, *Social Intelligence* (2006). His books belong to the category of pop science, as do Simon Baron-Cohen's *The Essential Difference: The Truth about the Male and Female Brain* (2003) and Louann Brizendine's *The Female Brain* (2006), to name just two of many.[2] This list may seem an incongruity at first sight. Though coming from different disciplinary backgrounds, these authors have jointly opened a discourse field on "sexualized brains," which not only laypeople but also scientists—working on the interplay of emotion and intelligence—have inhabited. Emotions are crucial parts of manifold academic concepts such as personality, morality, social stigma, unconsciousness, intelligence, survival of the fittest, and many others. And, of course, emotions are part of nonacademic public and private life. With

regard to the distinction between public and private life, and academic and nonacademic concepts of emotional life, their boundaries became more porous than ever,
particularly through the new brain research on emotions.

In contrast to previous studies on differences in brain weight and size, and in the
symmetry of men's and women's brains, and different grades of interconnectivity
between their brains' hemispheres, which are said to lead to different cognitive performances (Kimura 1999; see Schmitz 2006a for a critical overview), many of the
present studies on sex differences in the human brain are inspired by the idea that
individuals consist of brains which are *essentially* male/female. It is assumed that the
sexualized brain's essence is different with regard to both thinking and feeling. In
current emotions research of the neurosciences, the map of the human brain has a
new earth at its center (no sun), around which many planets, metaphorically embodying scientific approaches, are orbiting: the *amygdala*. Particularly social (cognitive)
neurosciences have been creating a new cosmic system around this small area of the
brain, and they hope to one day finally understand "it all": emotions, sexuality,
behaviors, attitudes, relationships, social norms, personal success, and more—in short,
the human and the society (in singular). However, this new anthropology which is
now on the horizon is still working with classical stereotypes. The female brain is said
to be good at empathizing, while the male brain is adept at systemizing (Baron-Cohen
2004, 2ff). Even if this sounds like an old story to feminists, the rhetorics and entities
recently have changed: It is not women and men, or their bodies and their brains,
but female brains and male brains.

One major step in this direction was taken with the neuroscientific idea that emotions can be found in the brain. The colored representations of emotionally active
areas, resulting from brain- and neuroimaging techniques, are, it seems, so persuasive
that their character as representations (i.e., representing something which has been
established in advance as an epistemic model, in order to serve a certain function) is
fading away in public discourse. It is worth noting that models are always models *of*
something and models *for* something. The same is true of image representations, particularly when they have been generated in scientific contexts (Köchy 2005).

The main model relevant for this new kind of emotion research is the "emotional
system" of the brain which is modeled as a composition of brain areas, regions, and
related structures of different order (see section 1.5). From an epistemological point
of view, the newly defined emotional system overlaps with former concepts like
"lymbic system" and "pain matrix." Neural processing of emotions engages diverse
structures from the highest to the lowest levels of the neuraxis, and this processing
is mediated by hormones and neurotransmitters. Areas like the hypothalamus and
the septal area, regions like the orbitofrontal cortex, and related structures like the
amygdala (an almond-shaped complex of related nuclei) and the nucleus accumbens
belong to the emotional system, that is, they function—though not exclusively—for

emotionality. According to Tania Singer et al. (2004b, 2006), they also function for morality, understood in this specific context as a category in which ideas of (economic) fairness, empathy, and the desire for punishment of "cheaters" are involved. Both emotionality and morality are potentials (Hubig 2006), which have to be instantiated to generate emotions (or morals)—a fact that is disguised by using the term "system." In pop science texts, the emotional system is often referred to as "the reptile mind," as parts of it are considered primitive in connection with evolutionary biology. In the experiments presented by the Singer group and others, men and women show significant differences in the neural activities of their "reptile minds." Again, female brains were found to be good empathizers (Singer et al. 2004a), but this time "women" were referred to explicitly. In the experimental setting of neuroimaging, where (presumably only heterosexual) couples were tested, results showed that women "experience"[3] the physical pain of a loved one all but as their own, though only part of the pain matrix is involved (see figure 1.1; color plate 1). In the article, published in the journal *Science*, there is no indication of a reverse experimental design, that is, in this study the empathic capacity of men was apparently not tested:

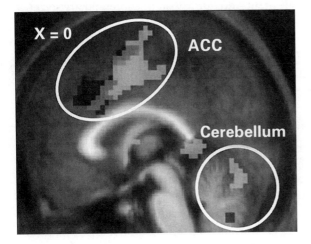

Figure 1.1
(color plate 1) Pain-related activation associated with either experiencing pain in oneself or observing one's partner feeling pain: activation in anterior cingulate cortex and cerebellum. Areas in green represent significant activation ($p < .001$) for the contrast (pain–no pain) in the "self" condition and areas in red for the contrast (pain–no pain) in the "other" condition. The results are superimposed on a mean T1-weighted structural scan of the 16 subjects. Activations are shown on sagittal slides. (Source: Singer, Seymour, O'Doherty, Kaube, Dolan, and Frith. 2004. "Empathy for Pain Involves the Affective but Not Sensory Components of Pain." *Science* 303, no. 5661: 1157–1162, 1158; reprinted by permission from the American Association for the Advancement of Science: *Science*, © 2004.)

We assessed brain activity in the female partner while painful stimulation was applied to her and her partner's right hand through an electrode. . . . The partner was seated next to the MRI scanner and the right hand of each subject was placed on a tilted board, allowing the female partner with help of a mirror system to see her and her partner's right hand. On a large screen situated behind the board, cues were presented in random order indicating whether she (self) or her partner (other) would get low (no pain condition) or high (pain condition) stimulation. We were especially interested in comparing pain-related brain activity . . . in the context of "self" and "other" (Singer et al. 2004a, 1158).

The boundary between the self and the other seems to be especially thin in women, reminding one of the old misogynous concept of the flexibility and assimilating abilities of women, rather than the rigidness of men (see, e.g., Weininger 1980). It might be that the motivation behind this kind of research is a desire to show the specificities of women's brains and, by the same token, to challenge the model of "the" brain because in terms of the history of science, it has usually been men's brains which have been scrutinized in the search for the ideal type of human brain (Hagner 2004); or the (questionable) aim might be to prove that women are—morally—the better humans, or mammals. However, what if good morals—an idea which Baron-Cohen (2004) also associates with the female brain—do not pay off in contemporary societies and market economies? As Singer et al. (2004a, 1157) put it, "Human survival depends on the ability to function effectively within a social context"—but what "human" and "survival" mean on the personal (rather than the species, population, and organism) level, or even what it means to "function effectively within a social context," remains obscure. As will emerge in due course, this special kind of research has a range of social, ethical, and socioeconomic implications related to exclusion, particularly concerning gender-related identities and the social division of labor.

The main arguments for "intelligent emotions" are supposed to be debated in the classical disciplines of psychology and biology, which have opposing theories of mind, cognition, and subjectivity, though, with regard to the soul (Greek *psyche*), contemporary biology has no theory of subjectivity at all. In the last decades, however, parts of biology and psychology have fused and established, for example, a *psychobiology* that focuses on hormones and neurotransmitters, a focus which is important for the emerging research fields of social neurosciences and pharmacogenetics (see, e.g., the findings of Hariri et al. 2002). Thus, when interpreting bio–psycho–scientific findings concerning the idea of the human, moreover the human person,[4] these sciences are in need of the humanities and the cultural and social studies in order to come to terms with the ontological and metaphysical hypercodes accompanying scientific modeling.

Nevertheless, they rarely adopt the findings of the latter, but on the contrary export their basic anthropological assumptions, which are often rooted in modern versions of Darwinism as well as in technofuturism (not infrequently related to research on humanoid robots and artificial intelligence in the cognitive sciences). Very often, emotions are important constituents of these assumptions, and they are reframed within special types of intelligence, as can be seen, for instance, in the recent book *Mating Intelligence* (Geher and Miller 2007), in which the authors, from the field of psychology, argue that there is something like a reproductive system in the mind. Of course, this system functions differently according to the different sexes, that is, only the two which are important for biology: men and women, identified by the well-established physical body capacities for biological reproduction. However, referring to the discourse field on EI, and by means of the associated techniques of brain- and neuroimaging (e.g., positron emission tomography and fMRI), which, together, allowed these new strategies for sexualizing the brain to emerge, scientists do not simply examine biological reproduction. They go much further, shaping the cultural understanding of what can be regarded as uniquely human, moreover uniquely female and male, in industrialized Western societies.

Claudia Wassmann argues that the brain became an icon as a normative instance especially in the years 1984–2002, due to several highly recognized TV programs on brain scans: "a gap has opened between the representation of brain imaging in the lay press and the properties brain scans acquired within the neurosciences. This gap has widened since the beginning of the new century" (Wassmann 2007, 153; see also Phelps and Thomas 2003). Within the same time period, the brain as icon has also become influential in the humanities and the social sciences. In all new disciplines which have emerged with the prefix "neuro" (e.g., neurosociology, neurophilosophy, neurotheology, neuroeconomics), the relationship between emotion and intelligence, the former topoi of the (potentially) irrational and the rational, are being (or already have been) reconfigured. According to neuroscientists (e.g., Damasio 1994, 2003), emotions now seem to have an original cognitive content and ensure rationality, at least in the brains of "normal" people. "Cognition," in the cognitive sciences, has a meaning which is quite different from its typical understanding within philosophy (i.e., a conceptual and propositional structure). Rather, in the cognitive sciences, it is "used for any kind of mental operation or structure that can be studied in precise terms" (Lakoff and Johnson 1999, 11). In this view, a "cognitive unconscious" exists, which, moreover, opposes psychological traditions and their ontologies of soul and mind. In recent years, models and terms from the field of neurosciences and cognitive sciences have colonized the epistemic cultures (Knorr-Cetina 1999) of many other disciplines, in the process transforming some of their ideas about what is normal, what is human, and, not least, what determines a functioning society.

In the meantime, EI, related to research on personality, has become an important issue in the discussion of creating *elites* in the business world. It was Goleman (1995, 2006) himself who drew the connection between brain research and mental training for better human relationships; according to him, both are needed to make a "better" society. This idea of improvement by both understanding and managing emotions can, described less dramatically and with less of a focus on the brain, also be found in, for example, the popular-science work of renowned psychologist Paul Ekman (2007). For Goleman, increasing the ability to understand and control emotions is seen as a crucial tool, especially for creating more effective organizations in a functioning society ("leadership").[5] At the popular level, "EI" has therefore become a buzzword in the discussion of behavioral issues in private, corporate, and public life. The compelling need for new solutions to many pressing problems, which Goleman describes as an "emotional crisis," ensured vast sales of self-help literature and sizeable participation in EI coaching seminars. Most of these problems, like social deprivation, drug abuse, aggressive behavior, and mental depression, are, it seems, driven by the isolation and self-centeredness of the modern subject. Goleman's answer to these problems is individual brain training and an emotional appeal for social commitment at various levels. In order to overcome the purported "emotional crisis," he offers a sort of turnkey solution and (though also educated in sociology) ignores not only the sociological patterns of reflexion but also the broader philosophical conceptions of mind, self, and subjectivity (see, e.g., Davidson 1989, Ricœur 1992, Godfrey-Smith 1998, Metzinger 2004, Searle 2005). These omissions are, at least to some extent, due to the pop-scientific character of his books, and due to the influence of contemporary cognitive science on shaping both a theory of mind and the category of mind reading by means of the concepts of behavior and cognition (e.g., Johnson 1987, Lakoff and Johnson 1999, Clark 2003).

However, providing a detailed analysis of Goleman's publications is neither our aim nor the reason behind this book. In fact it is the discourse field which the books on EI and related research fields have opened, that is, the assumed sex and gender differences—in the human brain and in the person's mind—and the underlying assumptions of, for example, social rank, leadership, empathy, mind reading, and their implications, that have inspired this book.

1.2   The Goal: Toward a Cultural Philosophy of Science

We want to contribute methodologically to a transdisciplinary approach, understanding scientific concepts, images, and narratives as cultural constituents in a cultural philosophy of science still to be developed, accompanied by sociology, history of science, and other disciplines (Karafyllis 2006b). For the discipline of philosophy itself, the term could be read in both ways, that is, that the classical philosophy of science which was mainly centered on experiments and theories generated within the laboratory setting is being challenged to become more oriented toward the life world of people's everyday experiences (Schütz and Luckmann 2003; see also Latour 1993) and that the subdiscipline of cultural philosophy is being encouraged to apply its concepts and theories (e.g., media theories) not only to society as a systemic whole, or a specific culture in the narrower sense, but also to the special context of doing science and stimulating the development of new disciplines (e.g., Latour and Woolgar 1986, Knorr-Cetina 1999).

In recent years, several outstanding books and articles leading in that direction have been published. Many of them refer to the theory modeling and integrating role of *metaphors* in science (e.g., Otis 1999, Keller 2002), while others explore the constitution of the assumed border between culture and science (Illouz 2008). Science can, on the one hand, be understood as a unique culture of its own and can be analyzed as opposing some sort of "other" culture, for example, culture of the life world. On the other hand, science itself consists of many subcultures and related disciplinary codes, many of them dealing with "the same" sort of problem, for example, EI. An example would be the disciplines of biology and psychology, partially fused and/or split into different divisions with various labels as, for instance, cognitive science, brain science, neuroscience, psychobiology, natural language processing, or even the science of artificial intelligence (AI; e.g., Minsky 2006). Looking closely at the models involved, one finds they do not in any way all deal with the same problem but with different ones. What makes them fuse is that they share metaphors and an overall sociopolitical background. For instance, when Goleman (2006) describes the interplay of neural-based and social emotions saying "we are wired to connect," he is employing a technical metaphor familiar from the source domain of robotics. And many uses of "mind" in the target domains of neuro- and cognitive science are related to the source domains of philosophy and psychology. Metaphors are also used to cross the border between science and pop science. The cross-border trade of metaphors takes place as well between society and science, challenging the very idea of a border (on the philosophy of metaphor, see Ortony 1993, König 1994, Karafyllis 2006a; in relation to gender, see Brown 2005).

Furthermore, all these subcultures intermingle with the life worlds of different individuals and their different cultural settings and historical traditions of understanding emotions and intelligence. For instance, in Western democratic and liberal societies, at the moment, it seems to be politically incorrect to speak of existing elites, or, worse, *the* elite (see section 1.4).[6] As historian Michael Hagner (this volume) points out, the term "elite brain" was first introduced in 1904 (in German: "Elitegehirn") and has had a strong relation to racial oppression. At present, this term is not explicitly used in scientific discourse. Looking at the pop science market related to EI, neuroscience, and leadership, deeply involved in a "therapeutic culture" (see Illouz, this volume), one gets the idea that this silence could soon be over. To put it bluntly, the well-known metaphor "class brain" is not suspected of being politically incorrect, as long as the brain remains an object of the imagination rather than of material representation of human capacities. Once "brain" is used in the sense of "essence," and connected to functionally interpreted qualities and quantities, it will "make" classes, that is, social representations. The ascription of sex to brains, in this sense, will also influence the structuring of society, related to both qualities and quantities. A quality would be the brain's capacity for empathy, which can then be interpreted, functionally, as relevant for service jobs or child care (see section 1.6). Moreover, it can be associated with both a quantity and a stereotype, for example, that female brains or women's brains have "more" of this quality. On the other hand, researchers state that men's blood has a higher level (quantity) of testosterone (quality), serving the evolutionary end of fighting against other male competitors to guarantee the survival of his genes (function) (see Sapolsky 1997, Baron-Cohen 2004, Brizendine 2006). Therefore it is not enough to stress—from a philosopher's point of view—that brain- and neurorhetorics imply naturalization, or biological determinism, which, moreover, are not necessarily the same thing. Neurorhetorics imply much more than that. Thinking further, the book titles, like Baron-Cohen's *The Essential Difference*, promising to analyze "the" essential difference between male and female brains contribute to the development of social classification; moreover, they bring a new sexual bias into social representations as will be shown in due course. Other than dealing with differences, in plural, they manifest the heteronomy of the two biological sexes of mammals, that is, heterosexuality. Perhaps the academic reluctance to imply such a broad range of consequences, triggered by the renewed sexualization of the brain, was one of the reasons why renowned psychologist and neuroendocrinologist Melissa Hines titled her recent book on sex differences *Brain Gender* (2004). She stresses that a relationship between a brain structure and a behavior does *not* confirm the argument that the behavior results from this structure (causality) or that the structure determines the behavior (determinism). Referring to the often-found deductions from the animal model to the human sphere (see Gruber, this volume), Hines' advice is that scientists should be more reluctant to make such deductions. While accepting the importance of gonadal hormones for the phenotypic sex differences, including genital ambiguity, Hines nevertheless votes in favor of flexible gender identity for neuroscientific reasons, as the brain is a highly responsive organ, and because of its plasticity, it is always open to experiences.

Argued quite similarly at first glance, the decrease in neuroplasticity from childhood to adulthood is the main hypothesis of Bruce E. Wexler's approach in *Brain and Culture* (2006), from which he draws some social implications, particularly related to migration and ethnicity (e.g., ethnic violence). The brain of an adult, according to Wexler, tries to piece the social environment together to fit the internal structure. Note that "the brain" *does* something, that is, it constructs its world. In contrast, a child's brain shapes itself according to environmental features, which Wexler regards as one of the reasons why children of immigrants adapt more easily to a new culture, compared to their parents. By changing the cultural environment, each generation shapes the brains of the next. In his approach, he merges intraindividual variability (i.e., variations within one person, especially occurring between childhood and adulthood) and interindividual variability (i.e., variations between both generations and cultures) of the human brain. Thus, Wexler votes for a cultural evolution of the brain—but it remains unclear how the term "culture" differs from "environment." In many neuroscientific writings, "culture" is reduced to "social environment." In Wexler's concept, however, culture seems to be determined by the spatial patterns of geography. Apart from its reductionism, this is interesting because the metaphors of cartography ("map") and navigation have been highly influential in brain research since the early modern period (Reddy 2001). Obviously, though, the mere focus on behaviors does not grasp the richness of symbols, narratives, and codes, which create cultural styles and are stored in cultural memories.

As language is able not only to cross disciplinary borders but also to overcome the somehow artificial border between science and society, it is worth thoroughly investigating this border and considering the market value of specific terms, for example, "emotional intelligence," "male/female brain," and "emotions." Moreover this view can contribute to gender studies of science (e.g., Haraway 1985, 1989; Harding 1991; Schiebinger 1993; Meinel and Renneberg 1996; Rouse 1996; Kourany 2002; von Braun and Stephan 2005; Ebeling and Schmitz 2006; Konnertz, Haker, and Mieth 2006; Wahrig 2006; Dickenson 2007), where linkages between dominant socioeconomic and elitist structures related to science have been pointed out most intensely. The traditional approaches, looking at scientific instruments, experiments, techniques, and machines, will not be neglected but will be placed in a socioeconomic and cultural setting with certain norms and values in which theories and experiments only then make sense.

Consequently, we editors bring together academic fields which seem to have nothing in common at first sight (e.g., the socioeconomic debate on elites and the popularity of brain research), and at the same time we want to separate the rhetorical alliances of fields which seem to have much in common (e.g., research on personality, research on the brain, and research on "the self"; sexuality in the life sciences and gender discourse in the social sciences and humanities). Our aim is to reflect on a new intellectual area. *The area encompassed could be described as the emotional brain culture of individuals who rationalize their "self" while still believing in their unique personality.*

1.3 Step 1: Reflecting on the Emotional Intelligence Hype from a Gendered Perspective

A short glance at one of Goleman's examples (1995, 44f; summarizing and interpreting findings of Berkeley psychologist Jack Block; Block 1995) for amendable emotionality offers a first hint at the high relevance of gender, social, and philosophical studies in this field:

The high-IQ male is typified—no surprise—by a wide range of intellectual interests and abilities. He is ambitious and productive, predictable and dogged, and untroubled by concerns about himself. He also tends to be critical and condescending, fastidious and inhibited, uneasy with sexuality and sensual experience, unexpressive and detached, and emotionally bland and cold.

By contrast, men who are high in emotional intelligence are socially poised, outgoing and cheerful, not prone to fearfulness or worried rumination. They have a notable capacity for commitment to people or causes, for taking responsibility, and for having an ethical outlook; they are sympathetic and caring in their relationships. Their emotional life is rich but appropriate; they are comfortable with themselves, others, and the social universe they live in.

Purely high-IQ women have the expected intellectual confidence, are fluent in expressing their thoughts, value intellectual matters, and have a wide range of intellectual and aesthetic interests. They also tend to be introspective, prone to anxiety, rumination, and guilt, and hesitate to express their anger openly (though they do so indirectly).

Emotionally intelligent women, by contrast, tend to be assertive and express their feelings directly, and to feel positive about themselves; life holds meaning for them. Like the men, they are outgoing and gregarious, and express their feelings appropriately (rather than, say, in outbursts they later regret); they adapt well to stress. Their social poise lets them easily reach out to new people; they are comfortable enough with themselves to be playful, spontaneous, and open to sensual experience. Unlike the women purely high in IQ, they rarely feel anxious or guilty, or sink into rumination.

Goleman, here, makes two purifications on a vertical level (1. pure IQ types, in contrast to—less pure—EI types; 2. women/men). Instead of robust empirical data, he simply provides two reasons for the suggested dichotomies: First, women in general never seem to reach important business qualifications, for example, productivity and ambition. Second, they do not climb the highest step of EI, that is, they never reach "pure" EI. IQ-type women are depicted as intellectually confident (but only as far as they are expected to be), thoughtful, aesthetically oriented, and passive–aggressive, whereas high-IQ men, while being ambitious and productive, are on the whole unerotic. According to Goleman, emotionally intelligent women learn to control their assumed outbursts, are playful, and are highly functional in coping with stress (see section 1.6). Unlike their male counterparts, they still do not seem to fully recover from their feelings of guilt and anxiety, no matter how emotionally intelligent they are.

Whether or not this caricature, reminiscent of the classic nineteenth-century stereotype of the "male intellectual" and the "middle-class housewife" (see also Fraisse and Perrot 1995), is due to the biological sex or the social gender role—sometimes referred to as the nature–nurture divide—is not discussed in depth, perhaps because in the real world no clear-cut differentiation is possible. There is no such thing as an isolated individual with an interior brain and an outer social environment (or "social universe"; see above); instead, there are social and cultural relations from the very beginning of existence. In any case, the ambiguity of these two possible explanations (with regard to the mind: internalist/externalist in a broad sense) gives the book the potential to critically reflect on imbalanced interpretations of why men and women think, feel, and act the way they are assumed to. Obviously, the sex matters for emotionality, meaning the potential of being "typically" emotional and having a life rich in sex-specific emotions. But how, and why? And does emotionality matter for the sex?

In the following passages, some crucial terms for the debates are clarified. According to the United Nations Educational, Scientific, and Cultural Organization (UNESCO), "Sex describes the biological differences between men and women, which are universal and determined at birth" (UNESCO's Gender Mainstreaming Implementation Framework [GMIF] 2002–2007, Annex 2, 17). Gender, on the other hand, refers to the roles and responsibilities assigned to men and women in families, societies, and cultures. Gender roles and expectations of how men and women typically behave (masculinity/femininity) are learned. They are not biologically predetermined nor permanently fixed. The concept of gender is a category of social analysis, which reveals the variations within and between cultures due to class, ethnicity, age, physical and mental disabilities, and more. Going beyond UNESCO's GMIF, we now add *science* to this list.

Rather than physical disabilities that are obvious, neuroscientific—like genetic—research focuses on phenotypic abilities which are still hidden and often remain hidden. The brain's *capacity* (e.g., to show effects when stimulated in a laboratory context) is not identical with a person's *ability* (e.g., to feel, understand, or do something)—and this is something we would like to state as a basic differentiation for the entire book. Depending on how the brain is modeled as an epistemic object in relation to certain functions (see Godfrey-Smith 1998; on philosophy of functions, see Millikan 1984), a capacity can appear as an ability; moreover, it can also appear as a mental disability.

Evelyn Fox Keller (1995, 80) has pointed out that the relation of gender and science can be analyzed in a threefold sense: (1) *women in science/as scientists*, (2) *science of gender*, and (3) *gender in science*. Our book stresses the relation between (2) and (3), that is, the (not only) neuroscientific construction of sex-related differences, and the cultural idea of gender stereotypes within the formation of scientific terms, models, and theories. Strategy (3), gender in science, especially allows for questioning prominent perspectives on research fields and, thus, the related ideas and ideologies influencing the scientific modeling of categories (2) by means of specific terms used for description and explanation. Subsequently, when one looks closely at scientific descriptions, they reveal a priori normative assumptions and challenge the idea that there is something like pure and objective knowledge, particularly regarding the science of gender. Related pop-scientific discourses essentially belong to the epistemologic level of gender in science, as many people (including peers from the humanities and social sciences, politicians, and other decision-makers, e.g., in science funding) inform themselves about recent scientific findings mainly through "easy to read" texts and by images which seem to show "obvious" differences. Both scientists and journalists writing pop science books thus play a mediating role in shaping science-related discourses, that is, here, regarding the neuroscientific findings on sex-related differences.

There are complementary approaches to critique, which this book will not explore in great depth. First, one could ask why Western societies in particular are so interested in finding gender (and other) differences, and why these differences are frequently inserted into a *binary structure*, for example, woman/man, black/white, and so forth. The movement endorsing "queer thinking" concerning gender issues turns to this question. Above all, this question was inspired by biological research on the causes of same sex sexuality, particularly male homosexuality—which has also given rise to previous neuroscientific research (LeVay 1991, Byrne and Parsons 1993; for a critique, see Hegarty and Pratto 2001).

Second, the methodological concepts, analyzable within the "science of gender" approach, offers many points which are also relevant for objections regarding the explanatory level of neuroscientific research (for details, see Schmitz 2006a). At this level of critique, one questions the methods of experimental design, measurement, mathematical calculation, and statistical interpretation (concerning, e.g., research on bilateral language representation in men's and women's brains; see Sommer et al. 2004) and the instruments and artifacts involved. Turning to the latter, the still questionable *comparability* of neuroimages, when resulting from different laboratories and different data processing by means of different visualization techniques and computer programs, challenges the idea that with respect to constructing sex differences by means of, for example, spatial orientation capacities, emotional capacities, and phonal processing capacities, the results could be aggregated for modeling "the" woman's or "the" man's brain. Thus, this approach attempts to defeat science with its own weapons, questioning whether sound science was produced. Third, analyzing the concepts of *visual culture* (Gombrich 2000), the shaping of what is actually seen and not seen in (neuro)images, is another highly relevant method for critique. For example, as in other in vivo representations of the interior body (most prominently, the human embryo), the black modeled background of most neuroimages suggests that the entity of attention (brain) exists context free, that is, has a life on its own.

Another interesting question to pose for art historians and media scientists would be "Is there an iconology of neuroimages?"—that is, do these images remind us of others already known (Boehm 1994; Bredekamp 1995, 2005; Reichle, Siegel, and

Spelten 2007). Speaking as laypeople, perhaps the fluorescent colors remind onlookers of a gloriole, related to religious iconology, or a map of unknown territory which can be marked as visited or even colonized. Otherwise, why would people from Western cultures understand the binary blue/pink color code in the artificially colored neuroimages as a signal for men/women (see figures 1.2 and 1.3; color plate 2, 3)? Neuroimages have also become part of the visual arts and have entered the contexts of biopolitics (DaCosta and Philip 2008),[7] for example, in the work of Portuguese visual artist Marta de Menezes.[8]

Last but not least, all approaches critical of neuroscience harbor the notion that there is both an interindividual and an intraindividual variability concerning what people regard as being human.

Research on emotions is deeply influenced by cultural norms and sexual stereotypes, and—not to be forgotten—by gender role types (Butler 2004). By relating gender in science and science of gender, we emphasize the ambivalent epistemic fields and levels of autonomy and control in which emotions are analyzed.

From a sociological point of view, not only are emotions related to the microlevel (the individual and the family) but they are also relevant at the mesolevel (corporations, institutions) and the macrolevel, where questions of social patterns and social systems crop up. We may ask, with a kind of Durkheimian approach, what these levels have to do with each other when self-help concepts like EI and research fields like social neuroscience emerge. This broad perspective may seem discouraging from an analytical point of view; however, we are interested in more than asking if EI really is a useful construct. Rather, we are interested in the cultural and scientific climate that produces scientific concepts of self-enhancement which are then disseminated to laypeople. Everyone wants to be "above average," and the fetish object brain will trigger related enhancement strategies, just as the fetish object body[9] did in years past.[10]

1.4 Step 2: Analyzing Refigurations of "the Self" in the Light of Elites

1.4.1 Society and Science

Before one can attribute emotions to someone or something, there has to be an entity which can have these emotions, that is, a self. The ontological question of where one self starts and ends, that is, how the boundaries of the self and the other are defined, is thus of critical importance. For instance, when EI is discussed as promoting leadership, one has to ask which entity is supposed to be more emotionally intelligent—the leading CEO, the sum of employees, the individual person, the person's brain? EI as a concept touches on both social and scientific ontologies, and, when it refers to the category of sex, also ontologies of nature. Ontologies always lend basic structures to

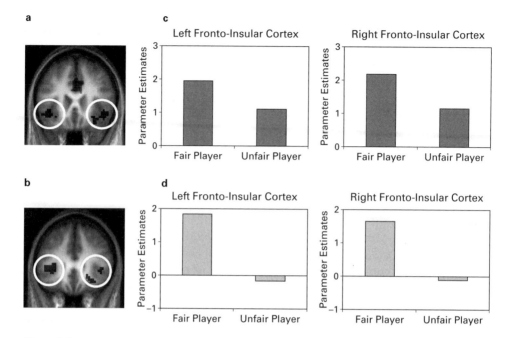

Figure 1.2

(color plate 2) Pain-sensitive activation networks to the sight of fair and unfair players in pain. (a, b) Conjunction analysis between the contrasts pain–no pain in the context of self and the fair condition at $p < .001$ for women (pink; a) and men (blue; b). Increased pain-related activation (asterisk indicates whole-brain corrected) for women in ACC* [9, 18, 27], left fronto-insular cortex* [–42, 15, –3], right fronto-insular cortex* [30, 18, –18], left second somatosensory area (SII)* [–60, –30, 18], right SII* [63, –30, 24], and brainstem* [3, –18, –18]; for men in left fronto-insular cortex* [–33, 33, 3] right fronto-insular cortex [42, 33, 3], and brainstem [3, –33, –30]. (c, d) Average activation (parameter estimates) in peak voxels of left and right fronto-insular cortex for the painful–nonpainful trials in fair and unfair conditions for women (pink; c) and men (blue; d). (Source: Singer, Seymour, O'Doherty, Stephan, Dolan, and Frith. 2006. "Empathic Neural Responses Are Modulated by the Perceived Fairness of Others." *Nature* 439: 466–469, 468; reprinted by permission from Macmillan Publishers Ltd.: *Nature*, © 2006.)

Painful trials in unfair — painful trials in fair

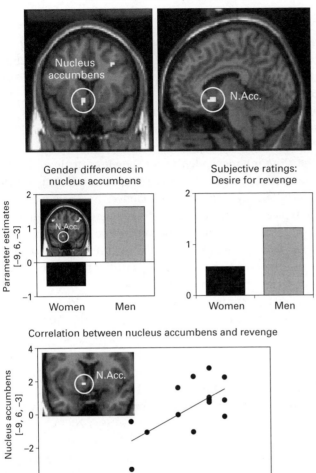

Gender differences in nucleus accumbens

Subjective ratings: Desire for revenge

Correlation between nucleus accumbens and revenge

Figure 1.3

(color plate 3) Gender differences in brain activity in nucleus accumbens (N. Acc.) specific to the perception of an unfair compared to fair player in pain. (a) Increased activity ($p < .005$) in nucleus accumbens [–9, 15, –9] for painful trials in the unfair/fair condition for men but not for women. (b) Average activation (parameter estimates) for women (pink) and men (blue) in left nucleus accumbens [–9, 15, –9] when testing for gender differences. (c) Men (blue) compared to women (pink) indicate stronger feelings of desire for revenge, $t(30) = 2.40$, $p < .05$, measured on a scale ranging from –2 ("not at all") to +2 ("very much"). (d) Correlation ($r = .68$, $p < .05$) of parameter estimates at peak of nucleus accumbens activation [–9, 6, –3] for the (pain in unfair–pain in fair) contrast in men with expressed desire for revenge in men. There was no correlation for women. (Source: Singer, Seymour, O'Doherty, Stephan, Dolan, and Frith. 2006. "Empathic Neural Responses Are Modulated by the Perceived Fairness of Others." *Nature* 439: 466–469, 469; reprinted by permission from Macmillan Publishers Ltd.: *Nature*, © 2006.)

the world and its entities existing in time and space. They constitute a sort of architecture—of society, of science, of human life, of biological life, of nature. This structure is often interpreted hierarchically and contains—metaphorically speaking—a basement, several floors, and a top floor.

In sociology, the top floor is often characterized as the "elite." However, this top floor has different apartments, since there is not only "one" elite but many, in different parts of society and in different parts of the global world. C. Wright Mills, in *The Power Elite* (1956), showed the close interdependencies of the elites in the different fields of economics, politics, and the military in the United States and contrasted their power with the disinterested "mass society." Although he claimed that the power elite is represented by men, he is typical of a large group of elite theorists because he neglected to do a gender analysis of the issue. Another open question for elite theorists is the relation of EI and the creation of elites. Moreover, feminist research in general is critical of elite theories because it tends to view itself as part of a liberation movement advocating an egalitarian society (Dackweiler 2007).[11]

With sociologist Suzanne Keller (1963)—in 1968 the first woman in the history of Princeton University to be granted a tenured professorship—we can differentiate between *strategic elites* who are important for society, because their decisions influence many of its members across different contexts, and elites who are only formative for special contexts, like beauty queens. Stardom regularly functions as a channel of upward mobility for individuals with low incomes. Similarly, Goleman's concept of EI in general nourishes the hope of becoming a star performer through individual brain training (see, e.g., Stein and Book 2000; Bradberry and Greaves 2005).

Strictly speaking, EI is a concept that serves strategic elites ("leaders"), particularly in the business world. According to recent data, women are still not adequately represented among strategic elites. This is a global phenomenon. One of the most important elite areas, the economy,[12] can be taken as an example. Research on the top 200 companies worldwide in 2004 showed that women comprise only 10.4% of the boards of these companies. Breaking this figure down into percentages by country, 17.5% of board members in U.S.-based firms are women, in Germany the figure is 10.3%, and the lowest percentage is found in Italy with 1.8%.[13] In addition to these facts, which form part of gender research on women's employment rates, there also exists a global "gender pay gap." The gender pay gap represents the relative difference between the average hourly pay for men and women before taxation. According to the latest figures from the European Commission's experts groups (2006, 2007), across the E.U. economy women continue to earn an average of 15% less than men. This figure has barely changed within the last decade, although the European Union tried to implement policy strategies for change, as this figure, so to say, insults the self-image of a democratic society. Asking why this figure has remained so stable, one of the experts' judgments is that women have lower wages not only due to unequal pay for equal work but also due to the different scales of evaluation of women's competencies in the labor market, particularly concerning jobs dominated by women rather than by men, though based on the same qualification levels deriving from school or college (e.g., the payment of nannies compared to car mechanics). Here, jobs considered "emotional labor" (see section 1.6) are addressed in particular. Statistics show that the pay gap grows significantly with age, education, and years of service. In the European Union, women with third-level education face a gender pay gap of up to 30%. Not surprisingly, the highest pay gap is found in the financial and business sector—that is, the sectors which are inspired most by the idea of emotionally intelligent leadership and individual brain training for increasing emotional quotient (EQ).

A differentiated perspective on elites helps to critically analyze where cultural concepts of science, sex, and gender influence elitist structures within society. Membership in "the elite" stands in close relation to having a position of strategic, financial, or some other form of power—as described in functional elite theory (e.g., Dreitzel 1962). There are, however, family structures where women are present as part of "the elite," as Tomke Böhnisch (1999) analyzes in her research on wives of members of the economic elites in German-speaking countries. Böhnisch shows that, although these women do not hold positions of power themselves, their self-images clearly consist of being "the female part" of an elite (Böhnisch 2003, 186). Wives can share their husbands' high social rank, though without sharing their husbands' power. Böhnisch also shows that this mind-set creates a social distance with respect to women who define themselves as "career women" to maintain or develop their social status—or simply because they have to earn money.

We can now try to connect the neuroscientific finding that there are two sexually stereotyped forms of an "extreme brain," as put forward by Simon Baron-Cohen (2003), with the idea that a person's brain condition is essentially relevant for gaining a top position. Assuming there is something like a male elite brain, making up a new functional elite, the wife's adoption of the elitist aura of her husband will become more difficult, because the woman has a brain of her own. Moreover, she is responsible for her own brain training and enhancement—or, if there is a corresponding concept of an elite female brain, specific functions have to be envisioned, according to which a woman can belong to a female elite.

One of the main criteria for analyzing elites is the access to and the recruiting of elites. Keller sees the primary recruiting principle for strategic elites as showing target-oriented capacities and corresponding achievements, whereas family and origin play only a secondary role. Is the recruitment of elites—at least theoretically—open to everybody who is adequately qualified? If yes, then elites also seem to be an acceptable construct for building a democratic society (Dahrendorf 1992). Merit and reward become central entry requirements for elites, and they are closely connected to education. Successfully completing an educational program is the basis upon which a meritocracy is built. However, there are three limits to the meritocracy.

One limit lies in the link between the socioeconomic power of individuals, their families, and access to education. In the United States, the book *The Price of Admission* (2006) by Daniel Golden, a *Wall Street Journal* deputy bureau chief and 2004 Pulitzer Prize winner, once again raised the issue of admission practices to Ivy League institutions of higher education. Golden reports that college admission offices are not only looking for high achievers in selecting their incoming students but also give preference to privileged wealthy candidates—a practice he criticizes. Therefore, although Ivy League schools try to convey the image that they are meritocratic institutions, Golden's analysis shows that this image is pretence.[14]

A second limit of meritocracy lies in the link between gender stereotypes and positions of leadership. The average school and university marks of many girls and young women (Macha 2004, 27) show that "girls out-perform boys," as E.U. Commissioner Vladimir Špidla recently declared in a press release (European Union, Brussels, no. IP/07/1115, released July 18, 2007). Given the additional fact that (in the European Union) more women enter the labor market with a university degree than do men, it is amazing (in the words of Špidla: "absurd") that these achievements are not adequately accounted for in elite recruitment in top positions—be it in the economic, political, scientific, or cultural sector. While the methods of measuring intelligence, in general, seem to need further development, the existing EI testing methods reveal that women score higher in the abilities which are often called "the soft factors" of leadership (see MacCann et al., this volume). These findings could transform the overall idea of leadership, while keeping in mind the open question of whether soft factors matter once you are a leader or in advance, in order to become one. However, it is mainly the sex differences which are measured here, not the gender differences. And it is mostly personality which is scrutinized for "soft factors," rather than emotions themselves. Unless there is a testing method which refers not only to sex but to gender roles, too, it will remain unclear how emotional styles ("female" and "male" and various mixtures of the two) influence the test results ascribing a certain level of EI to a person. This approach would also touch on the question of equal opportunities for lesbian and gay persons in the (business) world.

Obviously, there is no way for science to avoid typifying behaviors, reactions, and styles. This is due to systematic reasons: deciding which methods applied to which models (referring to theories and hypotheses) produce robust results and are, thus, agreed to produce scientific findings in a true sense. This decision also touches on the question of what can be regarded as knowledge, and its other, for example, nonknowledge and its various forms (Ravetz 1990, Beck 1999, Wehling 2006, Schiemann 2007). Scientific findings and the produced knowledge are reckoned universal, that is, the findings have to be reproducible and applicable within all laboratories working with the same standards. For science, the construction of distinct categories, abstract models, and artificial environments is a must. The problem we address here is that the universality claimed by science should be sufficiently valid for real life outside the laboratory, that is, for living practice (in the sense of the Greek *praxis*). On the other hand, outside the realm of pop science, it is possible for science to refrain from stereotyping and to explicitly stress that the findings refer to types and not to individual human beings (and this difference, after all, is mentioned in the final section of Baron-Cohen 2004).

Gender equality—understood as ensuring equal opportunities and living conditions for realizing full human rights for women and for men—obviously has not been achieved yet.

A third reason why there are limits to meritocracy lies in the link between *habitus* and elite positions. In taking up Pierre Bourdieu (1979/1984), we also argue that the habitus and its sovereignty are important elements for recruiting elites (see Illouz, this volume, for details), and it also plays a role in access to elite positions (Hartmann 2002). With habitus we understand the embodied social and economic conditions of an individual. However, although the habitus is embodied, it is, of course, socially constructed (Bourdieu and Wacquant 2006, 160). The idea of elite brains and their both innate and essential capacities, expressed as functionally interpreted abilities by means of the body (see also Pfeifer and Bongard 2006), would challenge this position. With regard to the theories of brain science, neither the habitus nor performativity is relevant. Embodiment would then mean, as in embodied robotics and AI research, that a body is the medium (here used in the sense of a mere "carrier") of functional expressions, which are internally controlled and externally decoded by a central processing unit.

The second point (sexual stereotypes as a barrier to elite positions) and third point (the habitus as a limit) are interlinked because these "fine differences" concerning the habitus are also of importance for success or failure in entering elite ranks and surviving in elite surroundings. Women and men have, own, and use different forms of capital. Differentiating between economic, social, cultural, and symbolic capital, Bourdieu emphasizes that these different types of capital influence each other: Economic capital and the right economic assets, for instance, ease the acquisition of cultural capital (Bourdieu 1979/1984, 189), as we have seen in the example of Ivy League schools. Even if women are endowed with equal economic capital, other types of capital which could make all the difference might still be lacking.

For instance, the cliché that girls and women are not interested in technology and its artifacts (Baron-Cohen 2004, e.g., 92), seen as a proof of the "femaleness" of their brains, is based on other than economic forms of capital. Australian "technofeminist" Judy Wajcman (2004) points out that nowadays there is much more gender equity in the use of technologies (PCs, mobile phones, etc.) than in decades and centuries past (of course, in reference to other artifacts). Nevertheless, she argues, at the design stage women still rarely enter engineering and information technology contexts, and once they have entered, they are less encouraged to continue than their male counterparts (see also Leicht-Scholten 2007). In contrast, and excluding the private sector, a recent study on German researchers' access to holding a professorship (i.e., for the German context: reaching the associate professor level) revealed that professors of engineering and computer science, a male domain, encouraged their few woman students and PhD candidates much more than did colleagues from language and cultural studies (where more than half of all graduate students are women), the humanities, and medicine (Löther 2006). The study's results show that the technology departments lost significantly fewer women during the qualification process, though women comprised only about 12% of the students.

When we understand Goleman's EI concept as a way of acquiring capital in Bourdieu's sense, it is still the failure to combine his approach with a social theory that makes it problematic. EI cannot be understood as a way of overcoming the limits of meritocracy because this approach to refiguring and improving oneself—as a man or a woman, with male or female behavior—leaves the question open as to how capacities, abilities, and functions are defined and who defines them. Meritocratic structures are always in a state of flux. Taking into account that members of elites are recruited not only due to their achievements but also because of a special habitus—which is different in the various areas of society (for the scientists, cf. Beaufaÿs 2007)—the notion of "elites" is also a social construct which must be evaluated and questioned from a gender perspective, especially in the wake of new neuroscientific findings concerning the "essential difference" between men and women, and being male and female.

1.4.2 Science and Society

In this book, the authors focus on some of the structures which underlie elite concepts and touch on feminist issues without explicitly identifying themselves as feminists. Research on "the" brain, particularly on "the female" and "the male" brain, will probably help to both create new elites and strengthen existing elites. At the moment, an expanding literature (e.g., Angier 2000, Brizendine 2006) which contributes to *feminalism*—trying to solve the "mysteries" of the woman's body and sexuality by means of "hard" bioscience, that is, neuroscience and genetics—ignores many ideas that are important in *feminism*, for example, considering the social construction of science and the fight for social and economic equality. Here, brain research is particularly engaged in "pleasure studies," for example, finding essential differences between female and male orgasms, sexual arousal, and the activation of the brain's reward center after orgasms and faked (female) orgasms, often combined with hormone research.[15] This faked orgasm is particularly important in brain research for methodological reasons. Comparing the brain images resulting during/after a faked orgasm and during/after "real" pleasure allows scientists to determine what—in a theoretical view—makes the "real" difference. The research field of sexual arousal and the brain, focusing on the various kinds of "sexual dysfunctions," is undoubtedly related to our book's focus, as there seem to be sexual elites as well: sexually omnipotent and easy to arouse, unaffected by any kind of stress resulting from the workplace or private life. However, the authors of this book will not explicitly discuss this topic.

Obviously, new questions concerning elitist thinking arise, starting with the following: How could definitions of elites change when they are related to brain functions, as Goleman and Baron-Cohen envision? Historically, especially in the nineteenth and twentieth centuries, there has been research on the topography of the brains of geniuses (see Hagner 2004; Hagner, this volume). Who can be regarded as a *genius* depends on a historically fluid understanding of "elite" and "idiocy" as the following example might elucidate.

The French pioneer of intelligence testing, Alfred Binet, introduced his classical paper "New Methods for the Diagnosis of the Intellectual Level of Subnormals"[16] (French original 1905, coauthored with Théodore Simon, transl. 1916) as follows:

Before explaining these methods let us recall exactly the conditions of the problem which we are attempting to solve. Our purpose is to be able to measure the intellectual capacity of a child who is brought to us in order to know whether he is normal or retarded. We should[,] therefore, study his condition at the time and that only. We have nothing to do either with his past history or with his future; consequently we shall neglect his etiology, and we shall make no attempt to distinguish between acquired and congenital idiocy; for a stronger reason we shall set aside all consideration of pathological anatomy which might explain his intellectual deficiency. So much for his past. As to that which concerns his future, we shall exercise the same abstinence; we do not attempt to establish or prepare a prognosis and we leave unanswered the question of whether this retardation is curable, or even improvable. We shall limit ourselves to ascertaining the truth in regard to his present mental state.

Binet writes quite precisely about the limits of his investigation and, though from today's point of view the text might give another impression, his motivation was first and foremost pedagogical. In his article, Binet rejects the concept of "idiocy," borrowed from "alienists" (an archaic term for one who treats mental illness, particularly a physician specializing in legal aspects of psychiatry, from the French *aliené*, meaning insane), as in the alienists' concept regarding children with a "rebellious disposition," that is, children who were called "moral imbeciles" at that time fall into this category. Binet reminds instructors not to treat children "whose character is not sympathetic with their own" as pathological cases. For this reason, he also feels the urge to remove the aura of idiocy and pathologization from those with an "inferior intelligence" (this is the term he suggests). Of course, his new testing approach implied a comparison

with what is "general intelligence" (*g*), that is, what is normal (on the different acceptance of statistical methods at that time, see Hacking 2005). Besides its content, Binet's
article is also noteworthy for the nearly vanished style of academic prose, which
reveals the intellectual's awareness of social problems, for example, with regard to the
societal "aptitude" of the different intelligences, which might be involved in his
approach from the very beginning: "Some have a good auditory or musical memory,
and a whole repertoire of songs; others have mechanical ability. If all were carefully
examined, many examples of these partial aptitudes would probably be found." As
a consequence, his method of testing intelligence(s) included tactile and other nonverbal abilities, which, moreover, shows deep insight into the phenomenal ontology
of the senses.

And there is another suggestion, concerning Binet's test, which would also be relevant for the present neurosciences and their image runs with follow-up questionnaires,
even if the volunteer is an adult: "Rapidity is necessary for this sort of examination.
It is impossible to prolong it beyond twenty minutes without fatiguing the subject."

Binet rejected physiological and craniometrical research on inferior intelligences
(on Binet, see also Hacking 1998, 97–99). Nowadays, neurobiological and neuropsychological research ascribes certain physiological events in the brain to certain kinds
of intelligences, attitudes, and behaviors.

For instance, in an interesting study entitled "The Good, the Bad, and the Ugly:
An fMRI Investigation of the Functional Anatomical Correlates of Stigma," Anne C.
Krendl and her colleagues (Krendl et al. 2006) analyzed how feelings of disgust toward
socially stigmatized groups are represented in neuroimages with reference to the
brain's capacity for controlling this disgust. We have explicitly chosen this study to
exemplify how transformations of models and terms from both sociology and the
social world take place in the laboratory of the social cognitive neurosciences, as its
experimental design is very thoughtfully conceived. Although these researchers are
particularly sensitive to the underlying biases of social neurosciences and are aware of
the impact of these biases on society, the study shows how difficult it is, methodologically, to keep to one's own normative premises.

The general hypothesis of this study is that control and disgust refer to two separate
neural systems. The amygdala, the "organ" of emotions, is involved in the areas
responsible for "feeling" disgust. The scientists were interested in both modeling
and understanding how the process of social categorization takes place. Twenty-
eight students, all right-handers, were recruited from Dartmouth College (in New
Hampshire); three had to be excluded from the experiments because of "excessive
movement" during imaging (and another three because of problems with data acquisition). "Excessive" here means more than 2 mm. The implicit architecture of the
experimental design, for example, regarding the level of students' familiarity with the
stigma type, which we will not discuss here, was quite challenging.

Photographs of persons who self-reported having any one of a group of specific attributes—*being obese, extensively face-pierced, transsexual, generally unattractive*—were selected and shown to students (both men and women) at random. The students were supposed to rank the intensity of their feelings of disgust for each face in the photos on a special disgust scale. Previously, a scale for general attractiveness ("likeability") had been developed for every single volunteer, based on individual evaluative ratings of photographs with "control faces," in order to compare the brain condition for each individual when looking at photographs of "normal" people with the condition which developed while looking at the photos of the stigmatized individuals. *That* these people are generally stigmatized was the scientists' decision (i.e., it was their categorization), even if Krendl et al. claimed that the chosen stigma categories are "widely acknowledged" (Krendl et al. 2006, 7). Their assessment was accompanied by the decision to take the photographs from social platforms of self-defined groups, such as Web pages of piercing artists or a dating Web site for overweight people. This means that they selected photographs of people who identified themselves as obese, pierced, transsexual, or unattractive, which does not necessarily mean that they view themselves as socially stigmatized.

In general, for social neuroscience the problem arises that if you want to measure the process of stigmatization (i.e., a categorization) in the brain, you must define a priori what stigma (i.e., a category) is and in which brain area(s) it might show up, for example, in the area responsible for feeling disgust. The neuroscientific approach is similar to scrutinizing whether, in the neuroimaging, a woman's brain proves to be empathic or not (see Singer et al. 2004a), except for the important fact that the category "woman" seems to be both *self-evident* and *normal*. Therefore, she becomes the volunteer and not the stigmatized.

Put in philosophical terms, in the study of Krendl et al., *acceptability* was modeled neuroscientifically, and the category of "stereotype," on which, according to Krendl et al., social stigma is based, was considered as given. Here, already, the terms used are important for modeling knowledge, as the experimental use of "stereotype" provides a reference to previous neuroimaging studies on stigmatization of race (to which Krendl et al. refer). This is what Ian Hacking—referring to Nicholas Jardine—called "calibration" of instruments within scientific developments (Hacking 1998, 98), that is, that every new method introduced for measurement has to be calibrated against the old one, including the evaluation of how adequate the old one was. In psychological terminology, the concept "calibration of instruments" (e.g., clocks) is known as validation (of tests and questionnaires, i.e., constructs), which leads to other problems. Obviously, there is no awareness among some scientists within the social neurosciences of the need to calibrate their instruments, meaning *social concepts* like stigma and stereotype, with sociology or philosophy. We argue that concepts like stereotype can be *instruments* in social cognitive neuroscience. They make it possible to technically generate hypotheses in the context of cognition and emotion, and these concepts differ from the concepts which result from the experiment. It is important to notice that this transformation differs from metaphorical use and the science/society cross-border trade of metaphors. How can concepts be instruments? Because within the experiment, their real meaning seems to be irrelevant. Instead, they just lend the experiment their linguistic skeleton, purified of metaphorical and social meanings and implications, for the purpose of social cognitive science. A cultural and social concept, like stereotype, which is binary coded can be an extremely useful instrument, because it can be combined with attributes which are also binary coded.

There is a clearly established cultural stereotype of black and white, likewise of man and woman. Concerning the "old" and still intensively used instrument, that is, the stereotype black/white applied in stigmatization studies of race, the concept of stereotype somehow made sense (this is not to suggest, however, that it made sense in all of the studies in which it was employed). However, a stereotypic structure is not obvious in fat/slim, extensively pierced/not at all or not extensively pierced, unattractive/attractive. They relate to aesthetic categories, which are highly heterogeneous. There is no objective beauty, moreover, which is not related to a type, and even the idea of ugliness does not contradict the idea of attraction. All chosen types involve *continua* and are not discrete attributes. Of course, black/white also involves continua of color, but color *can be more easily stereotyped* (see Berger 1999), for example, by scientists' choice of photographs, than attractiveness. And what is the binary other of transsexual? Not transsexual? Heterosexual? Same sex sexual? Taking a closer look, it appears that this study focuses not on stereotypes but on normality and its opposite, the construction of abnormality. This is a slight but nevertheless important difference. And it makes all the difference regarding the question of who shapes this normality—science or society, the scientist with her abstract categories or the individual within her life world of personal experiences?

During the experimental process, and by means of several abstractions and generalizations, predefined attributes of individuals' faces on photographs were converted into properties of members of social groups. On the other hand, the idea of a social group emerged because one single attribute was seen as principal and thus made the essence of this social group. The social world was remodeled. Within the laboratory context, the individuals in the photographs became "targets" of social stigma, whereas the members of the indicated social groups became "bearers" of social stigma. The volunteers in the laboratory became "perceivers" of social stigma, and the photographs themselves "stimulus materials." This setup is not an exception but the normal approach and terminology for social cognitive neuroscience.

According to Krendl and her colleagues, the disgust inspired by obesity is much more controlled within the students' brains than disgust toward transsexuality, that is, seeing a photograph of a transsexual feels more disgusting than seeing a photograph

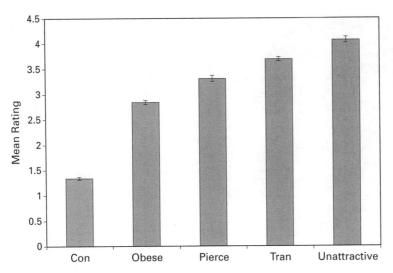

Figure 1.4
(color plate 4) Mean disgust ratings: post hoc individual ratings, reverse scored such that 1 = "not at all disgusting," 5 = "very disgusting." Con, control; Tran, transsexual. (Source: Krendl, Macrae, Kelly, Fugelsang, and Heatherton. 2006. "The Good, the Bad, and the Ugly: An fMRI Investigation of the Functional Anatomic Correlates of Stigma." *Social Neuroscience* 1, no. 1: 5–15, 9; reprinted by permission from the publisher Taylor & Francis Ltd., http://informaworld.com: *Social Neuroscience*, © 2006.)

of an overweight person. The most disgusting of all is to perceive general unattractiveness (see figures 1.4 and 1.5; color plates 4, 5).

We can explore Krendl et al.'s study a bit further, with regard to the methodology and epistemology of social neuroscience. They assert that their study is, first, inspired by the awareness that social neuroscience studies on social categorization and stigmatization have predominantly dealt with race differences (see Phelps and Thomas 2003 for a critical overview). Second, their study represents a critique of previous studies of social stigma which had resulted in the concept that theoretically controllable stigmas (such as obesity) lead to more negative feelings in the receiver than uncontrollable stigmas (e.g., blindness). Again, in philosophical terms Krendl et al. tried to reject the idea that *blame* and *guilt*, which have been lurking behind the concept of controllability, are involved in stigmatization. This complex field of guilt and visible stigma, which was analyzed in the laboratory, imported a specific Christian tradition into the scientific modeling. The differentiation between controllable stigma and that which is "given" has a long religious history, distinguishing a stigmatized person from others on the basis of a bodily wound (Goffman 1963, Harrison 1996, Menke and Vinkenly 2004, Fessler 2007). Having biblical origin, stigmata in the Catholic tradition refer to

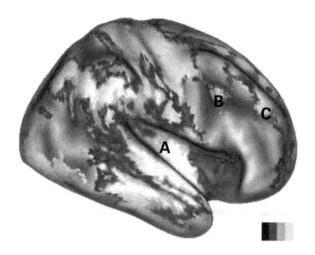

Figure 1.5

(color plate 5) Parametric modulation of disgust ratings: analysis conducted with individual disgust ratings modeled linearly as a covariate of interest. An inflated voxel-by-voxel cortical rendering of the right hemisphere with a minimum threshold set at T = 3.53 and maximum set at T = 7 for p < .001 uncorrected (Van Essen, Drury, Dickson, Harwell, Hanlon, and Anderson 2001). Region of interest analyses extracted activity in the right inferior frontal gyrus (A; BA 45: 53, 24, 18), right medial frontal gyrus (B; BA 9: 50, 8, 36), and anterior cingulate gyrus (C; BA 32: –9, 22, 35) activity. (Source: Krendl, Macrae, Kelly, Fugelsang, and Heatherton. 2006. "The Good, the Bad, and the Ugly: An fMRI Investigation of the Functional Anatomic Correlates of Stigma." *Social Neuroscience* 1, no. 1: 5–15, 10; reprinted by permission from the publisher Taylor & Francis Ltd., http://informaworld.com: *Social Neuroscience*, © 2006.)

marks on the body which resemble the wounds Jesus received while hanging on the cross—like wounds on the feet and hands. In religious tradition, stigmata are not a sign of guilt but show a cosuffering with Jesus Christ and the capability of bearing the sins of others.[17]

According to Krendl et al., they chose the attributes of obesity and transsexuality because these attributes are ambiguous, whereas piercings are clearly controllable, and unattractiveness is determined by genetics and is thus uncontrollable. The category of "control" is used variously in the social neurosciences: first, regarding personal and social behavior; second, regarding the control of emotions and emotional areas inside the brain by other, more "intelligent" areas (mainly the prefrontal cortex); and, third, regarding the social response (of groups) and emotional response (of individuals) to the perceived behavior of others.

Something else that is typical of social neurosciences is the lost differentiation between bias that is unintentional and bias that is unconscious. Bias is an issue in the use of questionnaires, where the volunteers are supposed to answer questions such as "Do you like this person?" after being shown a photograph of a possibly stigmatized person. This procedure is always done after the image has been shown. Whereas intentional bias results from volunteers who purposely give wrong answers, unintentional bias is due to the fact that—because of social norms—some people do not want to admit that they dislike the person or that they have prejudices. The difference is not easy to detect, though it is possible to do so employing conventional methods from behavioral and social psychology, for example, by measuring startle reflexes (see Phelps and Thomas 2003). This type of unintentionality is amenable to consciousness.

Another concept of unintentional bias is now entering the arena of testing culture, and this is where cognitive neuroscience of emotions comes into play: the *unconscious bias*. Unconscious feelings are not amenable to consciousness.[18] Rather, they are labeled "automatic" (Krendl et al. 2006), giving shape and form to an old vision of cybernetics (Wiener 1961; for a cultural perspective related to the development of electroencephalography, see Borck 2005): the control of behavior as an instance for locating an identity between animal and machine. The automatic feeling of disgust is labeled as "automatic evaluation."

In other words, a scientific target of social neuroscience is to unveil political correctness rhetoric, or other forms of learned control, and to determine whether the evaluation given in the questionnaire (behavioral data) contradicts the neuroimages (fMRI data) or confirms them. These two different measurement methods are newly referred to as "explicit measures" (questionnaires) and "implicit measures" (neuroimages), thereby tacitly abolishing or at least reducing the implicit measurement methods referring to unintentional bias from psychology (see also Phelps and Thomas 2003, 756). Unconsciousness wins over unintentionality. In the end, this issue is about the definition of truth and which science holds the greatest claim to defining it. And since emotions still seem to evidence the innocent nature of the uncivilized animal in us, which cannot lie, the neuroimages are thought to represent the "original" and true feeling of the reptile mind. It's a jungle out there, in the brain. Of course, the wildlife of the amygdala can be tamed by the civilized brain areas responsible for evaluation and emotional learning. As a consequence, social norms seem to be inscribed in the brain, somehow governing its cruel "nature."

Not surprisingly, in the discussion section of their paper Krendl et al. offer the opinion that "Over the course of evolution, the avoidance of those possessing stigma may have been adaptive" (Krendl et al. 2006, 12).

We, the editors and authors of this book, after having investigated so many neuroscientific studies on emotions, and, sometimes, as in the case of the study of Krendl et al., having been impressed by the fine architecture of the hypothesis and experimental design, have always been inspired with a deep sense of disappointment at the appearance of the repeatedly recurring sentence, "Over the course of evolution X may have been adaptive." As neuroscience is rooted in biology, and biology in Darwinism, this phrase seems to be unavoidable. It is like the final scene in a Western movie: Regardless of the story, the cowboys are on their horses, riding into the sunset; their work is now done.

We, however, continue with more questions. In nearly all of the neuroimaging studies we investigated which came from outside the clinical context (of explicit diagnosis and therapy), the volunteers were recruited from university campuses. With reference to social categories, then, do students' brains mirror societies' brains—or rather "the brain" of society?

Do social norms light up in the brain? What does this idea suggest for the creation and recruitment of elites? Will the elites of the present adapt to certain brain functions, or will new elites inhabit the top floors in the future, for example, the high-functional autists (90% of whom are men) as Simon Baron-Cohen (2004) envisions? Have new research programs already been developed within clinical contexts, for example, concerning diagnoses of sexual and social dysfunctions, which resist the classical approaches of medical therapy or surgery? Does it matter that the technology for neuroimaging already exists, and that financial investments have to pay off, that is, that as many people as possible should be brain scanned? To what degree would brain-centered elites change society and society's ideas of pathology? Looking at the current status of science and technology, it will not be possible to answer all these questions in this book. For the present, it should be enough to simply put them on the agenda.

Elites form a part of a "corporate self," for example, a company, a university, a nation, or a global economy. They have power and hold leading functions. Therefore, they also shape the self-image of the corporate self (corporate identity) and act as its representatives. The primary aim might be to gain money and influence for the corporation, its individual members, and their families. Over and above the issue of power and status, it is the task of modern elites to represent and take social responsibility for society as a whole. It was Daniel Goleman, after all, who tried to stress social responsibility in his EI concept.

1.5 Step 3: Making the Sciences of "the Self" Emotional

In the following passages, we will see that the limits of "the self" differ according to the experts' theoretical backgrounds, especially when the spheres of rationality and emotionality intermingle. For some reason, the sphere of rationality is easier to handle, academically, than its emotional counterpart. Every discipline uses different methods, media, and techniques for mediating between these spheres, for example, photographs and questionnaires in psychology, videotapes and neuroimages in neurobiology, symbols and ideas in the humanities and social sciences. In social cognitive (neuro)science and developmental cognitive science, these different methods and techniques are being merged. What they all have in common is that they are motivated by the desire to clarify, intellectually, what emotions are, what they reveal, how they do it, and what end they serve. Accordingly, we find ontological problems (What are emotions?), methodological problems (How can emotions be made accessible?), epistemological problems (What purpose, or even end, do emotions serve?), and, finally, a normative problem: How can emotions be functionalized, and should we do that? All these questions relate to different levels of "the self," starting with the level of the individual human person, with respect to his or her brain. Emotions today have a physical place *in* the brain, as, for example, prominent neuroscientist Antonio Damasio argues, and we all seem to be emotional people who think *by* feeling (see also Wassmann 2007, 160).

In this book, we are not going to answer the question of what emotions are. Commonly, these five basic emotions are considered to form the core understanding of emotion: anger, anxiety, sadness, disgust, and happiness. Surprise is also often listed. Let us take a short look at the complexity of the field. The sciences search for the physiological basis and evolutionary function of emotions, based both on the anthropological category of "the human being" and on the biological category of "the human organism." Propositions on "human nature" are nowadays valid for all individuals who are acknowledged to fall into the biological category of *Homo sapiens*. A well-known example of a both physiological and evolutionary explanation for emotions is the hormone adrenalin, which causes high pulse rates and most often aggressive behavior. Both are useful in dangerous situations where combat might be necessary. Sex-related hormones like testosterone and estrogen also are said to serve evolutionary functions which guarantee the survival of the species. Biological explanations in general refer to the organism, the population, and the species (i.e., to models) and not to the individual human being, that is, neither to "personhood" nor to personality. The category sex stands somehow crosswise to the category of the species *Homo sapiens*, as it divides the species' population into two different types of human beings (man and woman), nevertheless serving one common aim: survival, that is, producing the next generation. Many scientists who shape the discourse field of biological sex differences and brain research (of emotions), that is, Robert M. Sapolsky (1997), Louann Brizendine (2006), and Melissa Hines (2004), use an endocrinological approach to the research field by analyzing the internal processing and the functions of the gonadal hormones (for a feminist perspective on the gonadal hormone concept, see, e.g., Fausto-Sterling 2000, Ebeling 2006; for a cultural history of gonadal hormones and anti-aging therapies, see Stoff 2004). Moreover, fMRI studies on hormone-related neural activities of nonhuman primates before mating (see Ferris et al. 2004) inspired neuroscientific research for finding also a human "mating intelligence" (Geher and Miller 2007). Emotions then aid reproduction via—philosophically speaking: the medium of—hormones. By the same token, emotions have been used in recent neuroeconomics (see Ulshöfer, this volume), though there the hormones as mediators are only of marginal interest. For neuroeconomists, the emotions represented "in" the brain, which are said to be relevant for rational decisions, are methodologically (economic theory) and practically (consumer behavior) important. They seem to complete the model human being, the *Homo oeconomicus*. Looking closely at the theoretical architecture of modern biology and economics, it becomes obvious that both disciplines share common ground regarding efficiency, functionality, and reproduction of their systems' entities. Both interpret nature with economic and technological models of regulation and control. The essential difference, in the true sense of "essential," is that biological entities necessarily have to be alive to be efficient, functional, and reproductive, and that their functionality shows *ex post*. Taking this argument further, living beings need to grow and develop to *become* efficient, functional, and reproductive (i.e., when grown-up), and recent research findings on the brain's plasticity show that only a brain which has already learned develops further potentials of plasticity, enabling it to learn more. This implies that, for characterizing living beings, it is not sufficient to only *behave* in a functional way. Even robots can do that (Haraway 1997), and in the history of science animals have also often been described as functioning like automatic systems (e.g., Wiener 1961; Rosenblueth, Wiener, and Biegelow 1943).

In contrast, human beings have to internalize the goals of their lives (and life's boundaries, above all, mortality) and the means to reach them in such a way that the resulting behavior makes sense to themselves and others. Therefore, it is not enough to have an "internal model" of consciousness (Holland and Goodman 2003). On the other hand, internalizing is a process in which both causes and reasons are involved, and reasons still remain in the sphere of subjectivity. Living subjects are not static but continue to reflect on their agency within a sociopolitical ontology (Marcoulatos 2003, Cole 2005). This will continue, even if brain research tries to model the category of personal experience, which is crucial for uncovering reasons which account for a subject's decision in terms of objectively measurable, intraindividual changes of neuronal networks (plasticity). However, the individual's modal space, provided by neuroplasticity, is, at the same time, described as limited by a fixed architecture which is both species-related and sex-related.

From an epistemological point of view, the emotional behavior one shows is not necessarily identical with the emotion one has.[19] This is a crucial problem for the sciences which try to make the subjective feeling accessible to objective reasoning. Neuroimaging is the main methodology for this, and its limitations and impact are currently being debated (see Hüsing, Jäncke, and Tag 2006). Moreover, the process of having and showing emotions ("way of feeling," "mood"[20]) differs from the content of the specific emotion felt ("the feeling" or "sentiment"). The distinction works in a way that is analogous to "thinking" and "thought." The single incident which causes a fast sensation is another relevant category, because in the laboratory fast results are of high value. For example, when you burn your hand with boiling water, you will feel the sensation of pain immediately and connect it to the incident. First of all, a sensation like this differs from long-term feelings which can last for a lifetime, for example, guilt or shame. Second, this incident is felt as experience and comprises a lived biography. You will never do it again.

In contemporary neuroscience laboratories, a majority of studies are devoted to representations of pain. Due to methodical constraints, related to experimental design, this is the case even when the real research interest seems to focus on empathy (note: Greek *pathos* means suffering). Results from several studies have shown that fear, conflict, and (what neuroscientists call) "social pain" lead to the activation of a common alarm system in the brain, which is localized in the anterior cingulate cortex (ACC; a part of the limbic system; see, e.g., Panksepp 2003, Eisenberger, Lieberman, and Williams 2003). These different kinds of pain share the same representation of pain within neuroimaging. If we have given the impression thus far that pain is an emotion, let us correct it. Pain is not an emotion. It remains a sensation and is simply an indicator of an emotion or a feeling, which is richer in content and which must be interpreted based on the particular context in which it occurs. By means of neuro-imaging, the hypothesis is put forward that humans may experience the same kind of feeling during their several modes of perceiving the world, even if the feelings have different causes and effects and are related to different senses and sensations. This misunderstanding is due to generalization and abstraction. However, the concept of perception (rather than cognition) seems to be underestimated in current cognitive neuroscience.

Therefore, emotions are a primary category of phenomenology, as they depend on the senses through which humans perceive and experience the world (see Karafyllis, this volume). Focusing on emotions in brains, that is, on looking "inside" the human head, we tend to forget that the primary organ of sensual perception is the skin, demarcating the boundary of what is "inside" and "outside" the body. Since the early 1990s, the pioneers of pervasive computing have tried to technically blur the skin's boundaries or, so to say, enhance the skin's capacities for perceiving the outside and inside world (including people's emotions) with intelligent clothes. The idea is to construct a sheath with optimized sensor components (see Baumeler, this volume). This research field is interesting, when reflecting on emotion research, because on the popular level it developed mostly without explicit reference to neuroscientific discourses, though it was nevertheless trying to control emotions from the very beginning.

In phenomenology, the perceptual contact with the world is prior to consciousness and cognition (Husserl 1922/2002). Emotions constitute the subjective spatiality and temporality of the body which only one single person owns and feels as being her own, the so-called *le corps propre* in the terminology of Maurice Merleau-Ponty (in German: *Leib*, which is different from *Körper*, i.e., the physical body; see Merleau-Ponty 1966). Moreover, in phenomenology sensually felt emotions ("feelings") are the media for creating an intersubjective relation for constituting the life world and are not causes, means, or ends (Schmitz 2007).[21] In a process view, they are regarded as personal drives which are not ends in themselves.

It is worth debating how far this media character of emotions is actually transformed in order to make emotions target-oriented means. In other words, the techniques for shaping emotions with regard to cognitive content imply normative assumptions at different levels of description and explanation.

In the humanities, there is a consensus that emotions can be reduced neither to desires nor to reasons and that they are essential to human life. Emotions somehow connect the sphere of sensitivity[22] and the sphere of what is going to make sense, and they are sometimes seen as dispositions. In his famous article "What Is an Emotion?," William James wrote "that the emotional brain-processes not only resemble the ordinary sensorial brain-processes, but in very truth are nothing but such processes variously combined" (James 1884, 188). He argues that "bodily disturbances" directly follow the perception (e.g., of something perceived as dangerous). The idea of disturbances refers back to the etymology of the word "emotion." They are the manifestations of emotions, from which then the feeling arises which is the emotion. James strongly disagrees with the opinion that it is the mental perception of some fact which "excites the mental affection called the emotion, and that this latter state of mind gives rise to the bodily expression" (James 1884, 189f). In short, James argues that there is no purified "mind-stuff," but bodily symptoms which necessarily belong to emotions and which are expressed quite consistently from an evolutionary perspective (e.g., by the contraction of the brow).

Antonio R. Damasio (1999) distinguished between emotions, defined as the body states caused by somatic markers, and feelings, which he defines as the conscious perception of emotional body states. To cut a long philosophical story short, this view refers to an interior map of representation and second-order representations which undergo further re-representations within the brain. In a simplified form, this idea was already put forward by Aristotle, who (in *De anima* 412b 5–9) used the metaphor of a wax plate situated within the human soul, enabling the soul to form concrete impressions while perception was being inspired by fantasy. It was a metaphor, though, and it was related to the cognition of a higher than empirical knowledge. In Aristotle's (and later Hegel's)[23] view, emotions were only alogical during childhood because they remained in the sphere of the lower appetites (related to the vegetative soul inside the human body), that is, what we call "drives" today (Freud 1991). However, they always contained the potential to be persuaded by rationality. During education, the child was taught to exercise self-control and to let emotions serve virtues for the sake of the human good (see Fortenbaugh 2002; Nussbaum 2001/2003; Elster 1999, 52–75). In the grown-up, the habituated and cultivated emotions enabled the individual to act properly even before reflecting on the consequences of the act, for example, in situations of war. In antiquity, emotions were related to both ethical and political theory, that is, they were practical and, if applied right, proof of prudence (Luckner 2005). With its appeal to social responsibility, one may well understand Goleman's concept of EI as a watered-down version of Aristotelian thought, adapted to modern times. Aristotle's list of emotions was long, compared to contemporary ones, ranging from mildness, love, and benevolence to contempt, shame, pity, selfishness, emulation, anger, and fear. This enumeration reveals that for Aristotle emotions concerned both the individual and family level (involving friendship; Greek *oikos*) and the community (Greek *koinonia*) and city (Greek *polis*) level, that is, emotions were always political (Sokolon 2006). It is noteworthy that Aristotle differentiated between emotion and emotional response (in relation to someone), a much richer version of the twentieth century category of behavior. There was, however, no special concept related to subjectivity such as consciousness, which would have allowed him to separate emotions from feelings.

The general dialectical structure of emotions, that is, possessing the potential to be both rational and irrational, and being situated between physical dependence and autonomy, has continued through the centuries. Influences from different cultural, religious, and political contexts reformulated the ontological architectures in which emotions were situated—above all, the potential of the human being to be actively good or bad.

One major question still debatable within present ontological architectures is whether the body or the mind is primary for having emotions. James, in contrast to Damasio, voted for the body. What for James was an emotion is, so to say, a feeling for Damasio. Damasio's idea of somatic markers in the brain is strongly inspired by neuroimaging, blurring the distinction between cause and representation. As a consequence, the mind, though immaterial, seems to be embodied a priori.

In the last decades, emotions have lost their primacy in the mind and in the body. In the past, they were responsible for the unmediated responses of human beings, while simultaneously representing authenticity and personality. In contemporary thought, they serve the intellect in different ways.[24] A well-known service function is named motivation. As a result, a feeling (a mental representation of an emotion) is not just a feeling; it can be right or wrong, it can be enhanced by mental training, and it can be provoked. The problem, similar to that with evolutionary theory, is that it is only clear afterwards which emotion would have been "right" to feel and express. The different disciplines involved in demarcating the line between rational and irrational choices "to feel something" lack a unifying fundament of rationality (Karafyllis and Schmidt 2002) due to the unclear ontological and epistemological status of emotion and of world. Emotions interact with cultural values, and the transformation of emotions by media cultures (see Fahlenbrach and Bartsch, this volume) configures culture-dependent emotional styles (see Reddy, this volume). On the other hand, there might be some invariant human facial expressions across cultures—a question Charles Darwin was already deeply interested in (Darwin 1872/1998) before it gave rise to a psychological research field, nowadays prominently represented by Paul Ekman (2006). This unclear status of emotions between nature and culture is but one reason why research on emotions has recently become prominent both in the sciences and humanities.[25]

When sociologists Gillian Bendelow and Simon J. Williams (1997) wrote more than a decade ago that Western intellectuals had neglected the study of emotions because they thought in dualisms like mind/body and nature/culture (on the latter, see Ortner 1972), they might not have imagined the outcome of today's research: a strong interest in emotions while researchers still cling to dualisms, even if the latter nowadays are more difficult to identify. Two of these dualisms which are sometimes difficult to detect in current neuroscientific writings are mind/brain and brain/body. When you subtract "brain," the old mind/body problem emerges again. It is obvious that, depending on what is to be explained or justified, the brain is modeled as belonging either to the sphere of the body or to the sphere of the mind. The commonly used term "embodiment" (Lakoff and Johnson 1999) makes understanding exactly what is embodied where, how, and why even more complex. Another dualism is emotion/ intelligence, or emotion/rational decision, and these dualisms all seem to have been merged into a monistic structure within some psycho–bio concepts of EI and social neurosciences.

However, in the academic world of psychology, EI's definition as a psychological construct is still in a state of flux, and there is disagreement about how EI is to be measured (EQ) and applied (Geher 2005, Murphy 2006). In the 1990s, psychologists John ("Jack") D. Mayer and Peter Salovey revisited and reconceptualized EI (Salovey and Mayer 1990, 1997). The idea of fusing emotions with intelligence is by no means new, and one of its forerunners is the concept of "social intelligence" (see Bechtoldt, this volume). In addition to concepts of multiple intelligences (as put forward by, e.g., Howard Gardner), the claim that there is an EI serving the "real," that is, rational intelligence, yields two hierarchical, heteronormative forms of intelligence which can easily be affiliated with the heteronormativity of biological sex—even if this connection was never intended by its originators.

From a cultural point of view, the brain has now replaced the heart, which until the early modern period had been "the" organ of emotions, while the blood was their carrier (once thought to produce different temperaments). The biologically interpreted ontic nature of the human being (i.e., in the neuroscientific context: the brain and its neural activity) seems to work toward useful ends, when viewed from a metalevel, but, in so doing, this approach to humans neglects the individual, practical, and social level of useful meanings. Humans, rather than the brain, take action. Moreover, the classic philosophical questions concerning the mind/body problem and intentionality (e.g., How can I think "myself"? Is there a free will?) are still unanswered and will probably never be fully answered.[26] Maybe it belongs to being human to live with unanswerable questions. Nevertheless, the stories of an overall *neuromythology* (Fuchs 2006/2007), imagined by brains which have attained the status of meta-subjects in modern—mostly Western—societies, linger on. Individual brains, we argue, have a status that falls between subjects and objects in contemporary science. They are hybrids (Latour 1993), or biofacts (Karafyllis 2007a, 2008e), and neither resist naturalization (objectivation) nor personification (subjectivation) (see Latour 2004, 47). As epistemic things, which are also said to be alive, they allow scientists and others to forget that the concept of life they represent is exclusively neurobiological, and that "alive" is reduced to a mere attribute.

Brain research, in general, operates on three epistemic levels. On the macrolevel, it offers functional descriptions and explanations of conceptualized areas, such as the cerebral cortex and the amygdala. The mesolevel deals with larger cell units and tissues, while the microlevel elucidates the processes of single cells and molecules. Most advances in the neurosciences are made at the macro- and microlevel, the latter having a strong affiliation with genomics and proteomics research programs. The general direction of related research is top-down, not bottom-up. Looking at the microlevel, you can find genes for expressing hormones that might be relevant for certain reactions, but you cannot find a gene for an emotion or emotionality in general. Processes on the mediating mesolevel are still rarely understood. In neuroscientific studies of emotion at the macrolevel, there is currently a strong focus on making the functions of the ACC visible by neuroimaging. The ACC seems to be involved in reward-based learning and emotional affects.

At the microlevel, a special class of cells occurs in the ACC regions of humans, whales, and great apes, the so-called *spindle neurons* (the Von Economo neurons; see Nimchinsky et al. 1999, Allman et al. 2002), which could be responsible for intelligence and emotion (in general) and adaptive responses to changing environments. They were already described in the nineteenth century but recently have been found to occur only in the most intelligent mammals. Strictly speaking, this view challenges the idea that the ACC forms part of a primitive region (see section 1.1). Spindle neurons seem to arrange the transit of signals exchanged between the cortex and distant parts of the brain. In people with "autistic" disorders (pervasive developmental disorders), the spindle neurons are suspected of having developed abnormally.

Up to now, the category of neurons called spindle neurons has primarily been described anatomically. In contrast, the second prominent category of neurons important for the field of EI has been described physiologically and thus has gained greater significance in epistemic contexts within the neuroscience of emotions (particularly related to empathy): the *mirror neurons*. In the 1990s, the research group around Giacomo Rizzolatti discovered that observing the action of others and imitating the same action activates a common neuronal network. They called this neuronal system the *mirror neuron system* (Gallese et al. 1996, Rizzolatti and Craighero 2004) and defined mirror neurons as a special type of visuomotor neurons. Empathy research at the macrolevel is, at present, intensely involved in mirror neuron research at the microlevel.

These explanations all sound very rich in presuppositions. It seems that when neuroscientific findings are exported to other explanatory contexts, they lose their theoretical backgrounds. On the other hand, the disciplines importing the neuroscientific propositions gain the aura of a scientific fundament, in the narrow, empirical sense of the word "scientific." The new neurodisciplines in the humanities, such as neurophilosophy, -sociology, -theology, and -economics reinforce the reductionist approaches to the complex world of everyday life and living practice. They more or less accept the basic assumptions transported with the neurobiological interpretations of the empirical data and artificially evoked effects and provoked phenomena (resulting from stimulation and context isolation) which result from experiments in the worlds of the laboratory and thus transform the ontological and normative theory backgrounds especially in the humanities and social sciences.

What is also forgotten, then, is that any biological interpretation always operates with historical assumptions about the development of life on earth, due to evolutionary thinking. Because of this, our objective is to provide the historians of science and culture with a platform side by side with the biologists and psychologists in order to narrate different stories about how the results of different studies of the emotions and intelligences were constructed. As is well-known in the history of philosophy, the humanities themselves have carried sexualized, sometimes misogynous concepts of human nature (e.g., concerning temper and character, from Aristotle in ancient times to Otto Weininger in modern times)[27] throughout the centuries. As science is part of the culture in which it develops, recent scientific models of male/female brains and behaviors necessarily are influenced by these cultural settings. At least for Greek antiquity, the existence of something in between, that is, hermaphrodites, was certain, moreover admirable, and the existence of intersexes and transsexual persons (see Nye, this volume) remains a challenge for brain and behavioral research today.

Moreover, psychology, with part of its theoretical background of subjectivity rooted in psychoanalysis, is one of the disciplines which has been put under great pressure by the neurodisciplines. When subjectivity is not reduced to mere personal behavior, psychology emphasizes the philosophically important point that individual identity is determined more by its temporal (biographical) than by its spatial (localized) constitution. Neurobiology still focuses primarily on the spatial dimension of the central organ brain, its areas, and regions ("neuroarchitecture"), although there have been recent efforts at historicizing localized dysfunctional emotions as "temporal injuries," especially in trauma research. Related to these findings is the distinction between primary (innate) emotions and secondary emotions, which are attached individually to specific objects and events. The terms "function" and "dysfunction," nevertheless, refer to biological and economic ends which seem to be fixed in a state of cultural vacuum.

1.6 Step 4: Analyzing the Equity and Equality of Emotions, as Well as the Impact of Brain Research

At first sight, emotions might seem to be a resource which everybody has plenty of—something that is obviously not true for intelligence, as has been demonstrated in the elaborate testing culture around the IQ.[28] When we look closer at the intertwined concepts in the sciences, this veil of equity and equality of emotions is a very thin one, with the old stereotypes and social stratifications still visible underneath.[29] Because of strong competition in the job market, a high value is set on scientific proofs of special qualifications for doing the right job (and doing the job right). Emotions are nowadays also interesting as additional qualifications for intelligent abilities, helping to fill out a person's rational capabilities and to acquire new ones. Only if a person is conscious of her abilities can these qualities be communicated and offered as capabilities. Women seem to have plenty of potential for "good" emotions in private life (e.g., empathy), while men may have potentially useful emotions for the workplace, connected with aggressiveness, competitiveness, self-assertiveness, and so forth.

Social neuroscience engages in research on job qualifications, as does research on EI within work and organization psychology. To cite but one example, neurobiologist Tania Singer and her colleagues tested which of the men's and women's brain areas lit up during fMRI scans while the test persons were watching physical pain stimulations to the hands of four complicit professional actors, that is, "confederates," some of whom had cheated in a game symbolically dealing with money—related to economic models of "altruistic punishment" and social preferences (Singer et al. 2006). The so-called primitive brain areas for reward lit up in the 16 men examined but not in the 16 women (see figure 1.2) when seeing the unfair "confederate" receiving a pain stimulus. Instead, women's "empathy centers" glowed.[30] After undergoing scanning, the volunteers were given questionnaires, asking, among other things, about the volunteers' empathy and desire for punishing the confederates for their unfairness. Astonishingly, women wrote that they did *feel* a desire for punishment, though this feeling did not show up in the neuroimages, in contrast to men (see figure 1.3; see also Ulshöfer, this volume, for further descriptions of this experiment). Interpreting these results, Tania Singer said in an interview with *The New York Times* (see below) that men "expressed more desire for revenge and seemed to feel satisfaction when unfair people were given what they perceived as deserved physical punishment." Her interpretation of the male reaction, which does not seem to be very sociable, is as follows: "This type of behavior has probably been crucial in the evolution of society as the majority of people in a group are motivated to punish those who cheat on the rest." Even though she states that there is more research to be done, she does not hesitate to make a recommendation which goes far beyond the biological setting: "This investigation would seem to indicate there is a predominant role for men in maintaining justice and issuing punishment" (all citations quoted in *The New York Times*, January 19, 2006, in the article "When bad people are punished, men smile (but women don't)" by E. Rosenthal).[31] Putting aside the ambiguous relation between perceiving and feeling something, and the desire for something and the actual emotion, as both systemic problems of the neurosciences, at this point let us ask some rhetorical questions. For instance, are male lawyers and policemen right for the job? How about men's lower ability to communicate the reasons for issuing their punishment (women in general show higher communication skills in experiments; see, e.g., Kimura 1999)? Or has the Stone Age become the new utopia for science, replacing the popular science fiction visions for assessment? Why not look at the present societies, for a change?

Seen through the eyes of a neurobiologist, individual cheating is obviously not useful for the so-called evolution of society, which is outlined in the quotations above according to models of population biology, moreover without hierarchical stratifications. This view challenges some of the approaches to EI, where various ways of individual cheating (on the rest), for example, pretending, can be a sign of EI and of being qualified for leadership.

Let's return to the question of who is right for which job. What is "right" is narrowly and functionally interpreted in the quotations above, and the definition of functionality moreover differs according to sex and dominant socioeconomic structures. Back in 1983, Arlie R. Hochschild analyzed, in her classic book *The Managed Heart*, the "emotional labor" typically reserved for the service sector. It is mostly women (and also a high percentage of gay men) who work in this field that is likely to be associated with neither elite thinking nor high wages. They seem to be "naturally" qualified, although they might culturally have adopted management techniques in handling their emotions depending on the social context, that is, what Paul Ekman calls "display rules" (Ekman 2007, 4). According to Nicky James (1989, 15), emotional labor is "the work involved in dealing with other people's feelings, a core component of which is the regulation of emotions." We editors do not know if there are studies in which the EQ of flight attendants, nurses, or wait persons has been tested. However, the jobs offered in service, caring, and child care depend on professional "warm hearts" (Bernard 1981, 215). Will they depend on "warm brains" in the near future, or on female brains, or can these, because of the glowing empathy centers shown in neuroimages, even be regarded as the same? When Goleman (see section 1.3) typified the pure female EQ type with the attribute of easy stress coping, he might have been thinking of the cultural reality that it is primarily women who actually are working in jobs of emotional labor,[32] connected with a special kind of stress (Persaud 2004).

In contrast to the neuroscientific Tania Singer group, psychologist Paul Ekman explicitly stated that during his research on facial expressions of emotions (e.g., Ekman, Friesen, and Ellsworth 1972), trying to determine whether they are innate or not, he searched for a culture which was still living in the Stone Age (Ekman 2007, 3f). Before changing his hypothesis, he showed photographs of white Caucasians with facial expressions of distinct emotions to U.S. Americans, Brazilians, Japanese, and others to observe their nonverbal behavior, especially their facial expressions, but wrote, "All the people I . . . have studied might have learned the meaning of Western facial expressions by watching Charlie Chaplin and John Wayne on the movie screen and television tube" (Ekman 2007, 4). This statement reveals why the questions put forward in this volume belong together: the different media (photographs, videotapes, professional actors, mirrors, etc.) used in experiments, popular culture (including media culture), and science are influential in shaping an emotion.

Among the five basic emotions, the semantic fields and indicators (e.g., pain) related to anger and anxiety have been examined most intensely in the neurosciences, compared to happiness, for example, as these emotions inspire the strongest reactions and responses. Referring to long-lasting feelings, guilt is one of the prominent candidates for research in psychology. However, empathy and love are currently receiving much scrutiny, though it is debatable whether this is for better or worse. Undoubtedly, gender and sexual stereotypes will continue to influence models and explanations of emotions.

1.7   Science and Emancipation—A Conflicted Relation

As we saw previously, sexual stereotyping has already had an impact on both the context of discovery and the context of justification of cognitive neuroscience. This means the normative dimension does not arise in the—"later"—context of application, where specific technologies and policies are developed, but already in the early stages. Even prior to theory development, the metaphors, models, and symbols play a key role in consolidating a new research field (Keller 2002). Certain technologies for representing a functional nature and a functioning "society," like neuroimaging, also shape new ways of intervening and canalize the development of both new tools and hypotheses. A cultural philosophy of science has to be sensitive to these early stages of a science (or its subdivisions) in progress, such as social cognitive science and the model of an "extreme male brain" (Baron-Cohen 2004).

In the philosophy of science, the question has arisen many times since the beginning of the twentieth century of whether there are possible alternatives to a value-laden science. A philosophy of science which takes the cultural dimension of science seriously has to put the implicit normative assumptions of science in relation to the values of the specific culture in which science is situated and in which its research problems and hypotheses are generated. This would also elucidate science's explanatory limits. Many feminists want more, however, and vote for a science that should not primarily serve explanation, but emancipation, as Noretta Koertge (2003) critically points out. A serious challenge to this idea of an emancipatory science would be, first, the restriction of a science that contributes to concepts like sex, class, and race,[33] and, second, the imperative to actively include emancipatory elements into science. This conventional enumeration of sex, class, and race, which is often found to generally address oppressed groups, is misleading. While the biological attributions of sex and race are more or less innate and, in general, not open for change, a person is born into a specific class, but it is a political and societal decision how rigid social strata are and if (and how) a certain status can be overcome. Even if sex, class, and race together have typically comprised a category of the disadvantaged, referring to social cognitive science they are not at the same ontological level. To be more precise, in a political ontology these categories may be identical, but in a "natural" ontology (thinking, e.g., of Aristotle's philosophy of nature, or the ontology of the senses, that is, that olfactory and tactile senses give rise to sensations "closer" than the visual sense) they are not—at least insofar as the properties of "class" are not regarded as hereditary, and as the class structure and morphology are not reduced to mere hierarchy. Binet (1905/1916) had already mentioned that the socially privileged might object to intelligence testing, as it might result in prohibitions against perpetuating privileges which seemed to be guaranteed by bloodline.

Note that when we speak of "nature" as a philosophical term for self-reflection, we are not addressing the category that has been established by anthropologists and biologists (Konner 2002), based on Darwinian thinking (Darwin 1859; Darwin 1874; on Social Darwinism, see Young 1973, 1990, Bannister 1979); the same should also be taken into consideration when we speak of "culture." This differentiation is important to stress because sex and race have been well-established and explicit categories of biological research for centuries, while class and gender framed these categories (class has been inscribed particularly in biological systematics).[34] This scientific tradition is still apparent in the fact that the majority of social cognitive neuroscience studies, when exploring the perception of group differences, dwells on either race or sex differences, whereas class and gender are thought to belong to the political sphere and not to science. The reason is quite simple: class and gender are not considered to be entities of natural selection but rather their result. They resist serious biological scrutiny. However, they have made their way into structures of various anthropological and biological concepts (Janich and Weingarten 1999).

Sex is a concept which is primarily employed in the research dimension of *science of gender*; class generally refers to *gender in science* (see section 1.3); with regard to race, no differentiation is possible, as races or cultures which are defined as inferior are often labeled "female" (e.g., regarding Western intellectual history about the division orient/occident). Race differences, like sex differences, have also been a topic of interest for neuroimaging (e.g., Lieberman et al. 2005), related to the neuroscience research of social stigma (particularly: same-race-face vs. other-race-face recognition by means of amygdala activity; for a psychologists' critique of this research area, see Phelps and Thomas 2003). Lieberman et al.'s study (2005) rejects findings from other studies, which had found race differences in the race recognition of others. This study reveals that the processes happening, while either saying "African-American" to volunteers or showing a photograph of an African-American to them, are controlled differently by the brain. Emotional responses to words are more amenable to learning. This finding would seem to stress the importance of political correctness (PC) in the written and spoken word. At the moment, the question of whether PC is useful or not seems to be one of the important political contexts for social cognitive neuroscience, and thus its experimental designs frequently mirror political opinions. However, the real problem might not be the concept of PC itself, but rather the growing impression that PC is mere rhetoric without any real belief in the underlying ideas of justice, thus reveiling a *Menschenbild* which is pessimistic by heart.

Racism, like sexism, is making its way back into scientific journals. For instance, in the paper entitled *Race, brain size, and IQ: The case for consilience* (Rushton 2003), author J. Philippe Rushton, professor of psychology at the University of Western Ontario (Canada) and editorial-board member of the international journal *Intelligence*, compares brain sizes between races and tells the age-old story that the average size of African-Americans' brains are smaller than those of Caucasians, and he therefore concludes that the latter have higher cognitive abilities, which have recently been exceeded by the Mongolian type (see also Rushton 2000). It implies the idea of a "national intelligence" (Cattell 1937, Cattell 1971; see also Dobzhansky and Montagu 1947) which plays a part in global competition, obviously focused on China at the moment (on Rushton's racist research, see, e.g., the critiques of Cernovsky 1995, Lieberman 2001). Since he used MRI to support some of his findings, Rushton managed to place the paper in the journal *Behavioral and Brain Sciences*. The equation, smaller brain = lower intelligence, has often been applied to womens' brains, as well, and sometimes still is (see Hagner, this volume; Schmitz 2006a). The recently revived questions, in the field of behavior and population genetics, about whether *g* is hereditable, and what has happened to human intelligence for the better since the Black Man left sub-Saharan Africa, allows neo-eugenics, for example, Beyondism and Jensenism (Jensen 1998), to emerge, moreover supported with economic data from "successful" economies, their racial profile, and the average IQs of races (Lynn 2006; see also Turner and Glass 1976). If fast breeding of high-priority human genes and behaviors is a potential goal for science, and for the society in which science is embedded, then women will have to be modeled as highly reproductive and available (for a social history perspective, see Schwartz 2006).[35] Thinking of genetics and neuroscience as "hard sciences"—as materialized if-then conditionals of pure causality, without having a cultural and social background in which they emerge, are applied, and make sense— makes it easier to say, "Just look at the data! The differences speak for themselves!" Perhaps a look at the last 200 years of related anthropological research would clarify the outcomes to which all-encompassing strategies in science can lead, how they arise, and how they can trigger various ways of oppressing or even eliminating "minorities" (Dobzhansky 1966, Stocking 1968, Chorover 1980, Tucker 1994, Stanton 1982, Stepan 1982, Stümke 1989, Harris 2001, Lieberman 2001, Jellonnek and Lautmann 2002, Tucker 2002, zur Nieden 2005a, 2005b, Weiler 2006). Alfred Binet's original idea of preventing discrimination (against individual children in school) through intelligence testing has been turned to the opposite purpose, though there are exceptions. When testing is done for reasons other than supporting the individual, that is, to help the individual achieve her or his own goals, such testing is better not done. After all, there should remain something like a property right to one's own "cognitive" unconscious. However, testing culture of humans, applied to humans, has traveled a long way down the slippery slope.

For both scientists and ethicists, it is important to understand how scientific modeling in advance sets normative benchmarks, which cannot be later erased by ethical evaluation if they are later detected at all. The previously mentioned case in which emotional processes in the brain were either labeled "automatic evaluation" or defined as "natural" stereotypes in the brain a priori, and where people were defined as stigmatized without asking for their self-understanding, is but one example.

As philosopher of science Ian Hacking (1998, 99) puts it:

Binet's great innovation, the testing of intelligence, made sense only against a background of shared judgments about intelligence, and it had to agree with them by and large, and also to explain when it disagreed. Who shared the judgments? Those who matter, namely, the educators, other civil servants, and Binet's peers in the middle classes of society. Despite the sometimes unattractive features of the history of intelligence testing, there was seldom a deep problem about calibration. This was because, at any time, there was a body of agreed judgments and discriminations of intelligence to which the IQ tests were calibrated.

Psychological research on intelligence, referring to educational backgrounds, necessarily focuses on class differences. "Class" in a political ontology has a structure parallel to the category of "gender," as the social gender role of many "women" can still be regarded as a disadvantage (e.g., from an economic or legal point of view). The role, however, is not a disadvantage in and of itself—as long as it is not biologicalized with the aim of transforming women into a *body of society* and making this altered role a reality in society (e.g., Tiger and Fowler 2007). The success of this will depend on how desperate the leading elites' desire is to become the *brain of society*.

So how should science serve emancipation? On the one hand, one may ask if such a political enervation of science would still be science and if scientists could then still function as a "small, powerful, well-educated group" (Koertge 2003, 229), that is, as an elite. Koertge is right to argue that prolonged debates would emerge about which types of hypotheses are actually politically progressive. She concludes, "We should make every attempt to keep politics and religion out of the laboratory." But what if they are already in the laboratory from the very beginning? Currently, there is a strong public and scientific interest in finding the neurobiological basis of religious feelings and spiritual phenomena, giving rise to a neurotheology (Goleman 1997b, Dalai Lama 1999, Newberg and Lee 2005). On the other hand, then, we have to answer the question of whether science in general can be "neutral" to political and economic developments. As the history of science (e.g., concerning military research and eugenics) has shown, and some of the contributors to this book also show, it obviously cannot. The laboratory world is not simply an isolated world of its own, though with regard to hypotheses and findings as mere sentences (propositions) within a theoretical framework of deductionism and empiricism it may appear to be one (Köchy and Schiemann 2006). It is doubtful whether an attempt at ideological purification would be feasible at all and, moreover, whether it would even be useful. Furthermore, one could ask how the border between the laboratory and society is constituted in a vision of a purely explanatory science. Nowadays, a culture of testing, therapy, and enhancement pervades many industrialized societies, which means that society itself functions as an extended laboratory (Krohn 2007; see also Cunningham and Williams 1992). Thus, philosophy of science has to engage with political philosophy and sociology because science itself engages with society and politics. It has always done so, as philosophers and sociologists can learn from historians of science. Therefore, there is a need not only for a philosophy of applied sciences but also for an applied philosophy of science. The laboratory, as a detached sphere of value-free experimenting geniuses which disseminates pure knowledge into a society, is a myth. Another myth is that in capitalistic societies, where huge amounts of money are invested in the funding of science by governments and companies, the two-phase approach of science—first, "undisturbed"/ "pure" science, and, then, ethical evaluation—will lead to better science in the normative sense (Düwell 2004). If ethicists really were given a veto right with regard to the context of the application of scientific findings, the possibility would then exist that some investments might turn out to be a waste of time and money. The pop science book market already adjusted to this mere possibility of ethical limits, as, for example, media activist John Brockman recently has been asking scientists, "What is your dangerous idea?" (Brockman 2006; see also Brockman 1996, 2004a). A waste of time and money is unlikely to happen due to economic rationality which, thus far, has been put forward to justify attempts to make scientific progress (and vice versa). In the long run, citizens and consumers will decide which scientific findings, technologies, and products are culturally relevant and lasting. And, last but not least, these decisions will depend on emotions and what sense they make in real life—not just in the jungle inside the brain.

1.8   Outlook

Science as such necessarily remains based on empirical data collection, solid analysis of the data, and theoretical scrutiny. In fact, the openness of this process as well as the accessibility to it has to be guaranteed, in order to observe and review this process from the very beginning. Consequently, we neither suggest that EI-related science is wrong, or even "bad" in general, nor do we claim that there is no such thing as sex-related differences in human beings. The problem seems to be the narrow construction of normality and functionality which is supposed to correspond to two unique sexes and one type of sexuality (heterosexuality), and that this one type is thought to be constitutive for any functioning society in general (see also Richardson 2000).

There are good reasons to support research on sex differences. Some feminist activists, for example, argue for a more "sexualized" medicine and an epistemology related to the female body, as many illnesses and maladies—heart attacks, for instance—appear in men and women with different symptoms. When medicine uses only the male body as a boundary object for diagnosis and therapy research, the health care of women is endangered, as illustrated by recent figures showing that fewer women recover from acute heart attacks because of incorrect and/or late treatment. What we can learn from the experts in this book is that gender research in the neurosciences is still in its infancy. It remains to be seen whether feminists—and others—will find good reasons for fighting for a female (and male) brain.

Finally, why not ask for the scientist's self-understanding, which is reflexively related to the self-image of science? When Koertge (2003, 232) criticizes Helen Longino's idea of a "feminist scientist" (1990) who is responsive to the ideals of a political community, she expresses doubts about whether science can simultaneously be made both more objective and more humane. Here we would like to add that science is practiced by human persons who must have motivation from outside the laboratory to find out "something" in order to explain it (and do something good) to "someone." This humanist interpretation of scientists and their ethos is not restricted to the scientist's sex. Ensuring gender perspectives in science will not "naturally" be guaranteed by recruiting more women scientists[36] but by employing people who are interested in scientifically acknowledging the pluralism of modern societies. With regard to neuro- and cognitive science as "hard science," "big science," and pop science, small scientific solutions and limited explanations currently do not seem to be *en vogue*. On the contrary, holisms of mind, brain, gender, and world might soon go out of fashion.

If science is understood in an elitist and thereby exclusionary way, and scientists are forced to choose between either "the true" or "the good," science will lose its relevance for cultural progress. There is no such thing as scientific progress without the assumption of cultural progress, whatever both mean in detail. For modern societies, the emancipatory element is fundamental as is the possibility to critically reflect upon it. This is but one of the reasons why the sciences and the humanities depend on each other.

1.9   Summary

To sum up: The modern cartography of the human brain describes areas which are said to perform thinking and feeling functions. By virtue of this topography, a neurobiology, a neurophilosophy, and even a neuroeconomics can be developed. In the context of these scientific and philosophical developments, questions of gender and sex become matters of critical importance: To what extent are specific types of intelligence—EI, for instance—restricted to female or, alternatively, male behavior or performance, or the biological sex? In contrast, to what extent do cultural and biological attributions of sex and gender define the topography both of the human brain and of society? Raising the question of gendering in relation to the neurosciences also enables us to ask, are specific forms of intelligence or performance socially and economically privileged? In terms of EI, are all brains equal, or are some more equal than others? Did and do we have "elite brains"? Can you train yourself to become "at least" emotionally intelligent, if not "really" intelligent? If some of the questions are answered with a "Yes," what are the consequences? Behind the social acknowledgment of elites one can find masterminds—and how masterminds are defined.

Acknowledgments

We are indebted to Stephen L. Starck for his continuous and invaluable help during all stages of translation. Thanks also to Carmen Baumeler, whose comments on a draft version have had an enormous impact on the finished product.

Notes

1. Goleman's first book on EI (Goleman 1995) was translated into 30 languages—for example, German translation *Emotionale Intelligenz* (1996), Dutch translation *Emotionele intelligentie* (1996), Italian translation *Intelligenza emotiva* (1996, transl. Isabella Blum), French translation *Intelligence*

émotionnelle (1999, transl. Thierry Piélat), Spanish translation *La inteligenca emocional* (1999, transl. Elsa Mateo), and a Japanese translation that appeared in 1998. Whereas in German and Dutch the acronym EI is used as it is in English, it is referred to as IE in the French, Italian, and Spanish literature.

2. Earlier examples of related books are Moir and Jessel (1992), Sapolsky (1997), Geary (1998), Kimura (1999), and Blum (2007, 1st ed. 1997). In this book, we focus only on those authors of both scientific and pop-scientific volumes who had an education in science or are still science practitioners, for example, Simon Baron-Cohen, Louann Brizendine, Paul Ekman, Robert M. Sapolsky, Doreen Kimura, and Daniel Goleman, though the last has spent the past 25 years of his life working as a science journalist, editor, and coach. For example, science writer and Pulitzer Prize Winner Deborah Blum's *Sex on the Brain* will just be listed to mark the discourse field but not considered here for a thorough investigation. We also do not touch on the issue of how sexual arousal is represented in the brain, although there is a close relation between functional magnetic resonance imaging (fMRI) of nonhuman primates—for example, marmosets, which showed neural activity in different brain regions (including those relevant for "decision making") after olfactory hormonal stimulation (see Ferris et al. 2004)—and the claim for a sexualized human brain (Brizendine 2006) and a human mating intelligence (Geher and Miller 2007).

3. In contrast to the study's authors, we would suggest "perceive" here.

4. "Human being" and "person" cannot be used interchangeably in the context of our book. As is known from philosophy, it is debatable what exactly makes a human being a person, for example, his or her biographical consciousness of temporality, forming an individual identity. This problem particularly emerges in bioethics—for instance, concerning the question about whether newborn babies, great apes, or coma patients are—already or still—persons or not.

5. "Outstanding leaders' emotional competencies make up 85% to 100% of the competencies crucial for success" (Goleman 1998, 187).

6. In Germany, there was a huge political debate in 2006 concerning whether politicians are allowed to use the word "Unterschicht" (literally translated: "understratum," meaning underclass) for addressing the less economically successful. The Friedrich Ebert Foundation therefore suggested the word "Prekariat." On the other hand, there seems to be no problem in emphasizing the special status of an elite university.

7. Both bioartists and bioscientists increasingly take part in "sci-art" programs, which are funded by the U.K. Wellcome Trust, among others. As Jens Hauser (2008) puts it: "One of the questions we may ask is whether artists engaging with biotechnologies can still choose the appropriate context for their action, or if they fulfill context's expectation of *usefulness* that can become a slippery terrain."

8. We thank Jens Hauser for this information. On endogenous design in BioArt, see, for example, Karafyllis 2008c.

9. Enhancement strategies concerning the body range from fitness training to cosmetic surgery, as well as pharmaceutical and biomedical treatments to achieve a perfect body.

10. One cannot only think of recent research in deep brain stimulation, which is trying to enhance the capacities both of remembering and of forgetting certain incidents. Recent approaches to neuroeconomics must also be kept in mind (see Ulshöfer, this volume).

11. For a broader view on the relation of feminism and liberalism, see Nussbaum (1999a) and Fraisse (1993; 2007).

12. We do not want to get into a discussion of the role of the economic elite area here (cf., e.g., Münkler 2006) and whether it is *the* leading elite; it is, in any case, one of the leading elites.

13. Quoted in the national report of the German Federal Government (2006) on women in leading positions in the economy: Die Bundesregierung. 2006. *2. Bilanz Chancengleichheit: Frauen in Führungspositionen.* http://www.bmfsfj.de/kategorien/Forschungsnetz/forschungsberichte,did= 69162.html (accessed May 4, 2007), 11.

14. In a national study on elites in Germany, Ursula Hoffmann-Lange argues that the social background exerts only an indirect influence on access and recruiting with regard to the chances of getting a good education (Hoffmann-Lange 1992, 129ff).

15. For the research field of sexual arousal, see, for example, Heath (1972), Park et al. (2001), Hackbert and Heimann (2002), Holstege et al. (2003), Holstege and Georgiadis (2004), Canli and Gabrieli (2004), Komisaruk et al. (2004), Maravilla and Yang (2007).

16. In the French original it is *anormaux*.

17. The use of the Greek word *stigma* derives from the Bible, where the sentence in Paul's letter to the Galatians reads: "I bear on my body the marks (τα στιγματα) of Jesus" (Gal. 6, 17). The idea of stigmatized persons developed in medieval times; the first extensively documented case (1224) was Francis of Assisi, Italy (Yarom 1992). The first stigmatized woman is thought to be Christina von Stommeln (who died in 1312) of Jülich, Germany, who had the wounds of the crucified Jesus on her body (Harrison 1996). From then on, the number of persons purportedly bearing stigmata increased.

18. Brain research, especially when related to cognitive science research (see LeDoux and Hirst 1986), now seems to offer a "more scientific" alternative to "understanding" the true rationality of emotions: the *cognitive unconscious* (Lakoff and Johnson 1999, 9–15).

19. In philosophy, this difference is referred to as the *"qualia* problem."

20. During World War II, Otto Friedrich Bollnow wrote the basic work on the essence of moods (Bollnow 1995), in which—strongly influenced by the philosophy of Martin Heidegger—he characterizes moods as preliminary to emotions and feelings. Moods thus are essential to human existence, making an individual self-aware and inhibiting or facilitating certain emotions.

21. This view includes sexuality, which Merleau-Ponty views as "sexual drama," rooted in the very dialectic of existence: autonomy and dependence (Merleau-Ponty 1962, 153f).

22. Historian of science Adelheid Voskuhl (2005) points out how sensitivity and (French) *sensibilité* as one of the leitmotifs since the late eighteenth century were constructed by the interplay

of music, machine (music playing female androids), and literature. See also Barker-Benfield (1992), with a focus on sensibility.

23. Hegel (1830/1970, § 396).

24. This idea goes back to Aristotle's theory of intellect (Nussbaum 2001/2003).

25. See DeSousa (1987), Stocker and Hegeman (1996), Hatzimoysis (2003), Prinz (2006), to name just a few. For an overview of research fields focusing on emotions in psychology, see Lewis, Haviland-Jones, and Barrett (2008). For the relation of emotions and sociology, see Bendelow and Williams (1997). For a recent philosophical approach to emotions, see Kochinka (2004).

26. For a historical analysis of how the "I" became materialized in the brain research of the nineteenth and twentieth centuries, see Breidbach (1997).

27. On Greek antiquity, see Föllinger (1996); on Otto Weininger's influential main work *Geschlecht und Charakter* (translation: *Sex and Character*), see Harrowitz and Hyams (1995), and for a broader perspective, especially on the relation of sex and sexuality, see Nye (1999).

28. Nathan Brody presents a useful overview of the problems of scientifically understanding "general intelligence" ("*g*") and mentions score differences in intelligence tests related to race and class. Gender differences are not examined. Brody argues that the influence of race and class is overestimated, writing that "tests are sometimes disliked by privileged parents because they serve as a barrier to the perpetuation of social privilege" (Brody 2006, 174). Ironically, he supports his argument with Francis Galton's book *Hereditary Genius* (1869), in which Galton argues for a genetic explanation "because he noted that many men of genius had modest family backgrounds" (Brody 2006, 173). Galton is known to be one of the fathers of eugenic science.

29. This can be seen in Brizendine (2006).

30. As mentioned above, in earlier experiments, Singer et al. (2004a) observed that the bilateral anterior insula, the rostral ACC, the brainstem, and the cerebellum were activated when subjects experienced pain but also when they saw (in a mirror) that a loved one was experiencing pain (see figure 1.1).

31. In the scientific publication (Singer et al. 2006, 469) the conclusion is this: "It is possible that our experimental design favoured men because the modality of punishment was related to physical threat, as opposed to psychological or financial threat. Alternatively, those findings could indicate a predominant role for males in the maintenance of justice and punishment of norm violation in human societies."

32. Emotional labor means professional labor in which the regulation of emotions plays a crucial part, whereas emotional work means the same structural element in private life.

33. Koertge (2003, 227) presents the example of psychologist Paul Ekman, who reports that when he began to study facial expressions, which are supposed to be invariant in different cultures and can be identified as related to identical human emotions, Margaret Mead and Gregory

Bateson advised him against this study. They feared that any sort of biological explanation of emotions would encourage eugenic thinking. A source indicating that Ekman asked them for advice before studying this field can be found in Ekman (2007, 2).

34. Sociobiological research is an important exception.

35. In the communist countries after Lysenkoism, the idea of testing intelligences was rejected, though not exclusively. For further readings see Eysenck (1982) and Davis (1983), particularly on Eastern Germany (former German Democratic Republic), see Friedrich (1981), Schulze (1986), and Hagemann (1988).

36. On the contrary, women's access to science is important with regard to the different opportunities offered them in society.

I Historical Analysis: Cultural and Scientific Forces

2 Genius, Gender, and Elite in the History of the Neurosciences

Michael Hagner

2.1 Introduction

On the 21st of February, 2006, the president of Harvard University, Larry Summers, resigned from his post.[1] There are a number of explanations for this resignation. Summers was not particularly liked by Harvard professors: His innovations were contested, and his less than charming manner met with considerable opposition. The latter developed into open animosity when, during a discussion in early 2005, Summers remarked that it was possibly no accident that so few women made it to the top in science. To make matters worse, he referred to women's biological constitution. No matter how vehemently Summers later protested that he did not mean to defend any kind of physical determinism—and that the lesser ability of women to succeed may well also be a result of chronic social discrimination—the damage was irreparable. Summers never recovered from this lapse, right up to the time of his resignation.

No doubt any male academic permitting himself such a remark would incur serious damage to his career. What made the Summers case particularly remarkable, though, and caused it to receive worldwide attention was the fact that it linked two highly contested issues: on the one hand, gender, and on the other, the elite. Harvard, as an institution, symbolizes the academic elite par excellence. It represents a concentration of talents, energy, and financial resources that is the object of worldwide admiration and emulation. Moral values are likewise a part of Harvard's image. Like the other elite universities in the United States, Harvard is supposed to be a place where political correctness and strict equality are painstakingly observed. Summers' remark was a blatant violation of this rule. When the president of an academic institution educating and representing "the" elite excludes women from this sphere, he is calling into question the implicit understanding that justifies the very existence of and striving for elite status: that it is, in principle, attainable for all. Even if—for whatever reasons—most people do not reach this goal, no social or biological group per se is excluded. In disregarding this rule, Larry Summers was thinking in stereotypes that stem from the nineteenth and twentieth centuries and are obviously still very much alive today, in spite of all the political and cultural changes of the past decades. Suddenly, all the old questions associated with those old stigmatizations return: Do women by nature have the same intellectual capabilities as men? Can they fill socially responsible positions as effectively as men? Do they have the same aptitude for advanced studies and are they as suitable for high academic positions as men? Whoever thought we had left all of these questions behind once and for all, and could turn to other matters, was mistaken. One passing remark, made by Summers on the occasion of a meeting that, in itself, was insignificant, recorded as if by accident and circulated around the globe, serves to show how quickly the old associations come up again, and how narrow the gap is that separates us from the past we thought we had overcome.

Larry Summers studied economics, so he does not come from the natural sciences, which is usually—rightly or wrongly—considered to be the bastion of such simplistic biological imputations. The prejudice is not entirely unfounded. Still, this seen merely as prejudice allows for an underestimation of the potential of the natural sciences, in particular of the cognitive neurosciences, for pulling the carpet from under the feet of such stereotypes. I am, in fact, of the opinion that brain research has not only the potential but also the responsibility for exerting a mitigating influence in this regard. It has the potential precisely because of the considerable difficulties that are involved in the task of comprehending mental processes in terms of neuroscience. In spite of claims to the contrary, brain research today has no definitive or even satisfying answers to questions about human emotions, capabilities, and talents. In this weakness, however, lies a strength that should not be underestimated. Neuroscience has something valuable to say about the relationship between knowledge and ignorance, between the possibilities and the limitations of brain research that is conducted in a reasonable manner. If neuroscience were to express its view of itself today, it would neither promote an unchecked naturalization or *cerebralization* of mental phenomena nor would it boastfully pose as a leading science. It would define its place among the human sciences even more critically and thoughtfully than it has in the past. Whether or not cognitive neuroscientists are indeed prepared to take on this task remains, however, an open question at this time.

Brain research also has an obligation to help dispel scientific myths about the nature of human capabilities and gifts. To an extent that is far from negligible, it has in the past been guilty of legitimizing and spreading stereotypes like those above. Prominent brain researchers, invested with the authority of science, have used the results of their studies to delegate women to a subordinate social role. This is not to suggest that the skewed relationship between the sexes was invented by brain researchers. However, they did make a decisive contribution to the hardening of the stereotypes that still inhabit too many minds today, as the example of Larry Summers shows.

2.2 Gall's Organology, or: The Invention of Cerebral Biography

In the following, I would like to focus on this historical dimension. I have tried to argue in a number of studies that since becoming an object of scientific research in the early nineteenth century the brain has developed into an object laden with psychological, moral, cultural, social, economic, and political meaning (Hagner 2004).[2] Long before the present-day discussions about free will and cerebral determinism began, fundamental anthropological questions about freedom and necessity, primitiveness and civilization, autonomy of the subject and mechanically interpreted behavior and cognition and feeling (formerly referred to as understanding and disposition) were being discussed with regard to the brain. There is nothing new about the observation that the brain is an entity contaminated by symbols. However, there is a not altogether helpful tendency to view this as a purely cultural problem, which doesn't directly concern the natural sciences. For too long, people have been content with a simple division of labor, according to which the natural sciences produce facts and knowledge, which are then culturally consumed in one way or another. In contrast to this claim, I would like to pose the following question: What are the historical situations that have given rise to certain theories and value judgments in the cognitive neurosciences? The historical examples I will present in the following are drawn mainly from German sources, but similar cases are also familiar in French, British, and U.S. brain research.

Modern cognitive brain research began with the *Organology* of Franz Joseph Gall.[3] Gall was the first scientist to distance himself from the idea of a special organ located somewhere in the depths of the white matter of the brain and acting as the connecting hinge between the brain and the mind. Instead, Gall saw the brain as a distributive organ, in which more or less all the human characteristics were inscribed. The characteristics in question were those of the human being considered as an everyday being and no longer as a metaphysical being created by God. In this respect, Gall was following the bourgeois values and attributions that prevailed around 1800, and accordingly he postulated independent faculties such as sense of color, sense of sound, logical strength of argument, language sense, religious sense, charitableness, miserliness, sex drive—30 faculties in all. He delegated each of these faculties to a certain region in the brain and called each region an organ. According to Gall, these organs were located almost exclusively on the cerebral cortex, which in itself already constituted a radical epistemological break with the past, for the cortex had until then been considered to be either a protective coating or nutrient substance for the inner, nobler parts of the brain.

Gall set up a number of different criteria for his localizations, but there was one thing he did not do: He never placed a drive, the sex drive for instance, next to a cognitive faculty, like, for example, the faculty of computation. In this regard, he

respected the division of psychological faculties, current in the bourgeois society of
the time, into intellectual faculties, feelings, and drives. Gall assigned each of these
three faculties to a separate region of the brain, placing the intellect in the front, feelings in the middle, and the drives at the very back. Another thing Gall did not do is
to make any distinction between male and female brains. This lack is all the more
remarkable because he believed he was able to recognize criminals or geniuses by the
pronounced development of one or several brain organs. And by that time, it had
long been considered psychologically and physiologically legitimate to contrast male
understanding with the female disposition (see Honegger 1991, Schiebinger 1993). We
have no reason to believe that Gall rejected such a polarization of the sexes, yet he
did not make use of it in his organology.

2.3 Systemizing the Convolutions: Imbeciles, Women, and "Twilight Peoples"

The distinction between male and female brains was not made until a generation later
by one of the most vehement critics of Gall, the Romantic physician, anatomist, and
artist Carl Gustav Carus. Carus developed a theory of the brain that aimed to diffuse
the feared materialist implications of Gall's organology. Already, early on in his work,
Carus had ridiculed Gall's division of the psyche into a great number of faculties, "so
that, in the end, not a single remnant or fiber of the brain remained that was not to
be regarded as the special organ of some specific mental power" (original: "um endlich
kein Läppchen und Fäserchen des Hirns übrig zu behalten, was nicht als ein beson-
deres Organ einer gewissen Seelenkraft zu betrachten wäre"; Carus 1814, 301). According to Carus, brain research was not a matter of finding the whole gamut of human
behavior reflected in 25 or 32 different brain centers. Instead, Carus distinguished
three large regions from the front to the back: the cerebral hemispheres, the midbrain
and medulla oblongata, and the cerebellum. This tripartite division echoes the division
of psychological faculties followed by Gall. This is confirmed by Carus' work on psychology, in which he identified "knowing, feeling and willing" as the basic psychological faculties from which one could derive "some indication about the individuality
of a person" (original: "einen Fingerzeig über die Individualität des Menschen"; Carus
1841, 7, 9). But more than Gall, Carus was committed to contributing to an anatomy
of difference, which inscribed the parameters of race, sex, criminality, and madness
in the head and in the brain. He claimed to have observed, for example, that the
middle region of the brain was particularly developed in imbeciles, women, and the
"twilight peoples (Mongols, Malays, and Americans)," the hind part in the "night
peoples (Ethiopians)." It goes without saying that he found the frontal region to be
primarily developed in (intelligent) males and Caucasians, that is, in the white race
(Carus 1841, 12). In order to translate these abstract differences into the concrete evidence of visual representation, Carus drew several skull contours one on top of the

other, creating an image that was supposed to clearly distinguish the "mental individuality" of a Friedrich Schiller or a Charles-Maurice de Talleyrand from that of an inhabitant of Greenland or a cretin (see figure 2.1; color plate 6). These skulls show a "beautiful and complete harmonic development of all three head regions for the German poet Schiller, a predominance of the front and the hind parts of the head for the French statesman Talleyrand, a stunting of the front part of the head in the case of the Greenlander" (original: "schöne und volle harmonische Entwicklung aller drei Kopfwirbel bei Schiller, das Vorherrschen des Vorderhauptes und Hinterhauptes bei Talleyrand, die Verkümmerung des Vorderhauptes bei dem Grönländer"), and a general absence of development in the case of the cretin (Carus 1843–45, vol. 1, commentary on plate IX). Carus was heavily criticized by his scientific contemporaries for

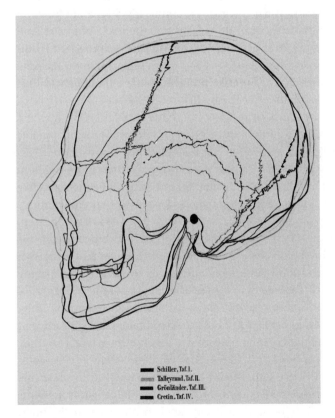

Schiller, Taf. I.
Talleyrand, Taf. II.
Grönländer, Taf. III.
Cretin, Taf. IV.

Figure 2.1
(color plate 6) Carl Gustav Carus, facsimile drawing of four skulls. (Source: Carus. *Atlas der Cranioscopie oder Abbildungen der Schaedel- und Antlitzformen beruehmter oder sonst merkwürdiger Personen.* 1843–1845, table IX.)

his Romantic symbolism of the mind, the details of which I cannot enter into here, and his cranioscopy did not find many followers. Nevertheless, the functional distinction between a hind cortical region associated with the feminine, the primitive, intuitions, and drives, and a frontal region representing the more highly developed and rational, masculine qualities was widely accepted in the nineteenth century.

In the years that followed, scientists began to search for parameters other than a rough division of brain regions, which would permit a quantitative and physiognomic determination of psychological differences. From the mid-nineteenth century on, attention turned increasingly to the weight and the convolutions of the brain. Gall had identified the cortex as the essential part of the brain, but it was left to his successors to try to make sense of the apparent chaos of its convolutions. At first, they directed their efforts toward refuting Gall's organology; later, in a complete reversal of their original intentions, they pursued the goal of identifying a separate function for each convolution. An important figure in this regard was the Jena anatomist Emil Huschke. The work he carried out over a period of many years, summarized in his 1854 book, *Schädel, Hirn und Seele* (*Skull, Brain, and Soul*), was remarkable for its exact measurements and careful presentation. Huschke fulfilled all the requirements of his time for an exact and objective anatomy of the brain.

It was an accepted principle of comparative anatomy that a correlation between the number and furcation of brain convolutions and mental abilities was only permissible among animals of the same genus or family: The convolutions of a wolf were less developed than those of a dog, those of a cat less than those of a lion (note: wolf and dog share the same genus, cat and lion the same family, but differ in genus). Huschke applied this principle without further ado to humans and claimed that convolutions in "Negroes" were less developed than in "Caucasians" (Huschke 1854, 135). In itself, this discriminatory assessment was not new. However, Huschke differed from his predecessors in that he combined his stereotypical ranking of the races and sexes with measurements and a systematization of the convolutions of the brain, thus paving the way for a physiognomy of the cerebral cortex. Huschke read the labyrinth of convolutions like the physiognomists read the face. His studies were supported by countless measurements, expressed in the form of figures and tables. This meant that they fulfilled the requirements of scientific objectivity, but it also meant that they could serve to legitimize assumptions and claims that were not really accessible to quantification. In actual fact, Huschke's interpretations of the branching, meandering, and size of the brain's convolutions relied not only on quantitative measurements but also on his physiognomic intuition. Thus it appeared to him that in the brain of Africans, the Sylvian furrow—one of the two main furrows of the cerebral cortex— was only slightly less crooked than in chimpanzees, whereas it was horizontal in Europeans. In Africans and women, he found the third frontal convolution to be extremely wide in comparison with that of European males, and the hind convolutions most certainly more pronounced "even if not very finely structured" (original: "wenn auch gerade nicht sehr fein gegliedert"; Huschke 1854, 155f).

Why should we occupy ourselves with this kind of furrow reading at all? The fact is that Huschke, with his measurements and tables, is representative—at least in the German-speaking world—of the transition from the older cranioscopy, organology, and morphology to a new style of brain anatomy that counted precision, quantifications, and objectivity among its virtues. Huschke's racist and sexist physiognomy of the convolutions of the brain did not quite live up to these standards, but he painted a rosy picture of the future, when a more individualized brain research would succeed in examining the brains of persons "whose natural mental abilities are precisely known, and this all the better, if they are one-sided individuals, with one prominent mental ability" (original: "deren geistiges Naturell genau bekannt ist, um so besser, wenn es einseitige, mit Einer hervorstechende Seelenkraft versehene Individuen sind"; Huschke 1854, 184f).

Buoyed up with a vision such as this, one could afford to be philosophically modest. In the politically sensitive times after 1848, one could turn against the politically suspect materialism and maintain a bourgeois, conservative stance that sought to immunize itself against social change. A particularly striking example of an attitude of this kind is provided by the Munich anatomist Theodor Bischoff, who began in 1864 to carry out elaborate studies of brain weights. Bischoff was no ignoramus weighing and measuring brains in a blind fury. He knew the basic rules of statistics, but when it came to applying his studies to the crucial social question of the admission of women to academic study, he forgot his scruples. In an infamous treatise about the study of medicine by women, he flatly dismissed the intellectual and academic capabilities of the feminine sex and substantiated his judgment by citing the lower average weight of women's brains (Bischoff 1872, 16–19).

Besides being surely one of the most embarrassing papers produced by an academic in the nineteenth century, backed by the full authority of science, this treatise also clearly demonstrates the logic that made a lapse of this kind possible. It was certainly no isolated case. The only response anthropologists like Bischoff, Huschke, and many others could muster to the changes in the relation between the sexes that were beginning to make themselves felt in the demand for equal voting rights for women or for free admission to the university was to insist upon the social status quo with the whole weight of their academic authority. All the measurements and mathematical operations that Bischoff carried out on his total of 559 male and 347 female brains produced meager results at best. The numbers were big enough to satisfy the statistical requirements, but the individual variations made these studies virtually meaningless. In regard to female brains, Bischoff was not prepared to consider even for a moment the complexity of different factors such as body weight or size. The methodical carefulness he otherwise demonstrated reached its limits precisely at the point where the demands for the legal, political, and social equality of women became impossible to ignore.

It would be a misunderstanding to regard Bischoff's studies of the brain and his resulting interpretations as an isolated mistake in an otherwise model scientific career. All of the scientists doing brain anthropology in the second half of the nineteenth century demonstrated a typical dichotomy between scientific skepticism and prejudice. Even the politically progressive materialists referred without any scruples to the results of the anatomists and anthropologists with opposing worldviews. In contrast to phrenology, interpretations of brain convolutions and even of brain weight were taken seriously scientifically. On the basis of these findings, anatomists began in earnest to explain all the human mental faculties like thinking, feeling, and imagining in terms of qualitative and quantitative developments of the different regions of the brain.

2.4 Physiognomic Images and Value Conflicts

The price to be paid for this trend toward explaining everything in terms of cerebral structure was that brain research became the stage for a conflict of values. The bourgeois conservative worldview was characterized by an unquestioned belief in the unity of the subject and the immortality of the soul as the fundaments of a well-ordered society. This belief began to waver after 1848. The cerebral determinants of mental life came onto center stage exactly at the moment when the social and cultural order began to be transformed due to the rise of socialism, the women's movement, and increasing urbanization. At the same time, and seemingly paradoxically, freedom of the will and the immortality of the soul were mobilized as a last defense against these massive changes. The lines of battle were drawn.

When the Neo-Kantian philosopher Jürgen Bona Meyer took both materialism and Darwinism to task in 1870, he also touched briefly on Huschke's studies. While acknowledging the thoroughness of his measurements, he carefully tallied up the inconsistencies in his results. He then went on to give free reign to his mockery of the materialists, remarking that "many a woman's brain is more capable of clear thinking than [Ludwig] Büchner and his consorts" (original: "manches Frauengehirn noch klarer zu denken im Stande ist als [Ludwig] Büchner und Consorten"; Meyer 1870, 164). Much as one may sympathize with this (rare) disqualification of the misogynist brain measurers, it is important to note that Meyer directed all of his fire in just one direction. It was not the materialists, like Ludwig Büchner, who had weighed women's brains and found them to be inferior, but rather their opponents, Huschke and Bischoff. Yet the Neo-Kantian Meyer drew a close connection between materialism and the denigration of women. Misogynists from the conservative camp, however, did not become the target of his criticism.

So far now, the issue of the weight of the brain and its problems is settled. What about the convolutions of the brain? Toward the end of the century, there was a veritable boom in the physiognomy of brain convolutions, accompanied by plenty of metaphorically laden terminology—ample material to further fill the pigeonholes of race, sex, criminality, and intelligence. Two of the most telling terms coined in this connection were *"Raubtiertypus"* ("predator type") and *"Affenspalte"* ("monkey fissure"), both of which played a dubious role in the history of anthropology. *"Affenspalte"* referred to the merging of two furrows, the lateral-occipital and the parieto-occipital fissures. The Viennese neurologist Moritz Benedikt, who coined the term, claimed that the merging of furrows was characteristic of a primitive brain, whereas separate furrows characterized a nobler, more highly developed type of brain. He was not alone in this view. Bischoff's student, Nikolaus Rüdinger, set about going through the collection of brains in Munich on exactly the same assumption. The carefully designed illustrations of his treatise show, in chronological and also hierarchical order, "Brains of monkeys," "Brains of women," "Brains of men," and finally "Brains of scholars," with the famous chemist Justus Liebig at the top (see figures 2.2–2.4; color plates 7–9). The illustrations are notable not only for their absolutely unabashed and unquestioned racism and sexism but also because they show how the physiognomic method, formerly applied to outer body features such as the skull, the eyes, the nose, or the jaws, was here applied to the brain to an extent that had hardly been encountered up to that time. These physiognomic cerebral images were meant to represent specific human profiles. The purpose of these profiles was to secure identities, either by means of classification according to ethnic group, gender, or profession or, in the case of the scholars, by naming the names.

This is the constellation that put individualized brain images, and the attribution of a spiritual and moral significance to the brain, on the agenda. The visual representation of the brain of someone like Liebig was part of a hagiographic process, the idealization of the memory of one of the leading scientists of the nineteenth century. The brain images of a servant girl, a black African woman, or a Jew were part of a process of stigmatization. They were supposed to become fixed in the collective consciousness, but differently from the way in which skin color, noses, or facial profiles were. The latter were primitive signs that practically anyone could recognize. With the brain, things were more complicated. It was not expected that everyone would be able to read these signs; one was just supposed to recognize that they were there and that a professionally trained observer could interpret them.

2.5   Helen Gardener, or: The Fight for Examining Brains of Outstanding Women

How did women react to such impertinence? I will limit myself here to one example, which shows just how powerful the scientific discourse about the brain was at the

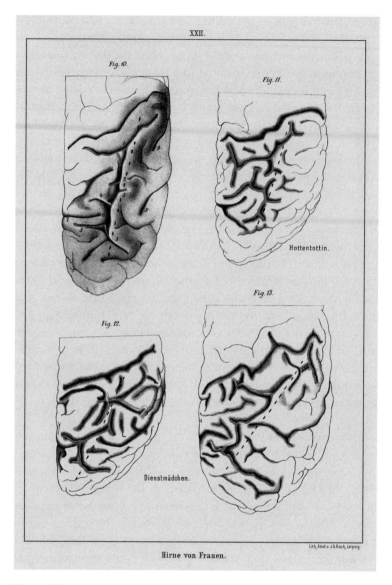

Figure 2.2
(color plate 7) Nikolaus Rüdinger, brains of women. Hottentottin, Hottentot woman; Dienstmädchen, handmaiden. (Source: Rüdinger. Ein Beitrag zur Anatomie der Affenspalte und der internen
Interparietalfurche beim Menschen nach Race, Geschlecht und Individualität. In *Beiträge zur
Anatomie und Embryologie als Festgabe Jacob Henle zum 4. April 1882 dargebracht von seinen Schülern.*
186–198. 1882, table XXII.)

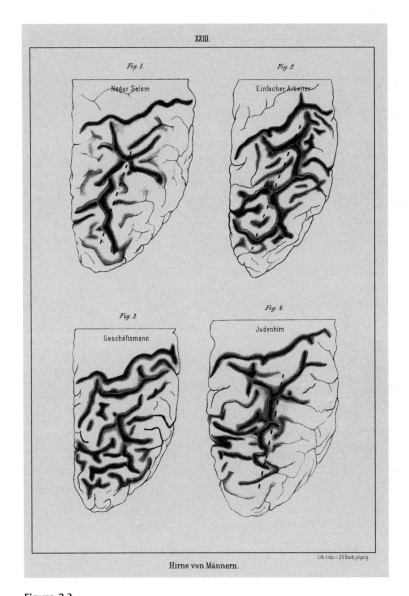

Figure 2.3

(color plate 8) Nikolaus Rüdinger, brains of men. Neger Salem, Negro Salem; Einfacher Arbeiter, unskilled worker; Geschäftsmann, businessman; Judenhirn, brain of Jew. (Source: Rüdinger. Ein Beitrag zur Anatomie der Affenspalte und der internen Interparietalfurche beim Menschen nach Race, Geschlecht und Individualität. In *Beiträge zur Anatomie und Embryologie als Festgabe Jacob Henle zum 4. April 1882 dargebracht von seinen Schülern.* 186–198. 1882, table XXIII.)

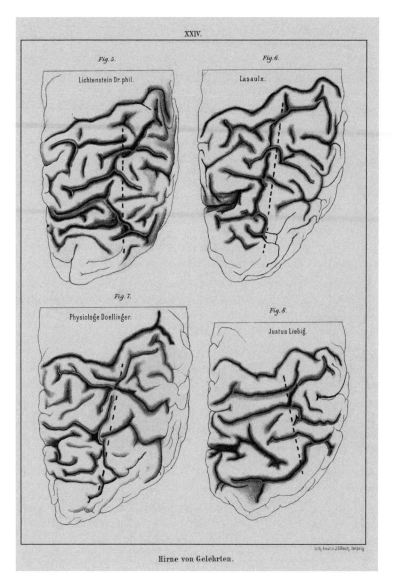

Figure 2.4
(color plate 9) Nikolaus Rüdinger, brains of scholars. (Source: Rüdinger. Ein Beitrag zur Anatomie der Affenspalte und der internen Interparietalfurche beim Menschen nach Race, Geschlecht und Individualität. In *Beiträge zur Anatomie und Embryologie als Festgabe Jacob Henle zum 4. April 1882 dargebracht von seinen Schülern*. 186–198. 1882, table XXIV.)

time. Around 1890, a vehement controversy arose between the U.S. army surgeon William Hammond and the women's rights activist Helen Gardener. Hammond had parroted the ideas of his European colleagues about the *inferiority* of the female brain, and for Gardener this immediately aroused the fear that efforts toward the social and professional emancipation of female members of the white middle class could be undermined.[4] However, since the acceptance of scientific knowledge was part and parcel of this emancipation movement, Gardener did not question the connection between brain structure and intelligence. Rather, her concern was to prove the equal ability of women by means of brain examinations. Consequently, she called for examinations of the brains of outstanding women—analogous to the studies that were being carried out on the brains of outstanding men (Gardener 1887/1893, 100, 104, 122–124). This project never materialized, but the fact that it was suggested shows us that a leading women's rights activist like Helen Gardener and her followers fully subscribed to the scientific brain discourse of the late nineteenth century. Brain examinations were the accepted criterion for deciding whether or not differences between the sexes existed. The fact that the examinations demanded by Gardener were not carried out also shows that this was a male domain. Women did not occupy the academic positions that would have allowed them to undertake such a project. Men, on the other hand, were prepared to examine the brains of their own academic colleagues but not those of outstanding women. The reason for this cannot have had anything to do with neuroanatomy. Rather, brain research societies functioned according to strict social codes that had nothing to do with scientific content.

Helen Gardener died in 1925 and donated her brain to the Cornell University collection. Two years later, James Papez published a study in which he reported that the brain of this extraordinary woman was in no way inferior to those of extraordinary men (Papez 1927). Although this finding did elicit some public attention, the tide of the examinations of scholars' brains had by that time subsided in the United States.

2.6 Rise and Decline of the "Elite Brain"

Up to now, I have made no mention of elite brains, and for good reason. Prior to 1900, the French term *élite*, which originated in the realm of trade and the military, hardly played a role in the German language. It is perhaps no accident that Richard Weinberg first employed the term "elite brain" (*Elitegehirn*) in an article published in 1904 in the journal *Politisch-anthropologische Revue*. This journal, founded in 1902, was among the first to provide a forum for racial anthropologists and promoters of racial hygiene. The results of brain research published here and in the *Archiv für Rassen- und Gesellschafts-Biologie* were followed with great interest, and even the question of brain weight, which the anatomists had long taken leave of, was discussed (Weinberg 1904–1905, 697). All of this is not to say that brain research was at the center of the eugenics movement. Nor does it follow that the examination of elite brains was necessarily carried out with populist intent. However, the close connection between elite brain research and eugenic goals did lead, in the 1920s, to a large-scale attempt at a political program of brain research.

The names most prominently associated with this undertaking are those of the Berlin brain researcher Oskar Vogt and his wife Cécile. They directed large institutes for brain research in Berlin and in Moscow, in which the brains of Lenin and other significant personalities, but also those of criminals and persons judged to be mentally inferior, were studied. The Vogts made use of a new technique of microanatomy called "cytoarchitectonics," which I cannot enter into a discussion of here (see Hagner 1994). Suffice it to say that these anatomic studies, in combination with methods of individual psychology, were elements of an all-encompassing program to "precisely determine the capabilities and behavioral tendencies of the individual members [of society, M. H.]" (original: "die Fähigkeiten und Betätigungstendenzen ihrer einzelnen Mitglieder [der Gesellschaft, M. H.] genau feststellen"). It was hoped that this determination of the individual capabilities of a person, and the localization of these capabilities in the brain, would furnish "the long-awaited scientific basis for controlled breeding, the racial hygiene of the future" (original: "der willkürlichen Zuchtwahl, der Rassenhygiene der Zukunft, die schon langersehnte wissenschaftliche Grundlage"; Vogt 1912, 313). In this scenario, the analogy drawn between the division of labor in the brain and the division of labor in society provided the key to the idea that brain research was to function as the center of gravity for the medically, socially, and pedagogically motivated human sciences.

What role did women's brains play in this context? The answer may seem surprising: none at all. Asked by the women's rights activist Agnes Zahn-Harnack about the validity of the older claims that women were less capable of high mental performances due to the structure of their brains, Cécile Vogt replied that parameters such as brain weight and the number of convolutions were irrelevant for the mental performance of an individual. She drew attention, rather, to the importance of the microstructure of the brain but admitted that this research was still in its beginning phases and had not yet begun to consider possible differences between the sexes. Therefore, women could not be excluded from any profession "on the grounds of brain research as it stands today" (original: "auf Grund des heutigen Standes der Hirnforschung").[5] Of course, a position such as this left all the options open for a future investigation of the differences between male and female brains, but the fundamental affirmation of equality fit with the Vogts' Social-Democratic societal model. A ranking of the sexes on the basis of brain anatomy had no place in their research, something that distinguished them from many other brain researchers (Satzinger 1996, particularly 75f, 79). The idea of an elite—in the Germany of the 1920s that referred to those who were supposed to bring Germany back into the circle of world powers after the disastrous outcome of World War I—was, however, further pursued until in the year 1933 a kind of elite came into power in Germany that was quite different from anything the Vogts might have dreamed of. The research on elite brains came to an end in Germany, and after 1945 the idea of an elite was unheard-of for decades. The term only resurfaced again in public discourse a few years ago. This return does not mean much for the moment. Nevertheless, I believe that a special challenge arises in this connection for brain research, and with that I return to the thoughts sketched at the outset.

2.7 Outlook

Today, brain researchers openly admit that we still know astonishingly little about the workings of cognitively relevant processes in the brain. *The Manifesto of Brain Researchers* (*Manifest der Hirnforscher* 2004), which, at least in Germany, received a lot of public attention, even states that the "brain theory" of the future will be developed in a language different from that employed in the neurosciences today. What this language will be, the Manifesto does not say. And with good reason: No one knows it as yet. With all of this well-justified modesty, it is all the more astounding that, at the same time, the Manifesto calls for a new idea of humans ("*Menschenbild*").

It is more than legitimate for brain researchers today to take part in the public discourse, but like their predecessors they have not yet found an intellectually satisfying way to deal with their ignorance. This is even more unfortunate in light of the fact that the natural sciences have a great deal of experience in mapping out and reflecting upon the individual steps of the acquisition of knowledge. They have developed a clear methodology that allows them to arrive at results that are generally reliable. Of course, the system is in no way perfect, nor is it always immune to all sorts of tainting that could render it unfruitful or lead it astray. Nevertheless, no other system of knowledge is in as favorable a position to determine the boundary between knowledge and ignorance—even if this boundary can never be absolutely determined, is always changing, and may be particularly difficult to define in individual cases. True, the scrupulousness with which the natural sciences carry out this exercise in methodological skepticism often leaves much to be desired. Undoubtedly, this has to do in part with the undue expectations society places on them, intensified by enormous economical investments that do not exactly encourage epistemological reliability.

Many unanswered questions remain, beyond even those listed in the *Manifesto*. We have no exact knowledge of how the nerve cells in the cerebral cortex are connected, nor do we have an adequate idea of their relative functional importance. And how the enormous plasticity of the brain goes hand in hand with the relative stability of our perception of the world and of ourselves remains a complete mystery. As in the past, neuroscientists diverge widely, both in their interpretation of results that have already been published and in their assessment of the possibilities and limitations of brain research. In light of this situation, there is no meaningful contribution to be made by the cognitive neurosciences to the discussion of the relationship between elite and gender, except to affirm that, from the point of view of neurological science, there is nothing meaningful to be said. Certainly, no society acting responsibly will have any use for a premature push to convert uncertain scientific knowledge into socially relevant fact. In this regard, brain research has fared pretty badly in the past. Of course, one cannot compare the present situation with that of the nineteenth and twentieth centuries, when racism, sexism, and the postulated existence of so-called criminal brains were an integral part of brain research. The shadow of the terrible events of history will remain over us for quite some time and continue to have a preventative effect against the return of such notions. So too will the new results of brain research itself. Key concepts in this respect are the plasticity of the brain, already mentioned above, and the complex interplay of genes and the environment, which is just beginning to be understood. It is therefore advisable, at a time when disastrous educational experiments and a bizarre longing for a new elite seem to have made us susceptible to simplifications, not to give way to the tendency for simple, all too simple answers.

Acknowledgments

The author thanks Ursula Froese for translating the text.

Notes

1. Harvard University, the Office of the President, Lawrence H. Summers. "Letter to the Harvard community." February 21, 2006. http://www.president.harvard.edu/speeches/2006/0221_summers.html (accessed January 12, 2007).

2. This book is the source for the historical examples in the present text. See this book for an account of the wider historical context in which the relationship between elite brains and gender has developed.

3. On Gall, see Hagner (1997).

4. On this controversy, see Russett (1989, 35–39) and Kern (1996, 104–112), whose interpretation I am largely following here.

5. Cécile Vogt to Agnes Zahn-Harnack, 15. 1. 1927, in *Cécile und Oskar Vogt-Archiv* (COVA), folder 91 (H) (original in German language). Zahn-Harnack then asked for permission to include this letter in her book *Die Frauenbewegung: Geschichte, Probleme, Ziele* (1928), which she did, although it seems Cécile Vogt was rather irritated about the fact that Zahn-Harnack had not played with an open deck from the beginning and only asked for permission to publish after she held Vogt's statement in her hands.

3 The Biosexual Foundations of Our Modern Concept of Gender

Robert A. Nye

3.1 Introduction

Nowadays we seem to be increasingly uncertain about the differences between what we mean by "sex" and what we mean by "gender." I refer here to "sex" not as a verb but rather as a noun referring to male or female. One can find numerous examples, often in the same text, of the words "sex" and "gender" being used interchangeably to refer to men and women and male and female. In contemporary journalism, it is particularly striking that "gender" is often favored in headlines, and, when it appears at all, "sex" is buried in the small print.

The ambiguous use of these terms extends even to the technical science literature. In a recent issue of *Science* devoted to Women's Health, one article, entitled "Gender in the Pharmacy: Does It Matter?," mixes the terms together in consecutive sentences: "Clinicians still don't always analyze data on women separately, and more research—and better research tools—may yet reveal more serious gender differences, they say. Even subtle sex differences may be important in an era of personalized medicines" (Kaiser 2005, 1572). This is not an isolated example. David Haig, an evolutionary biologist, has searched 30 million academic articles published between 1945 and 2001 for occurrences of the words "sex" and "gender" and has found that "gender" was used sparingly and usually in the sense of a grammatical category at the beginning of this period but in the social science, arts, and humanities categories now outnumbers the usage of "sex." In the natural sciences "gender" is now used half as often as "sex." When the terms "gender difference" and "sex difference" are scanned in all categories, the former term has been dominant since 1994 (Haig 2004, 87–90). When Haig asked working scientists why they chose to use "gender" rather than "sex" in biological contexts, they responded they wished to signal sympathy for feminist goals or "to avoid the connotation of copulation" (Haig 2004, 95).

It is likely these same motives operate throughout Western societies, particularly in puritanical North America, where, in common parlance, "sex" means "sexual intercourse" and where political correctness filters most public speech. Politics is also involved in this development. Science and social science grant writers to National Science Foundation and National Institutes of Health review boards have learned to use the term gender because conservative watchdog groups have search engines that are instructed to pick out the word "sex" in grant applications, which are then subjected to the undesirable scrutiny of congressional oversight.

The very fact that the word "gender" can be substituted freely for "sex" nowadays is also a product of feminist theory, which began to use gender to pry loose socially constructed ascriptions of men's and women's roles from male and female bodies in the late 1960s and early 1970s. They wished to make it clear that a woman could transcend her biological nature and should not be discriminated against legally on account of it. Thus, when the Education Amendments to the Civil Rights Act of 1964 were passed in 1972 (Title IX), they banned any discrimination on the basis of "sex" at any institution receiving federal funds. However, an important follow-up study of the effects of Title IX conducted in 1992 determined that much more needed to be done in the way of "gender equity." This proactive, one might say "affirmative action," aspect of the term "gender" also appears in the program statements of the United Nations Educational, Scientific, and Cultural Organization's (UNESCO's) "Gender Mainstreaming Implementation Framework," which baldly states that "The concept of gender is vital because, applied to social analysis, it reveals how women's subordination (or men's domination) is socially constructed. As such, the subordination can be changed or ended. It is not biologically predetermined nor is it fixed forever" (UNESCO's Gender Mainstreaming Implementation Framework 2002–2007, Annex 2, 17).

In view of this activist dimension of the term "gender," it is not surprising that there is a certain degree of political valence attached to preferences for one term or the other. Thus, conservative Supreme Court Justice Antonin Scalia has written: "The word gender has acquired the new and useful connotation of cultural or attitudinal characteristics (as opposed to physical characteristics) distinctive to the sexes. That is to say, gender is to sex as feminine is to female and masculine is to male." Note here that Scalia's usage distinguishes between the two, but makes sex the determinant of gender. By contrast, according to one legal expert, liberal Justice Ruth Bader Ginsburg uses "sex" and "gender" interchangeably so that "the word 'sex' would not appear on every page" (Diamond 2000, 53–54), which seems to be the organizing principle of anyone writing about men and women.

Conservatives readily appreciate what is at stake in this linguistic turf battle. They have sought to retain "sex" as the operative term for discussing men and women generally. One of the last official documents approved by Pope John Paul II was the letter to the bishops of the Catholic Church "On the Collaboration of Men and Women in the Church and in the World," released from the Offices of the Congregation for the Doctrine of the Faith (CDF) on May 31, 2004, and signed by

Joseph Cardinal Ratzinger (now Pope Benedict XVI).[1] It deplored the opposition encouraged by some between men and women: "In order to avoid the domination of one sex or the other, their differences tend to be denied, viewed as mere effects of historical and cultural conditioning. In this perspective, physical difference, termed sex, is minimized, while the purely cultural element, termed gender, is emphasized to the maximum and held to be primary. The obscuring of the difference or duality of the sexes has enormous consequences on a variety of levels." The document goes on to list the dangers of homosexuality and threats to the "natural two-parent structure of mother and father." More aggressively, the Catholic Bishop of Buenos Aires, Hector Aguer, defended the elimination of the term "gender" and its replacement by "sex" in the national educational curriculum by saying that the word gender was "intended to provoke an ideological shift and to generate a new conception of the human person, of subjectivity, marriage, the family and society. In short what is proposed is a cultural revolution."[2] On this, at least the proponents of these rival terms are in full agreement.

This terminological battle is not likely to end anytime soon, but in the long term it is likely to end up being moot, because common usage, as we have seen, is moving to compress the terms, not distinguish them. What is happening, as I see it, is that while "sex" continues to be useful to scientists and is not likely to disappear anytime soon, "gender" has taken on some of the characteristics that were formerly reserved to sex as a biological category. "Gender," in short, now has a biological dimension that feminist radicals never meant it to have when they popularized gender as a socially constructed category of analysis in the 1960s and early 1970s. I have discussed some of the reasons for this linguistic slippage above: political correctness and the progress of feminist analysis. In this chapter, I wish to draw attention to another historical reason why "gender" has become more biological, or at least more substitutable for "sex" than it has been in its short history as a nongrammatical term.

3.2   Old Sex and New Gender

"Gender" as a term that applies to the analysis of masculine and feminine roles in society is very new in English, entering everyday language in the mid-twentieth century. Other Western European languages have not yet found as simple a way to distinguish the social dimension of the biological. The term *Geschlecht* in German means both sex and (latterly) gender, and *genre* is only making slow penetration into French usage (Scott 2005, 56–58; Waniak 2005, 48–68). Gender has since been applied retroactively, as it were, to analyze historical societies and explain the extraordinary variability of men's and women's roles over time, though this variability has inevitably expressed itself in a dichotomous and hierarchical form throughout history. Before "gender" emerged, "sex" explained most of these social arrangements, both to contemporaries and to modern scholars. The word "sex" as an essential category of difference has been around as long as language itself. Though, as I will argue, the term was not fitted out in its characteristically modern form of biological determinism until the eighteenth century, it was the way that people made sense of differences between men and women.

This model aimed at reducing (what we now think of as) gender and (what we now think of as) sexuality to more or less direct expressions of male and female sex. In that model, though in language and causality appropriate to the times, male sex produced masculinity (virility in the old denomination) and the desire for vaginal intromission, while producing femininity in females and the desire to be penetrated. This orthodoxy was undergirded first by religious and philosophical and later by scientific authority in ways that preserved a remarkable degree of continuity. Both kinds of authority recognized the existence of intermediary sexual forms and corresponding expressions of (what we now think of as) gender and of sexual desire, but they were, according to the usage, unnatural or pathological, infrequent, and providentially sterile.

Until very recently, contemporary historians and social scientists have generally preferred to bracket "sex" as a thing apart, either an inscrutable "matter of biology" (Rotundo 1994, 1; Connell 1995, 3–5) or something unchanging whose meaning varies according to the (social) circumstances. In this view, sex is a hardwired foundation for the interpretive work that we perform on the mutable superstructures of gender and sexuality. Biological research agendas have inclined toward the exploration of sex difference from the XX/XY of the chromosome to cognitive style; scientific commentary on this sort of work characteristically concludes that sex differences are ultimately complementary in ways that assure the harmonization of males and females and are useful to society (Nadeau 1996). The former president of Harvard University, Lawrence Summers, has been crucified recently for uttering such opinions in the very heart of politically correct America (see also Hagner, this volume).

Londa Schiebinger has rightly observed that many biologists confuse matters by referring to gender as the secondary sexual characteristics of animals and humans; she astutely warns humanists and social scientists about contributing to the muddle by using gender "improperly as a PC code word for 'sex'" (Schiebinger 1999, 16f). Some biologists have self-consciously resisted the confounding of sex and gender and are exploring the processes by which sex itself has been and is being constructed by evolutionary theorists in molecular biology labs and in medical practice. The biologist Anne Fausto-Sterling argues for the complexity and against the either/or nature of sex. As she writes in her recent synthesis, "The more we look for a simple physical basis for 'sex' the more it becomes clear that 'sex' is not a purely physical category. What bodily signals and functions we define as male or female come already entangled in our ideas about gender." However, she also makes the more radical claims that beliefs about gender "affect what kinds of knowledge scientists produce about sex in the first place" and, secondly, that we literally "embody" in "our very physiological being" elements of the social and cultural milieu in which they exist (Fausto-Sterling 2000, 4–6).

I will take up this point later. But first, we must admit there has been a historic persistence in most cultures of binary sex and gender categories that have been replicated in religion, culture, language, and science. Why this persistence? It has been suggested that the mammalian model of reproduction has served as the template for male/female dimorphism in human societies. It is equally certain that human groups have made powerful investments in fertility to ensure survival in an environment of competition for resources. There is a rich archaeological record of fertility rites and goddesses and a regular equation of planting and harvest activities with human reproduction that testifies to the near-universality of these beliefs. Conversely, as Angus McLaren has shown, there is evidence to suggest that even very ancient societies acted to limit fertility when population outstripped prospects (McLaren 1990). Since in either case the management of procreation was the key to ensuring the prosperity, not to mention the survival, of individuals, kinship groups, and entire societies, a high premium was placed on the procreative capacities of males and females and on the sexual practices that ensured or regulated births.

3.3   The Biological Construction of Sex

Genitalia and sexual function have always figured prominently in assessments of these capacities, but though erection and ejaculation in males and menses, pregnancy, and lactation in women have been necessary features of cultural assessments of reproductive ability, they are only a part of the huge variety of ways that human societies have characterized males and females as men and women and as more or less masculine and feminine versions of their sex. It might seem reasonable to conclude from the crucial importance of procreation to human survival that (a biological) sexual capacity is primordial and gender is a secondary, cultural effect. However, in fact the opposite is more nearly the case. Despite the many forms it has assumed in human societies, gender appears to be the stable and persistent category while the sexed body and its sexuality have been more changeable and adaptive. The gender arrangements of most societies have dictated what is valued and permitted in the domain of sexual identity and behavior and have done so for the most part within binary male/female orders that have historically reproduced themselves as systems of male dominance. Though they can be studied on their own terms, sexual ideologies, sexual practices, and representations of the sexualized body are deeply influenced by the gender norms that prevail in political, cultural, and economic life. In a sense, gender makes a *social virtue* out of the necessity of biological sex, policing the boundaries of the sexually permissible, nourishing ideals of sexual love, and dictating norms of sexual aim and object.

On the whole, the great religions undergirded patriarchal gender orders, subordinated or segregated women, devised rituals of purification surrounding menses, and proscribed sexual deviations, especially same-sex sexuality and adultery. In effect, sexuality was more a public than a private matter, policed by communities and kin, governed by an economic logic, and divided everywhere into two great and generally opposing categories: *procreative* and *nonprocreative* (Foucault 1980).

At some point during the seventeenth and eighteenth centuries a schism appeared that would separate Western and Eastern sexualities for much of the next two centuries. In Europe and North America rapid economic development expanded and diversified prosperous *elites*, particularly the urban middle classes, causing rapid population growth and improved prospects throughout all levels of society. With sufficient assets couples could choose careers, marry, and plan families with greater certainty. As child and maternal mortality rates finally began to decline, couples were able to make emotional investments in one another and in their children, which strengthened the affective bonds of family life. Romantic love took flower from this more stable soil, and new forms of individualism emerged that encouraged people to cultivate personal distinctiveness in feelings and attachments (see Reddy, this volume).

Ironically, as individual and private selves, including sexual selves, became more common, scientists and doctors were busy discovering universal laws that ordered and regulated sexual bodies. In this way, too, Western and Eastern societies diverged. Scholars have shown that until about 1750 anatomical and physiological representations of male and female bodies in Western and Eastern medicine relied on a single, androgynous body with differently positioned but homologous reproductive organs in each sex, the vagina being an inverted and internalized penis and so forth. Physiological differences were explained by relative humoral balances, heat, or measures of yin and yang (Laqueur 1990).

By the eighteenth century, however, Western scientists were increasingly persuaded that women's and men's bodies were primordially different, particularly in skeletal structure and in reproductive function, but also physiologically. Women's wider hips, menstrual cycles, and weaker musculature, and their putatively changeable emotions and weaker reasoning, were regarded as naturally determining women's domestic and procreative functions, while men were believed better equipped for the rigors of social struggle. Male and female bodies were described as incommensurable but complementary, with physical attraction depending on the relative differences in masculine and feminine traits (Nye 1998, 57f). Children born with ambiguous genitalia were no longer thought to be punishments for collective sin—a violation of God's moral order—but rare outliers on a natural spectrum of pathology and norm (Daston and Park 1998, 103, 181, 329–363).

The consolidation of what Thomas Laqueur has termed a "two-sex" system in the mid-eighteenth century essentially locked men and women into a modern discourse of *biological determinism*. Coincident with this materialization of gendered bodies, women's and men's sexualities were held by medical specialists to be markedly different. Women were characterized as passive, inorgasmic beings, men as aggressive, opportunistic ones. These views confirmed and legitimated women's confinement to the domestic sphere at a time when greater numbers of middle-class folk could live on the husband's income alone and when claims for political rights were first expressed in a discourse of rational "capacity."

In this scheme, sexuality, sex, and gender (in our modern sense) were conflated. Victorians believed that sexual desire was a wholly procreative force (which they preferred to call "love") that brought the sexes together, which were otherwise separated by huge differences in biology and social role. It was regarded as an aberration for women to work in men's jobs or have sexual desires that did not have as their end the bearing and mothering of children. Biological sex, it was believed, determined every (normal) expression of men and women's behavior.

The most important conceptual revolution in the history of sexuality took place in the last decades of the nineteenth and the first decades of the twentieth centuries: the discovery of the "perversions" (Nye 1999, 212–310). In the medical schemata of the era, perversions were excesses or deficiencies of normal organic functions. Excessive heterosexual libido led to nymphomania in women, satyriasis in men. Sadism (named by the sexologist Richard von Krafft-Ebing after the Marquis de Sade) was an exaggeration of normal sexual aggression and dominance; masochism—pleasure taken in being dominated—was its contrary, passive expression. Deficiencies in what was believed to be the innate aim of sexual libido—to have intercourse with the opposite sex— produced attractions to inappropriate objects or bizarre actions that fell well short of full heterosexual intercourse. This list was long indeed, including all varieties of fetishism, exhibitionism, bestiality, and particularly inversion, which was the preferred term for an unnatural attraction to someone of the same sex (Oosterhuis 2000, Laqueur 2003). Inversion, which eventually came to be known as homosexuality, was the perversion that aroused the greatest concern among specialists and the general public.

Two things about this classificatory system are noteworthy. First is the fact that the desired norm against which all the perversions were measured was procreative heterosexual intercourse. Second, the entire logic of the effort to identify and cure the perversions depended on the gender orthodoxies of Western societies. The pathologization of the perversions was to a great extent a response to a perceived *crisis in traditional gender roles* and widespread fears that "normal" sexual drives were being deflected from their rightful ends. Women were taking jobs and entering the professions in increasing numbers; some were even bold enough to demand equal rights and the vote. In the years leading up to World War I, some European statesmen were convinced that the growth of perversions had lowered birthrates and weakened their nation's defenses. This explains the popularity of the sadomasochistic perversions that characterized women as whip-wielding dominatrices and men as groveling slaves, a subversively precise inversion of the gender hierarchy (Noyes 1997, 105–139). All perversions were by definition sterile; the entire family of fetishes violated the gender order by focusing on objects or on the "wrong" sex, the love that men and women owed spouses and children.

At virtually the same time, physicians and surgeons were employing new techniques to help identify the "true sex" of individuals who were known at the time as her-maphrodites. Alice Dreger has argued that, despite laparoscopic and microscopic evidence for the anatomical and physiological complexity of some of these individuals, doctors insisted on placing even the most complicated cases in one sex or other, according to the *gonadal evidence*. As she writes, the adoption of "The gonadal definition of sex was driven not by a strictly 'scientific' rationale but instead for the most part by pragmatism: it accomplished the desired preservation of clear distinctions between males and females in theory and practice in the face of creeping sexual doubt" (Dreger 1998, 153).

In the course of the twentieth century, science exercised a more important influence on the understanding of sexuality than at any earlier time, confirming existing prejudices in some cases and unsettling them in others. Evolutionary biologists sorted out the nature of genetic inheritance around the turn of the twentieth century. In some of the theorizing since that time, many biologists assessing the evolution of the "higher" species have concluded that sexual reproduction between distinctly "male" and "female" gametes conferred an evolutionary advantage on the species that employed it by ensuring natural variability and hence adaptability (Low 2000). Many of the early scientists who observed human gamete union under the microscope wrote rhapsodically of the active and vigorous sperm and the passive, nurturing egg, the "romance of the egg and sperm" ridiculed recently by feminist scholars (Tuana 1989) To many contemporary observers, including Charles Darwin and his contemporary critics of sexual selection, the evolution of sex nonetheless confirmed the advantages of contemporary gender arrangements and the logic of bodily dimorphism.

On the microlevel of scientific discovery, scientists in the 1920s and 1930s gradually pieced together the powerful role hormones played in human sexuality. Dubbed the "sex hormones" for their influence on sexual development and libido, estrogen and later testosterone were developed and manufactured in laboratories. As scholars of these developments have pointed out, it made no sense to label testosterone "male" and estrogen "female" as we still do today, because they do not originate exclusively in the male or female gonads and, in any event, exist and perform functions naturally in both sexes (Oudshoorn 1994). Similarly, Marianne van den Wijngaard has shown how, in the 1970s, organizational theorists investigating the role played by hormones in prenatal brain development could not resist identifying androgens as the hormones that produced so-called "masculine" mounting behavior in the male rat and "appropriate" sex object choice. Subsequent work has shown that estrogens are crucial to these developments, but the tendency of brain and behavioral investigators of sex and sexuality to employ a gendered language of either/or is clearly evident here (van den Wijngaard 1997, 40–43). The recent work on the developmental neurophysiology of the brain integrates the influence of the environment on neuron formation in order to bridge the nature/nurture divide, but the questions that drive this research continue to be oriented toward explaining "sex-specific behaviors" (Brizendine 2006, 26). This tendency to overlay physiological events with gendered language has also been noticed by historians and analysts of the immune system such as Emily Martin, who has found abundant evidence of "masculine" T cells and "feminine" macrophages in the modern immunological literature (Martin 1994, 53–62).

On its face, the discovery of the complex chemical and genetic underpinnings of sexual desire and the sexed body should have ultimately weakened the gender orthodoxies inherited from the past by drawing our attention to the extraordinary variability in the anatomy and physiology of sex. In reality, the story is more complex. It was in this context that a biomedical conception of gender emerged that has been crucial to our contemporary usages of the term. In the 1950s, the biologist John Money and his colleagues at Johns Hopkins developed a way to analyze the various ways that nature and nurture shape intersex individuals by way of providing sex assignment guidelines for physicians and parents. They came up with ten categories, including genetic, gonadal, and fetal hormone sex, internal and external morphology, sex of assignment, pubertal sex, and gender identity. As Haig has confirmed in his scan of the ISI Web of Science, Money was the first to use the term "gender" in a nongrammatical sense (Haig 2004, 91). He was importing a term that essentially built on the meaning of "sex role" as used by Talcott Parsons and Margaret Mead in the 1940s.

Though Money's original idea was to lay great stress on the gender identity that would emerge by the child's being raised either male or female, Anne Fausto-Sterling has pointed out the irony that, other things being equal, the baby's penis size was the ultimate basis for either rescuing the child for masculinity or excising it in favor of the "default" sex. By insisting on either/or in the traditional way, Money was policing sex and sexuality in behalf of traditional gendered certainties (Fausto-Sterling 2000, 57–73; Meyerowitz 2002, 117–120).

3.4 Sex Deconstructed

Since the 1950s, new surgical techniques, combined with powerful doses of the appropriate hormones, have made it possible for surgeons to remake the bodies of intersex individuals and perform transsexual operations on individuals who have been diagnosed with a condition dubbed "gender dysphoria," where "true" gender does not correspond to anatomy. Such operations have been performed on thousands of individuals, but the procedure retains an unsavory status in the medical community, and it has been legally established only in the face of entrenched resistance by jurists in the 1960s and 1970s who have used extant marriage law to insist on unions between individuals who had the requisite genitalia and heterosexual sexual and reproductive capacity. It should not surprise us that though transsexual activists have in recent years sought to promote an identity unique to them, the majority have simply wanted to square their bodies with their internal sense of gender, down to the last anatomical detail (Meyerowitz 2002, 141–167; Hausman 1995, 141–174).

Most male to female transsexuals await with some impatience the moment when surgery will complete the journey that began with their feeling they were trapped in the wrong body. As Anne Bolin has written about such individuals, they often celebrate their final surgeries in dual rites of passage of incorporation: into their new bodies and into our deeply gendered society in which they can finally live in peace (Bolin 1988, 179–181). The surgical obstacles to fully satisfactory sexual lives for female to male (FTM) transsexuals are far greater, but FTM individuals are similarly unwilling to capitulate to their incorrect bodies. As one FTM individual has written about his sexuality: "So the dildo was a compromise. For now. It assuaged that inner urge that compelled me to accentuate my maleness; it was a step toward matching my body to my gender. Furthermore, *it deepened my determination that my own destiny was not to be set by biological patterns*. I refused to accept such a biological dictum" (italics in original, as quoted in Califia 1997, 43f). The sociologist Holly Devor, who studied a substantial group of FTM individuals, has learned to characterize the practical relation of sex, gender, and sexuality by delinking sex and sexuality and arguing that "all sexualities are gendered." As she writes, "Thus most non-transsexual persons identify their own genders and those of other people on the basis of sex statuses when they are known to them. However, transsexual persons often use their gender identities as the basis of their sex identities" (Devor 1997, xxiv–xxv; see also Hüsing, this volume).

In the same vein, we are obliged to note that certain illnesses and the simple advance of age have made "hormone replacement therapy" extraordinarily common in the industrialized world. Estrogen treatments now come in many forms, as do testosterone therapies, and men and women use them in increasing numbers to simply maintain sexual health and vigor in the absence of any discomfort or pathology. As for the new range of drugs that promise improved sexual function, the ease of obtaining them via the Internet makes it impossible to know accurately how widespread their use might be, but the little blue Viagra pill has become as important a part of a man's sexual kit as his condom, and Mike Ditka's enjoining men to take Levitra to "get in the game" has already become a National Football League advertising icon.[3] And what are these therapies and medications but the effort—by men and women alike—to reestablish or reinforce the "typical" sexual characteristics of gender and of sexual desire and function?

Thus, notwithstanding growing uncertainty about nature's plan for the sexes, experts have continued to find evidence that confirms the natural distinctiveness of men and women and the advantages of heterosexual sexuality. Political and sexual liberation movements of the 1960s retained profoundly gendered and hierarchical structures. Prostitution and pornography that degrades women have prospered in the new era of relative decriminalization, not disappeared. Sexual panics driven by challenges to gender norms are very much still with us, even in the 21st century. The initial response to the HIV epidemic illustrates the extraordinary capacity that sexual deviance has always possessed as a symbol in moral panics and purity crusades against minorities or exotic sexual practices. In modern times, as Angus McLaren has pointed out, social upheavals or challenges to gender norms are often *read* as sexual rebellions or as crises in sexuality (McLaren 1999, 45). This was so with the fears of masturbation when adolescence emerged as a distinct new phase of childhood, with the challenges of both first- and second-wave feminism, with the linking of communist subversion with (homo)sexual deviance in the 1950s, or the obsession with the innocence of children in our increasingly sexually explicit society that has led to the persecution of day care and Sunday school teachers. We have seen that the specter of same-sex marriage has provoked a wave of legal and political resistance to this alteration of the "natural" or, alternatively, "sacred" character of marriage and the family.

3.5   Conclusion

In short, science and medicine have successfully destabilized the biological foundations of sex that gave earlier generations a material and ideological structure of male and female difference and that explained and justified the gender arrangements of society. We have thus learned that it is gender, and not sex, that determines the standards by which we value, reward, and judge men and women. Gender has not become biology yet, but it has become so much like a "natural kind" that the boundaries between social construction and nature have been profoundly blurred.

Consequently, transsexual, transgender activists like Kate Bornstein have concluded that to finally eliminate the pernicious requirement that we be one sex or the other, we must abolish the gender categories that drive that need. As she writes in *Gender Outlaw: On Men, Women and the Rest of Us*: "The differences are only what we decide they are. By focusing on so-called 'inherent differences' between men and women, we ignore and deny the existence of the gender system itself, and so we in fact hold it in place. But it's the gender system itself—the idea of gender itself—that needs to be done away with. The differences will then fall aside of their own accord." (Bornstein 1994, 114). For Bornstein, the facts of chromosomal sex, reproductive capacity, and genitalia are always interpreted through the distorting and oppressive lens of gender. If we could dispense with gender we could then all be free to choose our pleasures, our identities, and live comfortably in our bodies. Bornstein's cavalier dismissal of the biology of sex has been challenged by other sex radicals, but the notion of taking a vacation from gender, as Pat Califia has said, especially *"other* people's gender,"* remains a widely shared fantasy (Califia 1997, 277).

The "gender system," however defined, seems to be a remarkably resilient thing. Has the relatively recent scientifically grounded notion of gender identity as the foundation of sex and sexuality triumphed over the feminist-inspired notion of gender as a socially constructed category? When we use "gender" today in the former sense, we must ask ourselves have we really liberated ourselves from the determinisms of biological sex, or have we simply rechristened these determinisms with a new name?

Notes

1. The Congregation for the Doctrine of the Faith. "Letter to the Bishops of the Catholic Church on the Collaboration of Men and Women in the Church and in the World." http://www.vatican.va/roman_curia/congregations/cfaith/documents/rc_con_cfaith_doc_20040731_collaboration_en.html (accessed May 25, 2007).

2. "The Vatican and the Gender Wars." Reprinted from the Jan/Feb 1996 issue of the North American Congress on Latin America report on the Americas. http://inquirer.gn.apc.org/catholicgender.html (accessed September 12, 2006).

3. Both Viagra (sildenafil citrate), marketed by the company Pfizer, and Levitra (vardenafil), in the United States comarketed by GlaxoSmithKline and Bayer Pharmaceuticals, function as PDE5 inhibitors and are used as drugs to treat male erectile dysfunction (impotence). Since 2005, due to patent rights and E.U. regulation, GlaxoSmithKline is using the name Lavanza for the same product on European and many other markets outside the United States.

4 Emotional Styles and Modern Forms of Life

William M. Reddy

4.1 Introduction

In the long history of Western emotional styles, the idea that certain emotions are natural has gone through many variations. As thinking about natural emotions has changed, one might expect that such shifts would be quickly reflected in emotional practices. When new "cultural" or "discursive" material gains a footing, it is reasonable to suppose that action will follow. As virginity became more prestigious, late Roman Christians founded celibate monasteries for monks and nuns. As notions of absolute rule were elaborated in seventeenth century Europe, kings became more arbitrary. Of course, cultural change is never this simple. Conflict, contradiction, and miscues always play a role. However, in the case of emotional change, difficulties of quite a different order arise.

In the late seventeenth century, for example, romantic love was endowed with a new prestige. As the new science induced reconsiderations of human nature, love emerged as a possible natural impulse responsible for the formation of families, just as gravity was responsible for the equilibrium of the solar system. As the Earl of Shaftesbury put it in 1711, "It is impossible to suppose a mere sensible creature originally so ill-constituted and unnatural as that, from the moment he comes to be tried by sensible objects, he should have no one good passion towards his kind, no foundation either of pity, love, kindness or social affection" (Cooper, Third Earl of Shaftesbury 1711/1999, 178).

The successful British magazines of the early eighteenth century, *The Tatler* and *The Spectator*, both favored love marriages over marriages arranged solely with an eye to the advancement of status and fortune. Love, said *The Spectator*, is the "cement of society" and ought, therefore, to be conducted "with the same sincerity as any other Affair of less Consideration."[1] However, these prestigious magazines did not say how to reconcile conflicts between love and the duty of obedience to a domineering father or a status-conscious mother.

In English conduct manuals of the period, a new consensus emerged: A good marriage was suffused with love, and love enlivened obedience. Loving daughters must marry only with parental consent. Once married, they must love, and out of love, obey their husbands (Tague 2001). However, like *The Tatler* and *The Spectator*, conduct manuals did not advise young women as to how to respond in cases where their parents refused to grant them liberty to marry for love or where their husbands were not loving.

In this period of early sentimentalism, containment of one's feelings within the bounds of moderation was still considered important. The Roman Stoics were widely admired. As a result, individuals faced frequent contradictions and ambiguities, when enacting the new emotional norm of love. Women were expected to love and obey, men to lovingly guide; both were nonetheless expected to offer respectful obedience to their parents, and women to offer obedience to their husbands. All were expected to express emotions in a moderate, self-contained way.

However, as is always the case with emotional norms, there was a deeper difficulty, which was the question of how to command feeling and how to know if one's feelings were, indeed, the ones commanded.

With so many confusing injunctions, it is no wonder that plays provided an important aid in interpreting and applying new beliefs about feelings. The young Lady Mary Pierrepont was translating the works of Epictetus when her friend Joseph Addison (who, with Richard Steele, would soon found *The Spectator*) sent a draft of his new tragedy, *Cato*, to her in 1710. This play became, in time, a turning point in European theater, the earliest of a new kind of sentimental drama. From such a source, and its later elaborations, individuals could begin to learn what it looked like to be a "sensible creature," as Shaftesbury put it, filled with "good passions."

In this play, two sons of Cato, the ancient Roman Stoic, love the same woman. One, Marcus, expresses his feelings with unbridled fervor. He expostulated about his suffering, demanding that Lucia release him from his pain. Lucia was put off: "Marcus is over-warm," she complains to a friend,

his fond Complaints
Have so much Earnestness and Passion in them
I hear him with a secret kind of Dread,
And tremble at his Vehemence of Temper (Addison 1713, 15).

But Marcus' brother Portius kept his feelings for Lucia under strict control. He told no one but Lucia. And with Lucia, he was careful not to complain of his suffering. He urged his brother to do the same: "I wou'd not urge thee to dismiss thy Passion," he told Marcus,

... but to suppress its Force,
Till better Times may make it look more graceful (Addison 1713, 33).

Lucia found Portius' measured behavior far more attractive.

O Portius, thou hast stol'n away my Soul!
With what a graceful Tenderness he loves!
And breath's the softest, the sincerest Vows!
Complacency, and Truth, and manly Sweetness
Dwell ever on his Tongue, and smooth his Thoughts (Addison 1713, 15).

The young Lady Mary Pierrepont admired Addison's creation, and, in her secret correspondence with Edward Wortley Montagu, she seems to have modeled her behavior on Portius. Mary chatted frequently with her friends of their hopes to marry for love, but, in the end, she was the only one who did so. Even her courtship was fraught with difficulties. Edward, although himself a friend of Addison's, and a contributor to the *Tatler*, was not prepared to model his behavior on Addison's Portius. If anything, his behavior came closer to that of Marcus. The result was painful miscommunication.

"[Y]ou would have me say I am violently in love," Mary wrote to Edward on 22 August 1710, but this would only "give you a just cause to contemn me. . . . I am Afraid I shall be allwaies so barbarous to wish you may esteem me as long [as] you live" (Montagu 1997, 35). Mary was impatient with his jealousy, but Edward persisted. "Could I see into your heart," he wrote on 17 November 1710, "and find in it a partiality to me, I might break thrô all difficulties . . ." (Montagu 1997, 40).

"I am sensible," she wrote back, "that what I say makes no impression on your mind, but I will once more talk truth to you. . . . Tho' your thoughts of me are far from what pleases me, I think so well of you as to trust my ruine in your hands by telling you I am not entirely satisfyd with the proceedings of my Family [that is, her father's rejection of Edward's proposal], but—tis my Family . . ." (Montagu 1997, 41f).

"My Schemes of Happynesse are pritty near what I have sometimes heard you declare yours," she wrote again on 10 February 1711 (Montagu 1997, 43). This lukewarm language, in a secret love letter, could not satisfy Edward. Edward was "obsessed, possessive, angry at his own helplessness," remarks Isobel Grundy, Mary's biographer (Grundy 1999, 40). However, Mary persisted. She was convinced that if a lady openly admitted she felt love for a man, the man inevitably must begin to feel contempt for her. She refused to use the word *love* until she was ready to break off with him: ". . . there is no condition of Life I could not have been happy in with you, so very much I lik'd you. I may say Lov'd, since tis the last thing I'll ever say to you. This is telling you sincerely my greatest weaknesse, and now I will oblige you with a new proofe of Generosity—I'll never see you more" (Montagu 1997, 53).

Young, articulate, acutely self-aware, the two correspondents sparred back and forth like this through most of 1710 and into the spring of 1711. Then they did break it off, for about a year. Later, once she agreed to elope with Edward, she made a complete about-face: "I am at this minute more enclin'd to speak tenderly to you than ever I was in my Life. . . . In this minute I have no will that does not agree with yours" (letter of 7 August 1712; Montagu 1997, 78). But she also had moments of panic: "I tremble for what we are doing. Are you sure you will love me for ever? Shall we never repent? I fear, and I hope" (Grundy 1999, 53).

After carefully weighing the evidence, Grundy remains uncertain whether Mary truly loved Edward or not. But this may be the wrong question to pose.

A fuller understanding of what in the West are called "emotions" suggests that we ought not concern ourselves with what individuals "really" feel. This is so, not because emotions are merely cultural constructs, merely the enactments of a hegemonic discourse. On the contrary, recent research suggests that emotions are a vital feature of cognitive processing; that, in many cultures, emotional life is governed by norms and ideals; and that the application of such norms, and pursuit of such ideals, is complicated by the strange interaction of self-perception and effortful self-alteration. These new perspectives open up the possibility of a very different reading of Mary and Edward's courtship.

4.2   The State of Play in Emotional Research

The modern idea of emotions as physiological arousal states had its origin in the seventeenth century. It may be finally set aside in the 21st. While most psychologists are not prepared to drop this idea yet, experimental evidence has forced them to treat emotions increasingly as a feature of cognition (rather than as an opposing or alternative kind of mental event as the old reason/passion dichotomy encourages one to believe).[2] However, once emotions are disconnected from physiology, historical and ethnographic research can have an important role to play in probing the possible range of human variation in "emotional experience."

As with intentions or perceptions, we have evidence of emotions in others only indirectly. Psychologists can measure slowed reaction times, misperceptions and slips, endocrine system states, arousal levels, even blood flows through the amygdala or neurotransmitters in the nucleus accumbens—but these are not emotions. Despite long effort, no one-to-one correspondence has been found between specific emotions and specific arousal states. The trend in psychological research for the last 15 years has been strongly away from regarding emotions as hardwired.[3]

Anthropological work shows that our local, Western emotional vocabulary does not translate well. Translating color terms is difficult but possible, translating emotion terms is simply misleading. Whether emotions ought to be considered something independent of thoughts or judgments or else as simply a special kind of thought or judgment is not at all settled.[4]

As emotions have become a subject of renewed interest, and of many new studies, a bewildering variety of new general theories of emotion have been brought forward.[5]

This is a necessary evil. Because there is no consensus about what they are, it is impossible to have a general discussion of emotions without trying to say, first, what one thinks they are. This goes for any consideration of the history of emotions as well.

In this chapter, I situate emotions in relation to a concept of "form of life," a notion that a number of scholars have proposed recently as a fruitful adaptation of Wittgenstein's philosophy to the understanding of human communities (see also Gruber, this volume). I suggest that forms of life must include particular "emotional styles." Emotional styles come and go, develop or decay, according to whether they work for communities. For an emotional style to "work," however, it is not sufficient that it be coherent with the cultural configuration—that is, with the common sense, the "form of life"—of its time and place. An emotional style's characteristic emotional expressions must successfully call forth, in participants, responses that they recognize as warranting these expressions. Such success is something that no culture or discourse can guarantee; the success of an emotional style is not constructed. Such success is also of great political and historical significance.

Viewed from this angle, Mary Pierrepont and Edward Wortley Montagu were not simply testing each other's love but were also testing whether certain new ideas about emotions, when put into practice, called forth appropriate responses. By their written and verbal declarations, by gesture and facial expression, they were engaging in a kind of self-exploration that was also self-alteration.

By the fate of such efforts, emotional styles rise and fall.[6] This is a history that we can make sense of, at least partially, and also a history that we can evaluate politically, if we are prepared to appreciate the complex ways specific emotional styles have helped and hindered, liberated and entrapped, enlightened and deluded, people like Mary and Edward.

4.3 Forms of Life

This is a time of flux for theory and methodology, in history as well as in other disciplines of the humanities and social sciences. Some say it is time to move "beyond the linguistic turn" (Bonnell and Hunt 1999). There is a widespread sense that a proper conception of "discourse" must include practice—or else that practice, or "performance," ought to supplant discourse as our prime matter of concern.[7] Agency— its proper conception and its role in shaping historical change—has engaged a large number of commentators.[8] It is in this context that emotions have gained recent prominence as a research topic. Neglected, as an explicit theme, by poststructuralists, and poststructuralist-inspired criticism and historiography,[9] the question of emotions arose out of investigations of the history of gender identities and sexualities[10] and examinations of social discipline of the type familiar from Norbert Elias' work on the "civilizing process" (Stearns and Stearns 1990).[11] It is increasingly evident that emotions must play a role in any attempt to reconstruct a theory of the individual that moves beyond the discredited concepts of subjectivity and reason.

Wittgenstein's thought has offered a way forward to some philosophers of the mind, social scientists, and humanists interested in social theory in recent years.[12] Among the members of this loose party, Wittgenstein's critique of rules (especially as explored by Kripke 1982) is deployed to show that actions are too multifarious in their unfolding, their character, and their consequences to be neatly characterized as rule governed.[13] This point has been asserted by Hilary Putnam (1997) and Jeff Coulter (1997) to discredit the pretensions of cognitive science. Veena Das (1998) has made a similar point in relation to anthropological notions of culture. Linda Zerilli (1998) has issued a sharp critique of the overly formal and linguistically rigid conceptions of gender that have characterized feminist theory (see also Duran 2002). From the Wittgensteinian point of view, artificial intelligence research, some feminist theory, and poststructuralism share the same defect. All start with rules (algorithms, semiotic systems) and only get back to life afterwards.

These scholars have espoused Wittgenstein's notion of a "form of life" as the ultimate antidote to reductionistic fashions in theory. It is the form of life that provides the frame or origin of conceptions of gender, varieties of cultural consensus, or the sense that a rule is or is not properly applied. Forms of life provide the criteria of truth that are applied in daily practice; such criteria cannot be subject to critical evaluation because they are not propositional in form, and no set of propositions is adequate to characterize these criteria (see Rorty 1995). It is in this sense that Steven Shapin and Simon Schaffer argued that Boyle's famous seventeenth century air-pump experiments established a form of "experimental life" (Shapin and Schaffer 1985). Likewise, Putnam's best effort to ground scientific induction in the present also goes no further than Wittgenstein's "form of life."[14]

From within a form of life, it is impossible to doubt its fundamental features. A Western scientist cannot be expected to doubt that nature is impersonal. But a Balinese village magnate, by the same token, cannot be expected to doubt that the unseen world is heavily populated with powerful personages (Wiener 1995, especially 328–330). In each case, the bare ideas, put into propositional form, are only fragments of a larger, collectively enacted order. However, this order exists only as enacted; it cannot be meaningfully reduced to a set of rules or a law code, no matter how many volumes the code fills. Das insists on the fragility and contingency of such forms of life and suggests that their breakdown may be so catastrophic as to undermine the very possibility of meaning, leading on to civil chaos and mass violence. What is certain is that determining the boundaries of a form of life or finding a language for talking about historical changes in forms of life pose problems familiar from a long effort to historicize notions of culture (Bailyn 2002).[15]

Nonetheless, this Wittgensteinian trend is consonant with recent developments in performance theory, as inspired by Judith Butler (1990, 1993) among others, as well as with practice theory, as developed by Bourdieu (1977), Giddens (1979), Ortner (1999), Sewell (1992), and others (Schein 1999). All can agree with Andrew Pickering's comment that "No finite set of rules can serve to explain practice and closure" (Pickering 1995, 198). In human life, the flow goes in the other direction, from practices to rules, and rules only make sense in the preconstituted contexts of practices that give rise to them. As rules go, so goes any effort, whether ethnographic or historical, to generalize about social life. The descriptions and explanations we write down are not the whole story.

Within the framework of a form of life, "emotions," and the array of practices within which emotions might come up, would represent yet another domain where critical reflection can be of little use. No one has yet observed an emotion; yet in Western locations, lay and expert alike experience them and talk of them as concrete commonsense objects. Thanks to numerous ethnographic investigations of emotions, we know this way of experiencing and talking about emotions is quite local and contingent (Reddy 1999). Yet most experimental psychologists continue to speak of affect as if it were a self-evident reality.

A history of emotions inspired by the Wittgensteinian notion of forms of life might well represent an improvement, in certain respects, over histories guided by notions of culture or discourse. Within the Wittgensteinian framework, a modern emotional form of life might be said to have arisen in the Early Modern period, alongside the "experimental life" described by Shapin and Schaffer.

However, in spite of all the fruitful consequences that a Wittgensteinian turn in the writing of history might bring, treating the domain of emotions as part of a form of life is incomplete. Similar problems arise in attempting to contain emotions within theories of performance or practice. This is because emotional expression may involve what could be called, quite bluntly, feedback. By "feedback" is meant here an incomplete and unpredictable reflexivity. To make this claim clear, it is necessary to characterize, first, how emotional feedback differs from that self-aware self-evidence, beyond doubt because beyond propositional expression, that adheres to forms of life. Emotional "feedback" must also be distinguished from that intense self-reference of the performative—in John L. Austin's sense: the "I do" of the marriage vow, a kind of utterance that names the act that it is (see Karafyllis, this volume). Emotional feedback can best be understood in relation to the issue of attention, as conceptualized by experimental psychologists in recent years—an issue which philosophers have almost completely neglected.[16]

4.4   Attention in Experimental Psychology

Emotional feedback, as examined in experimental psychology, becomes available to view only within a form of "experimental life," that is, the form of life of modern scholarship, made up of reliable witnesses who share observations and explanatory schemes in a disenchanted world. However, there can be no question of our leaving this form of life behind or pretending it is not our own. As it turns out, recent research on attention by experimental psychologists offers some support for Wittgenstein's conception of forms of life. But it also offers reasons to go beyond this conception or at least to complement it with a notion of "emotional feedback."

In research on word recognition, for example, such as that of psychologists Jean Vroomen, Beatrice de Gelder, and their associates, semantic processing has been shown to begin well before the words in a stream of speech are even isolated, much less identified. These researchers find that (at least in certain languages) strong syllables in the stream of speech, no matter where they fall within the actual words that are being pronounced, trigger a search for lexical matches, which search activates semantic material. English-speaking subjects who heard the sentence "The carpet is worn out" would subsequently recognize the word *automobile* more rapidly. The strong syllable *car-* in *carpet* initiates a search for lexical matches that "activates" the word *car* and, in turn, the "meaning" of the word *car*.[17] Subsequently, while this activation lasts, the word *car* is more readily available to attention, as are "semantically" associated words, such as *motor, road, driver*, and so on.[18] In this research, lexical processing not only activates (at least fleetingly) a wide range of semantic material but also sends information back to aid the process of segmenting the stream of phonemes into discrete words. Word discrimination itself is based on metrical cues (e.g., the initiation of a strong syllable) and lexical processing (lexical candidates competing to establish a match with the whole set of phonemes found), modulated still further by semantic processing. This is a striking example of what cognitive psychologists call "parallel" processing—several distinct types of processing are initiated, coordinated, and unfold simultaneously. The rapid activation of material at successive levels renders this material more readily available to attention—even though most of it is not, in the end, useful to the task at hand.

Thus, before one knows what phonemes are being pronounced, one has already isolated two or three likely understandings of the whole sentence. However, what gets into our attention, in the end, is only a small segment of all the activated hypotheses, at different levels of encoding. A further filtering or resource allocation process of some kind controls this access, but theories of how this final stage of door-keeping operates are still fragmentary.[19]

Nested code searching of this kind, sometimes referred to as "cascade" processing, is an increasingly common feature of current cognitive processing models.[20] Stephen Kosslyn relies on it heavily in his theory of visual imagery (Kosslyn 1994). In an early experiment, Kosslyn asked one set of subjects to "look at" the stern of an imaginary boat and then asked if the boat had an anchor. He asked a second set of subjects to "look at" the bow of an imaginary boat and asked them the same question. The first set of subjects responded more slowly. They had to move their focus from the back of the imagined object to the front. The slowed reaction time was the same as in cases where actual pictures of boats were displayed. By Kosslyn's theory, coded memory traces of objects are sent down to a visual buffer, both when one is trying to recognize an object and when one is trying to imagine or remember an object. Once in the visual buffer, these rich mappings of objects can be inspected, just as real objects in our visual fields can be inspected, and new information gathered from them. Visual recognition of an object entails successful matching, in the visual buffer, of an array of visual inputs with the features of a remembered object that have been retrieved and sent to the visual buffer. The two are seamlessly "perceived" as one concrete thing. Kosslyn believes that the large number of efferent (i.e., outgoing) neuronal pathways (equal in number to the afferent ones) that link the various locations of visual processing in the brain are conduits for sending material down to the visual buffer.

Pain research in recent years has uncovered similar feedback structures that undermine what has come to be called "specificity theory." "Specificity theory," writes Mark D. Sullivan in a recent review,

makes two false claims. First, the amount of pain experienced is claimed to be proportional to the amount of tissue damage in the body. But clear proportionality between the strength of the stimulus and the severity of pain is unusual outside of controlled laboratory conditions. . . . Second, specificity theory holds wrongly that nervous activity relevant to pain travels only in one direction, from the body to the brain. We are now aware of a sophisticated descending physiologic system of pain modulation that might account for these originally inexplicable findings about the variable relation between pain and injury. Neurons from the midbrain and brainstem project into the spinal cord to inhibit nociceptive neurons and produce analgesia when stimulated. Endogenous opiates and biogenic amines serve as neurotransmitters in this system. More recently, mechanisms for the sensitization of nociceptors (e.g., through inflammation) and nociceptive pathways (e.g., through repetitive stimulation) have been identified. There are therefore multiple well-defined physiologic processes that modify the amount of pain felt from a given injury. These involve pathways from the brain to the body as well as from the body to the brain (Sullivan 2001, 149).[21]

Pain, therefore, is not so much sensed as interpreted, like boats or sentences, in a multilevel procedure involving activation and cascade processing.

The initial paradigm of cognitive processing was linear; processing was believed to be automatic, for the most part, delivering a finished product to attention. However, processing is now considered to be massively parallel. Increasingly researchers have also recognized that access to attention is highly sensitive to strategies that derive from attention's own current focus. These strategies influence processing far beyond the range of things one could expect a person to articulate in language. Similarly, it was once thought that anything in attention could be reported verbally by a subject, but now it is recognized that verbal reports offer access only to a very limited range, and, depending on context, a peculiarly limited range, of what comes before attention or influences its sensitivity (Schooler and Fiore 1997).

Research shows that attention and activation play an important role in emotional arousal. When subjects are asked to make certain facial expressions or assume certain postures, when they are asked to breathe according to certain patterns, when exercise arouses their autonomic nervous systems, when distraction prevents them from attending to certain tasks, subjects report to experimenters that they feel emotional responses: anger, joy, fear, sadness, boredom.[22] In these instances, as with speech recognition or object identification, it must be supposed that cascade processing is providing probable interpretations of inputs and aiding in the constitution of commonsense objects (in this case, emotions) that are presented to attention almost fully formed. "Fake" laughter can easily stimulate "real" laughter. Subjects also tend to respond "contagiously" to emotional expression in others (Chartrand and Bargh 1999).[23]

As the linear paradigm has broken down, so has the idea that there is a sharp line between cognitive processing and affect. Affect was once thought to be, and is still often spoken of as, a factor exogenous to both cognition and attention, which could interfere with processing, divert it from its course, delay it or speed it up. But *affect*, many now recognize, is simply a word for one subset of the many ways in which activated though material interacts with attentional strategies.[24]

Current models of cascade processing involve (1) the multiplication of levels of processing (a separate code for each level) and (2) the idea that each level relies on results from higher levels to speed its work. However, these models also underscore the profoundly important work of "translation"—as I have called it elsewhere (Reddy 2001, 75–96)—that must go on at the top of the chain. This high-end "processing" is little studied and tends to be treated as a black box into which anything not currently under examination is tossed. Translation coordinates inputs involving a variety of sensory modalities and codes—including the nested codes of imagery and word recognition—as well as a variety of action registers, that is, of remembered procedures and acquired skills: such as pushing a button in a psychologist's laboratory or using the proper formula of politeness for a high-ranking guest.

In principle, however, such translation ought to be subject to all the uncertainties that philosophers since W. v. O. Quine have identified with any process of translation.[25] It is doubtful that any algorithm will be found to help us see such central translating as a kind of "process." When English speakers come to use words such as *orange*, *headache*, or *fear* appropriately, therefore, they have accomplished something that is contingent and tentative. Cognitive psychology, pursuing its special kinds of "matters of fact" through experimental research, is running up against limits to its progress that we might have predicted, if, indeed, experimental research is just another "form of life," another domain of practices beyond skeptical challenge. The higher cognitive processes are, after all, the same ones that psychologists deploy in elaborating theories and evaluating evidence—that is, in living "experimental life." If Wittgenstein was right, models of such higher processes will never be more than approximate and suggestive.

Nonetheless, the special vocabulary developed to model experimental findings (terms such as *attention, activation,* and *cascade processing*) can be of great value. This vocabulary is only tangentially related to the traditional Western vocabulary of the self (including the "faculties" of reason, will, imagination, memory, passion). This vocabulary offers a fresh way of talking about what is sometimes called "discourse." However, this vocabulary does not attribute too much power to language. Language is just one code among many; language itself can be broken down into several series of nested codes, as can hearing, vision, touch, pain, muscular coordination, or memory. It is in the coordination of all these codes, at the highest level, in the black box of intention and practice, that "forms of life" take shape. Yet they do not do so in a vacuum. Puns, slips, tricks of memory, habituated procedures (such as those of speech recognition or those involved in putting on clothing) limit and shape what forms of life we can establish just as much as do, say, our need for a certain minimum daily calorie intake. If a specific "affect" represents a complex configuration of attention, arousal states, and activated thought material, then we can treat that affect as an experimental fact that influences the kind of action a person can engage in, and, by extension, influences the forms of life that take shape in a community.

For example, I may believe, in common with my community, that my severe stomach pain can be relieved by a certain herbal remedy. However, my belief is not, itself, sufficient to ensure that the remedy will work. This is true even though the "specificity theory" of pain also fails to account for my response to the herbal remedy. The outcome depends on a third factor: the unpredictable fate of the outgoing, modulating signals that my "belief" gives rise to. In this sense, my belief in the remedy is not the mere holding true of a proposition, it is not a mere fragment of a discourse, but it is a complex state of mind, implicating a number of cognitive habits. It is subserved by activated thought material outside of attention in one or more codes. It is what English speakers might call an "emotional" commitment to the remedy's power; its character reflects, in part, the place of such beliefs in the form of life of my community. The specific configuration of attention, arousal states, and activated thought material that results from my trial of the herbal remedy is an example of what I propose to call "emotional feedback."

Neither my exact belief in the remedy (which I pick up from the form of life of my community) nor the impact of its emotional feedback on the efficacy of the remedy are within the reach of immediate intentional action.[26] Nor are they the effect of any mere "discursive" structure. Both my belief and the collective "form of life" of my community are put to the test when I try the remedy. The degree and frequency of cures, and the kinds of feedback that the cures give rise to, are partially exogenous factors. The overall working of such factors sets definite limits, determining which forms of life will work for a community and which will not. From the interaction of such limits and such forms is born history and cultural variation. The same might be said for a person's tendency to shed tears at weddings: This is not a piece of discourse or belief; a package of thought material, likely to be activated under proper circumstances, makes certain utterances readily available to attention ("She looks so beautiful") and also stimulates tears.

4.5   Emotional Navigation

We are not able to say, yet, just how malleable the stuff that counts as "emotional experience" truly is. Ethnographic reports reveal a wide variety of affective vocabularies and practices. Varying interpretive schemas, this research shows, can have a profound impact on what people "feel," and the research on emotional feedback, mentioned above, provides a plausible account of at least part of the mechanism of such variability. Moreover, the following points from the ethnographic literature are noteworthy:

1. Despite great variations in the way the emotion domain is defined and parsed, local communities invariably have strongly held ideas about emotional norms and emotional ideals.
2. Emotions, however they are named or spoken of, constitute *a domain of morally and politically significant effort*; all are expected to participate in this effort.
3. Severe sanctions are often imposed on the emotionally deviant.

In tables 4.1 and 4.2 are gathered some examples of specific terms, from a wide variety of cultural venues, for naming emotional control concepts and emotional ideals, and in table 4.3 are listed some salient strategies for penalizing emotional nonconformity reported in the ethnographic literature. Ethnographers and historians have collected this evidence, but they have failed to see the common pattern of normative emotional governance found wherever affect has come under investigation. This evidence strongly suggests the likely utility of a political and historical approach to emotional regimes.

If intentional expression of emotion—verbal, facial, gestural, autonomic—creates emotional feedback, it is not unreasonable that emotional expression should be a matter of great political concern. Emotional expression undoubtedly exercises a powerful influence on arousal states. It can do so simply because of the range of thought material that is "activated," and becomes available to pop into attention, when one rehearses an emotional expression (one's own or another's). Speech recognition is set in motion by one's own speech as well as by the speech of others. Similarly, one's

Table 4.1

Emotional control concepts

Local Term	Translation	Source	Comment
'agl (Arabic)	"reason" that brings mastery of emotions	Abu-Lughod 1986, Lavie 1990	
bēya (Ilongots, Northern Luzon)	"knowledge" that allows elders to temper the *liget* of youths	Rosaldo 1980	Neither *liget* nor *bēya* come with birth; both are achievements, grow together.
ihuma (Inuit)	moderating force that outweighs anger	Briggs 1970	
repiy (Ifaluk atoll)	"social intelligence"	Lutz 1988	Enables individuals to feel *fago* (love, compassion, pity).
sinniligur (Faeroe Islands)	"even temperedness"	Gaffin 1995	"A person who does not become 'angry' (*óndur*) at being the brunt of a taunting joke, prank, or verbal attack is 'even-tempered' (*sinniligur*)" (Gaffin 1995, 153).
save (Gapun village, Papua New Guinea)	"knowledge about appropriate behavior and speech"	Kulick and Stroud 1993	"*Save* is a metaphor often used in Gapun to mean social sensitivity and solidarity." A wife criticized for not making dinner: she "*nogat save*" (Kulick and Stroud 1993, 44–45)
maa (Nukulaelae atoll, Tuvalu)	"shame"	Besnier 1995	
kunta (Pintupi, Western Australia)	"embarrassment," "shame," or "deference"	Myers 1986	Metasentiment that sanctions failures of compassion.
angirrup or akalup (Baining of Papua New Guinea)	"shame"	Fajans 1997	Reaction to violation of proper boundaries between public (social) and private (natural) domains.
"blowing off steam" or "talking it out" (20th century United States)	"ventilation"	Stearns 1994	Makes possible ideal state of freedom from strong emotions.

Table 4.2
Emotional ideals

Local Term	Translation	Source	Comment
mue cedang (Bali)	"bright face"	Wikan 1989, 1990	"Balinese are always concerned to see if the face is clear, and go by numerous, culturally elaborated signs which I will not expound upon here" (Wikan 1989, 302). **Also a control concept.**
Bhaw (Fiji Indians)	"built feelings"	Brenneis 1990b	Among Fijians of Indian descent, *tamashabhaw*—amity—or *prembhaw*—love—are examples of emotions "built" through collective effort. Anger is "the solitary emotion": it is not "bhaw" (Brenneis 1990b, 119). **Also a control concept.**
Rasa (Hindu tradition)	"sap" or "necktar"—generalized, impersonal feelings, collectively performed	Dimock et al. 1974, Lynch 1990	Central to Sanskrit poetry and drama as well as much bhakti ritual. **Also a control concept.**
amae (Japan)	"sweet dependence"	Doi 1973	Wishing to be lovingly indulged by another, or enjoying such indulgence.
liget (Ilongots)	"anger"	Rosaldo 1980	Positive energy; joyous, aggressive self-confidence; enables throwing off of grief.
gham (Paxtun)	"grief"	Grima 1992	Women among this Muslim people express grief elaborately, develop autobiographies of grief; its intensity brings them honor. **Also a control concept.**
ekimi (Mbuti)	"quiet"	Turnbull 1965	Mbuti concept of joy is "powerful quietness." Joy is engendered by "rejoicing the forest," by singing (song being cool like quiet) (Turnbull 1965, 289–290). **Also a control concept.**
ngaltu (Pintupi)	"compassion"	Myers 1986	"a judgment of sorrow or concern for another, a kind of compassionate empathy" . . . "the goal of considerable childhood training" (Myers 1986, 113).
apatheia (ancient Stoicism)	"absence of feeling"	Rist 1977, Veyne 2005	**Also a control concept.**
disinvoltura, sprezzatura (Renaissance Italy)	"nonchalance"	Castiglione 1528	Grace, and absence of self-consciousness of the perfect courtier. **Also a control concept.**

Table 4.2

(continued)

Local Term	Translation	Source	Comment
sensibilité (18th century France)	"sensitivity," a natural capacity for love, pity, generosity, gratitude	Baasner 1988, Maza 1993	Can be enhanced by means of novel reading, melodramatic plays, paintings, and so forth.
feaalofani (Nukulaelae atoll, Tuvalu)	"mutual empathy, interpersonal harmony"	Besnier 1995	

Table 4.3

Penalties for emotional deviance

Type of Penalty	Where Practiced	Source
Gossip	Awlad 'Ali, Fiji, Guadeloupe, Ifaluk, Nukulaelae, Paxtun, Zinacantan	See above, *plus*: Brenneis 1990a, Besnier 1990, Bougerol 1997, Haviland 1977
Exclusion, shunning	Bali, court of Louis XIV, Faeroe Islands, Ifaluk, Japan, Western professional and occupational contexts	See above, *plus*: Saint-Simon 1947–1961, Hochschild 1983
Angry criticism	Ifaluk, Nukulaelae, Pintupi	See above
Feud, duel	Ilongots, Jivaros, Awlad 'Ali, Europe	See above, *plus*: Descola 1993, Billacois 1986
Black magic	Bali, Guadeloupe, Jivaros, Awlad 'Ali	See above

skill in recognizing the meaning of facial expressions, posture, gesture, or breathing patterns can be engaged as easily by one's own behavior as by others'. Thus, in the process of thinking about something, if one puts it into words and utters the words, or puts an attitude into motion through a raised eyebrow or gesture of the hand, a much wider range of thought material associated with the subject becomes available to attention.

This secondary, proprioceptive, and imperfect activation—an approximate and changeable interpretation of the meanings of one's own behaviors—is characteristic of emotional feedback. Often, when one expresses a feeling, a confirming flood of associated ideas reinforces the expression (Duclos and Laird 2001).[27] I have elsewhere suggested, therefore, that emotional expressions be called "emotives," by analogy with John L. Austin's notion of "performatives," but with the difference that the fate of an emotional expression is determined not by syntax, nor by its "happy" performance in an appropriate context, but by the precise character of the feedback it gives rise to. When we express emotions, as when we utter performatives, we are doing something to the world, but the outcome is variable, changeable.

As a result, emotional expression becomes a powerful, if somewhat unpredictable, tool for shaping the self. It is unpredictable for three reasons:

1. Activation of thought material is automatic, not intentional. Activated thought material is not yet in attention; it is simply more likely to come into attention.
2. Attempting to avoid certain thoughts or feelings—including any attempt to focus attention closely or exclusively on a single concern—is fraught with uncertainty; the forbidden content must be "activated" in order to be filtered out. Thought avoidance can therefore have "ironic" emotional effects.[28]
3. Our goal-directed expressions of emotion can end up changing the goals that direct our expressions. After insisting I am happy, I may break down in tears. After insisting that I love my new job, I may resign the next day.

For these reasons, it is preferable to speak of emotional "navigation" instead of emotional "management," as certain other observers have proposed.[29]

Local "forms of life" are therefore not only arenas where skeptical reason cannot reach but also arenas in which emotional navigation is shaped by a local emotional style, an emotional intelligence or common sense that entails norms, ideals, and sanctions. However, this common sense is also limited, shaped in its turn by practical familiarity with what works (when attempts to shape emotions are made) and what does not work, that is, by practical skills in the handling of emotional feedback. Such a common sense is inherently political. A coherent political order necessarily finds support in an accepted emotional style. Without such a shared style, individuals are emotionally incomprehensible to each other. It is also certain that individuals will conform to this style with greater or lesser success, because of the unpredictable character of emotional navigation.

There ought to be substantial analytical payoff to presuming that "forms of life" possess, or are possessed by, normative emotional styles. (And just as there may be subordinate, deviant, and marginal forms of life, so each will have its own emotional style.) Normative emotional styles that are backed up by socially enacted rewards and penalties could be called "emotional regimes." Three kinds of historical questions can be raised about emotional regimes:

1. Changes in emotional norms or emotional ideals must be accompanied by improvisation and trial and error. Norms and ideals cannot establish themselves solely on the basis of their propositional or discursive structure. They must become anchored in practice through emotional navigation efforts that are more-or-less successful over a period of time. Historians and ethnographers ought to be able to find evidence of such improvisation.

2. Emotional regimes are likely to display "errors" about their own nature, that is, about the nature of forms of life and of the emotional regimes that sustain them. For example, the eighteenth century sentimentalist doctrine that certain inherently virtuous emotions were inborn, and not the product of learning and repetition, was in "error" in this sense—with heavy consequences for the course of European history (Reddy 2001). Many individuals learned to react as "sensitive hearts," misinterpreting their own learned responses as "natural." Taking such "natural" movements of the heart as moral guides, they often acted capriciously or made misjudgments based on very superficial information. Such practical error might not be available to skeptical reflection in a given time or place (because it participates in a form of life). However, a historian or an ethnographer might be capable of glimpsing how such error plays itself out in history.

3. Emotional regimes may give rise to greater or lesser degrees of emotional suffering, and suffering may be distributed very unevenly across different roles. With each emotional norm there must correspond a kind of emotional sanction or penalty. Norms are, in many cases, more easily approximated by persons occupying privileged social positions. An ancient Roman senator, for example, was much better situated to engage in the demanding pursuit of *apatheia* than his wife or his slaves (Veyne 2005). Apart from the injustice, in some abstract sense, of Roman marriage or slavery as institutions, there is also the question of whether, and how, the emotional regime worked for various members of society. To be held to an emotional standard and yet deprived of the means of pursuing it may bring its own kind of emotional suffering. Such a "double bind" might be regarded as unjust. The study of emotional regimes gives rise to a conception of emotional liberty in this way.[30] Just as pain can be relieved by a better understanding of pain (through, e.g., moving beyond the specificity theory), so emotional suffering can be alleviated or attenuated by understanding how powerfully our expressive practices mold our "experience." (However, the words *powerfully* and *mold* in the previous sentence also mark the great distance between the theory presented here and a thorough-going poststructuralism, for which there is only discourse, and nothing for it to mold.) Unlike the bare notion of "discourse," or that of "form of life" unadorned, this framework has the advantage of being both historical and political.

Thus, the uncertainty and fumbling of Lady Mary Pierrepont and Edward Wortley Montagu during their courtship, and the miscues and anxieties that plagued them, have more than a personal significance. This couple was attempting to work out how the new emotional norm of the marriage of love could be realized in practice. This is just the sort of improvisation one would expect when history throws up a new emotional theory that is, in fact, in error—such as the idea that love is natural (and therefore not a part of a particular form of life, but universal). This is the sort of improvisation that will determine, by its relative success or failure—for it cannot completely succeed—

whether, and how, a new emotional norm will become rooted in a form of life or else thrown off in favor of something else. Such improvisation also suggests, by the distress and anxiety it occasions, the inequalities and differential sufferings that will characterize the emergent emotional regime. It is such questions, rather than whether Mary or Edward "truly" loved, that can be fruitfully posed of documents such as their rich and fascinating correspondence.

Notes

1. *The Spectator*, No. 4, 5 March 1711. The role of love in marriage is discussed in Nos. 149, 199, 268, 437, and 511.

2. Useful reviews of research include Russell, Bachorowski, and Fernández-Dols (2003) and Robinson (1998). Russell (2003) is extremely useful for historians and ethnographers. His approach resembles that proposed in Reddy (2001). See also a review of earlier debates by Parkinson and Manstead (1992).

3. Some useful starting points are Ortony and Turner (1990), Lang (1995), Drevets and Raichle (1998), Aharon et al. (2001).

4. Landmark studies in the ethnography of emotions include Rosaldo (1980), Abu-Lughod (1986), and Lutz (1988). Recent titles include Fajans (1997) and Ahearn (2001).

5. A few noteworthy recent examples (by two philosophers, a sociologist, a neurophysiologist, and a linguist) are Elster (1999), Nussbaum (2001), Katz (1999), LeDoux (1996), and Wierzbicka (1999).

6. This idea was anticipated by Baasner (1988).

7. On performance and performativity, see Schein (1999).

8. On the need to appreciate practice and agency, see, for example, Giddens (1979), Ortner (1999), Alcoff (1996), and Sewell (1992).

9. Rei Terada notes at the beginning of her recent work that "It may be difficult to imagine what the kinds of experience proposed by poststructuralist theory are supposed to feel like. Many readers have assumed that the very idea of strong emotion is inconsistent with poststructuralism." She goes on to trace a discussion of affect in the works of major poststructuralists. While she shows they have not ignored this issue, it remains the case that their comments have been scattered and, until her work, invisible to many (see Terada 2001). Over ten years ago, Catherine A. Lutz and Lila Abu-Lughod tried to correct what they regarded as a lacuna in poststructuralist thought by developing a poststructuralist account of emotions (see Lutz and Lughod 1990a; see also, in the same anthology, Abu-Lughod 1990).

10. See, for example, Barker-Benfield (1992), Pinch (1996), and DeJean (1991).

11. Both Elias-inspired and gender-inspired concerns are evident in subsequent work of Stearns and associates in, for example, Stearns (1994) and Stearns and Lewis (1998).

12. Agassi and Laor have criticized this "Wittgensteinian turn," in the work of authors such as Ian Hacking, Daniel C. Dennett, and Jonathan Lear (see Agassi and Laor 2000).

13. For further discussion, see, for example, Bailyn (2002) and Burns (2002).

14. Says Putnam, "I agree with Wittgenstein that 'the "law of induction" can no more be grounded than certain particular propositions concerning the material of experience,' and I further agree that '[the language game] is not based on grounds. It is not reasonable [vernünftig] or unreasonable. It is there—like our life.' Where I perhaps differ with Wittgenstein is in finding attempts like Reichenbach's of permanent value nonetheless" (from Putnam 1994, 131–148, quote from 146).

15. On efforts to historicize culture, see Sewell (1999, 35–55).

16. However, see art historian Jonathan Crary's (1999) recent attempt to develop an approach to this issue. See also, for some preliminary remarks by a philosopher, Robert M. Gordon (1995).

17. Terms such as *meaning* and *semantic,* as used in experimental psychology, have specific implications and raise specific problems that will be passed over here.

18. See Vroomen and de Gelder (1995), Vroomen, Van Zon, and de Gelder (1996), and Irausquin and de Gelder (1997).

19. See, for a review, Robinson (1998). Another overview is Camus (1996). Representative studies include Stolz and Besner (1997) and Massaro and Cohen (2000).

20. On the concept of cascade processing, see Bentin and Ibrahim (1996).

21. See also Pincus and Morley (2001).

22. See Damrad-Frye and Laird (1989); Duclos et al. (1989); Cacioppo, Berntson, and Klein (1992); Hess et al. (1992); Stepper and Strack (1993); Philippot, Chapelle, and Blairy (2002); and Sinclair, Hoffman, and Mark (1994).

23. For an earlier review, see Hatfield, Cacioppo, and Rapson (1994). See also the theoretical approach developed by Rimé (2005).

24. Douglas Barnett and Hilary Horn Ratner propose a new term, "cogmotion," in their review essay (Barnett and Horn Ratner 1997). On affect in mental control, see Wegner and Gold (1995), Wenzlaff and Bates (1998), Hollon and Kendall (1980), and Robinson (1998).

25. See the useful overview of Quine's and Davidson's views on meaning in Alcoff 1996, 81–114. The relevant essays are collected in Quine (1969) and Davidson (1984).

26. A useful discussion of the cultural shaping of pain and its treatment is Le Breton (1996).

27. Says Margaret S. Clark, "There is also some clear evidence that choosing to express an emotion or to cognitively rehearse it may intensify or even create the actual experience of that emotion while choosing to suppress it or not think about it may have opposite effect" (Clark 1989, 266).

28. This comment is based on the work of Daniel Wegner and his associates; see, for a review Wegner (1997). On ironies in the mental control of affect, see, for example, Wegner and Gold (1995) and Wenzlaff and Bates (1998).

29. Hochschild (1983) and Wikan (1990), for example, have argued for the importance of the management of emotions.

30. Discussed in detail in Reddy (2001), where emotional liberty is defined as the freedom to pursue those emotional navigation strategies that have the least effect on the freedom of others to pursue their own. Thus an emotional style that depends on the threat of capital punishment (to frighten people into hiding or ignoring improper responses to normative emotional expressions) is less free than a style that depends only on gossip as a sanction.

II Emotions in the Laboratories: Methods and Impacts

5   Technology Assessment of Neuroimaging: Sex and Gender Perspectives

Bärbel Hüsing

5.1   Introduction

Over the past decades, neuroscience has developed and employed a multitude of different methodological approaches to explore the human brain and its functions, one of the latest being powerful brain imaging methods. They have opened up unprecedented ways of exploring the human brain, especially its function in cognitive processes. The results of brain imaging are often presented as *visual maps* in which brain regions are highlighted in brilliant colors which have been specifically activated during the performance of a given task.

Neuroimaging has attracted great attention in the media and the public because the pleasing visual maps produced by neuroimaging lend themselves to popularizing research results from cognitive neuroscience (Racine, Bar-Ilan, and Illes 2005, 159). In recent years, even laypeople who usually do not concern themselves with neuroscience and brain research have increasingly encountered these pictures, which resemble photographs of "the brain at work."

As a consequence, we are now increasingly confronted with research results of cognitive neuroscience: The images (seem to) show in a convincing way how different the brain activation patterns are of various cognitive processes that take place in the brain, how similar or different these task-specific activation patterns are in men's or women's brains, and how "elite brains," that is, the brains of outstanding scientists or musicians (Wittmann, Frahm, and Hänicke 1999, 9–19; Münte, Altenmüller, and Jäncke 2002, 473–475) differ from those of people with average talents and gifts. Neuroimaging also visualizes what happens in the brain during sexual arousal and seems to trace deviant sexual preferences and behavior back to abnormal brain processes (Wolpe 2004, 1031–1033).

Neuroimaging is often perceived as a direct, intrinsically objective approach and as "hard science" (Farah 2002, 1127) and is often deemed superior to related disciplines, such as psychology, and those scientists conducting neuroimaging are accorded elite status within the scientific community. The often expensive, highly sophisticated high-tech instrumentation required for neuroimaging may contribute to this notion.

Against this background, this chapter provides an overview of the most important brain imaging methods and their contribution to the study of cognition and emotions in men and women. From a technology assessment perspective, it anticipates possible future applications outside the research context and critically discusses their achievability, identifies drivers for these developments, outlines possible impacts, and discusses frame conditions under which these research findings are, or respectively should be, generated and applied.

5.2 Neuroimaging Methods and Current Applications

Neuroimaging comprises a set of physical methods which make it possible to obtain data on brain anatomy or function. The unique features of neuroimaging, as compared to other methods used in brain research, are its noninvasiveness, its applicability in vivo, and the precise relation of structure and function to mathematically reconstructed parts of the brain: Before the development of noninvasive neuroimaging methods, examinations of the brain were mainly restricted to postmortem brains, which allow only structural and anatomical analysis, not functional analysis (see Hagner, this volume). Brain functions could be investigated mainly by means of psychological experiments or via electroencephalographic measurements from the human scalp. With modern neuroimaging methods, the brains of living persons became accessible in a new way.

In cognitive neuroscience, different neuroimaging methods are used (Hüsing, Jäncke, and Tag 2006, 5–50). Methods which allow the analysis of brain anatomy comprise computed tomography (CT) and structural magnetic resonance imaging (sMRI). Methods which make possible the analysis of brain functions are either based on direct measurement of neural activity, such as electroencephalography (EEG) and magneto-encephalography (MEG), or record indirect measures of neural activity, for example, positron emission tomography (PET), single-photon emission computed tomography (SPECT), functional magnetic resonance imaging (fMRI), and near infrared spectroscopy (NIRS). These neuroimaging modalities differ from one another in

- the underlying measuring principle,
- the achievable spatial and time resolution, the specificity and sensitivity of the measurements, and the signal-to-noise ratio,
- the requirements, sophistication, and costs of the required equipment, devices, and auxiliaries,
- the applications and uses.

As each of the imaging modalities has its specific strengths and weaknesses, the appropriate technique must be carefully chosen with regard to the scientific, analytical, or diagnostic question that is to be answered, and full information can often only be obtained by the combination of different modalities. All in all, the variety of different neuroimaging methods allows brain imaging on different spatial levels from gross anatomy down to genes and molecules. The method most often applied in cognitive neuroscience is fMRI, due to its good spatial and temporal resolution.

The results of brain imaging are often presented as visual maps which give the impression of "photographs" of the brain structure or of "the brain in action," respectively. However, these visual maps are the result of extensive raw data processing: In a particular experimental setup, quantitative raw data, based on the physical measures for the ongoing brain processes in the test person, are recorded by the respective neuroimaging devices; subsequently, these raw data are processed by sophisticated software in such a way that brain tissue is mathematically reconstructed and the measurements are spatially related to these reconstructed and defined parts of the brain. As the results strongly depend on the chosen data-processing procedures and the subsequent data interpretation, it is possible to obtain different representations of the same phenomenon or to pick out particularly interesting details. On the other hand, it is difficult, even nearly impossible, to interpret a given visual map of brain activity unless information on the experimental setting and the data-processing procedures is also provided.

The scope of actual and potential future applications of neuroimaging is broad (Hüsing, Jäncke, and Tag 2006, 91f). Most brain imaging devices are installed in clinical settings, both in hospitals and in radiologists' clinics. This is the largest market segment for MRI, PET, and CT scanners, so that the manufacturing companies design their products predominantly for these clinical applications. The most important applications to date are clinical diagnosis, monitoring of disease progression, and neurosurgery (Hüsing, Jäncke, and Tag 2006, 93–104). The majority of clinically applied neuroimaging procedures are anatomical techniques, whereas only a few functional methods have already been developed to clinical applicability. MRI is the most important diagnostic tool in neuroradiology, and approximately 50% of all clinical MRI procedures can be attributed to neurology. MRI has become an important standard tool, for example, in the differential diagnosis of various brain tumors, in detecting pathological changes of brain vasculature, and in supporting the diagnosis of multiple sclerosis, acute inflammation in the spinal cord, and infections of the central nervous system. In stroke patients, MRI is applied to assess potentially salvageable tissue, thus supporting the choice of appropriate therapeutic interventions (Chalela et al. 2007, 293). In multiple sclerosis, MRI is routinely applied to monitor the patient's response to therapies (Minagar et al. 2006, 165). For other neurological diseases, neuroimaging methods are used either as sources of supplementary diagnostic information or in the context of biomedical research but have not (yet) attained the status of a standard tool, for example, in treating Alzheimer's disease (Villemagne et al. 2005, 221). In neurosurgery, not only do brain imaging methods provide detailed information for neurosurgical planning but interventional MRI scanners can also provide MRI images during the surgical intervention and support and guide the neurosurgeon with unprecedented anatomical and spatial precision (Mittal and Black 2006, 77). In addition to these clinical applications, neuroimaging plays a significant role in basic biological and biomedical research, where it is used to elucidate the neurophysiological basis and mechanisms of brain functions and neurological diseases. Moreover, imaging is firmly established and still expanding in pharmacological research and drug development because the use of in vivo imaging biomarkers in all stages of the drug development process could considerably accelerate the drug discovery process (Beckmann et al. 2004, 35).

In research, neuroimaging has had, and continues to have, a significant impact on the study of *cognition*. Because brain imaging made it possible to study brain function in a new way, the biological basis of brain functions and dynamic brain processes became a focus of neuroscientific research in the 1990s. In turn, cognitive psychology, a major scientific discipline in the 1960s and 1970s, also experienced significant stimulation from brain imaging methods. As a consequence, the new research discipline, "cognitive neuroscience," emerged through the method-driven convergence of the formerly separated disciplines of neuroscience and cognitive psychology. Initially, the focus in cognitive neuroscience was the elucidation of the neural basis of motor and sensory functions, but it has now shifted to the study of increasingly complex cognitive and emotional processes (Hüsing, Jäncke, and Tag 2006, 127–134). Within cognitive neuroscience, neuroimaging can be employed as a tool to study human cognition and emotion and the similarities and differences between the sexes in these areas.

5.3   Contributions of Neuroimaging to the Study of Cognition, Emotion, and Sex

It is well established that biological sex has an influence on brain differentiation and brain function, due to sex chromosome effects and due to the differentiating effects of sex hormones during prenatal and postnatal development, and that the hormonal status at the time of testing may also have an effect (Institute of Medicine 2001, 79–116; Arnold et al. 2004, 1057; Becker et al. 2005, 1650). As a consequence, male and female brains differ not only in the brain regions involved in reproductive tasks but also in other regions. Moreover, sex differences in human behavior, such as cognition and emotion, are well-known from psychological investigations: for example, women, on average, perform better in verbal tasks, whereas in visual-spatial tests which require spatial orientation, mechanical abilities, or mathematical abilities, men, on average, perform better than women (Weiss et al. 2005, 588–591). With respect to emotional behavior, women, on average, retain stronger and more vivid memories for emotional events than men, and men tend to be more interested than women in visual sexually arousing stimuli (Canli and Gabrieli 2004, 325f; Hamann 2005, 289).

Neuroimaging studies have only recently started to examine sex differences in cognition, emotion, and sexual behavior, aiming to contribute to the emergence of a more comprehensive picture of the important similarities and differences between men and women (Fiske 2004; Hamann 2005, 293) and to address the question regarding the extent to which the different brain structures and functions of men and women are correlated with different behavior. A key challenge in this context is the operationalization of the complex constructs "cognition," "emotion," or "sexual behavior" in a way that they become amenable to brain imaging studies which only yield interpretable results if the traits under investigation are well described at the psychological level and if experimental paradigms, developed and validated in cognitive psychology, are employed. Interdisciplinary cooperation with cognitive psychologists is indispensable here (Hüsing, Jäncke, and Tag 2006, 279–289). Moreover, how a given cognitive ability is operationalized for neuroimaging measurement may significantly affect the result, and thus the comparability with results from other studies, for example, behavioral or neuropsychological studies. If this challenge can be mastered, a straightforward and oft-chosen approach to the study of sex differences with brain imaging is a two-group experimental design in which test groups of male and female study subjects perform a given task while their brain activities are recorded with appropriate brain imaging methods. In this way, differences in brain activity in male and female brains have been observed which relate to the brain regions involved, the level of activity in a given brain region, and the temporal and spatial pattern of activity. It has to be noted, however, that despite these—statistically significant—differences, the results of such studies in general show a marked overlap in the cognitive abilities of males and females, and the similarities in the activation patterns gleaned through neuroimaging far outnumber the differences (Wager and Ochsner 2005, 87).

However, the temptation to jump to far-reaching conclusions as to what these observed differences in brain activation patterns really tell us about the biological "cause" of the behavior under study should be resisted. Rather, the enormous plasticity of the brain, which is significantly driven by environmental stimuli, must also be taken into account. As biologically influenced traits may also affect an individual's response to the environment or the way that the individual is treated by others (Institute of Medicine 2001, 89–90), different social experiences of men and women, which are clearly gender related, should also have a significant effect on brain responses. Therefore, experimental approaches are needed which also examine the mutual construction of cognition by physiology and by experience. In general, neuroimaging in this field has proven to be especially fruitful in the following:

• Gaining insight into the biological basis of these psychological phenomena. For example, the amygdala, a structure in the temporal lobe, was found not only to play a key role in emotional responses and emotional memory but also to mediate sex differences in emotional behavior and to show different levels and temporal–spatial patterns of activity during a given task. Moreover, it develops structurally at different rates in men and women and is significantly larger in male than in female brains (Hamann 2005, 289).

• Suggesting mechanisms for how psychological phenomena arise and helping to better understand the prerequisites for normal cognitive and emotional processes.

• Supporting, building, and refining existing models of cognitive functions, emotions, and resulting human behavior.

• Identifying and differentiating between alternative mechanisms, causes, and etiologies.

• Suggesting new hypotheses that could not be imagined without knowledge of the underlying processes, for example, that the observed greater prevalence of some psychological disorders (posttraumatic stress disorder and clinical depression in women, or voyeurism and autism in males) may stem in part from sex differences in amygdala responses (Hamann 2005, 288).

• Supporting decisions about the requirement, timing, and type of appropriate interventions to develop normal, or remedy impaired, brain functions.

• Monitoring the effects of interventions if they are not observable at the level of behavior.

5.4   Possible Future Applications of Neuroimaging in the Context of Sex, Emotion, and Cognition and Their Impacts

Many research groups today aim to identify and validate "brain markers" for cognitive abilities, emotions, and sexual orientation. The overall goal for future applications is hopefully to develop more sensitive, more specific, and more valid diagnostic procedures which make possible

• the (differential) diagnosis of cognitive or emotional disabilities and, potentially, discrimination between different causes or etiologies

• support for the choice of an appropriate intervention

• the monitoring of effects of the chosen intervention at the brain level if they do not (yet) translate into measurable altered behavior, and

• the assessment of the success of an intervention after completion.

Examples of such uses include examinations of persons with specific reading or calculation disabilities (Goswami 2004, 175–183; Goswami 2006, 406–413) or attention-deficit/hyperactivity disorder (ADHD) for diagnostic purposes and to monitor the effect of interventions on brain level in addition to behavioral level. In a similar way, neuroimaging could perhaps be used as an additional diagnostic tool for determining the "proper" sex in transsexual persons prior to surgery or for analyzing whether therapy of sexual offenders has resulted in reduced arousal after exposure to specific sexual stimuli. In the United States, neuroimaging has also been brought forward as evidence in court several times, for example, in order to support the defense attorney's argument that the accused showed anatomical brain anomalies in the prefrontal cortex which prevented him or her from controlling emotions and behavioral responses to provocation, thus pleading mitigating circumstances (Romanucci-Ross and Tancredi 2004, 61–73; Yang et al. 2005, 1103–1108; Eastman and Campbell 2006, 311–318).

While the above-mentioned examples apply to persons whose behavior obviously deviates from normal ranges, it can also be anticipated that such neuroimaging markers could be used on persons with unremarkable behavior. The purpose could be to obtain prospective information regarding the likelihood of future behavior, with the aim of giving the persons studied adequate support to develop their full potential or compensate for existing disadvantages or to be able to devise appropriate prevention strategies. Another aim could be to obtain information about cognitive and emotional abilities with a quality or effectiveness not possible with other methods. This also includes testing persons not able or not willing to cooperate as well as to uncover deceit and lies (Kozel et al. 2005, 605–613; Pearson 2006, 918f).

Possible applications could be the early screening and testing of the cognitive abilities of children, with the test results playing a significant role in the choice of school, career path, or access to remedial classes for pupils with special educational needs. In a similar way, it could be the aim to detect adolescents at high risk for violent and criminal behavior, for example, and to offer them specific preventive programs. Employers might be interested in obtaining prospective information on whether job applicants show the highest potential with respect to cognitive capacity, emotional intelligence, the ability to cope with stress and control emotions, and so on; it could report whether they are addicted to drugs or are at risk of developing addictions, what their cognitive perception of ethnicity and race is, or—for example, in the case of teaching and educational staff—whether they show pedophiliac sexual preferences. Easy-to-apply test systems to detect overload of cognitive capacity, stress, and waning attention might be of interest for staff in jobs where concentration and alertness are essential for performance and failure could have severe impact (airplane pilots, bus drivers, military staff, medical staff, and so on; Eaton and Illes 2007, 394). Insurance companies might be interested in brain-related markers which give information about future risk of occupational incapacity. Also individuals could have an interest in information about their cognitive and emotional state and their capabilities. In order to achieve their personal goals in private life, business, or sports, they might want to use this information or these methods, respectively, for interventions in order to compensate for predispositions and disadvantages, with the aim of achieving higher performance in alertness, attention, memory, and cognitive capacity, of attaining emotional control and stability, of improving sexual arousal and experience, or even of enhancing their capabilities beyond "normal" levels.

Underlying the possible applications outlined above is the tempting assumption that a large variety of complex cognitive abilities, disorders, and mental diseases, ranging from intelligence, dyslexia, and ADHD to schizophrenia or Alzheimer's disease, could be related to findings in a limited number of brain scans. Most experts dismiss this assumption as naive and simply not achievable. They regard it as highly unlikely that neuroimaging will—ever—replace established psychological test batteries and psychiatric diagnostic procedures. Rather, neuroimaging and genetic studies will complement tests for these traits in the foreseeable future. However, most biomarkers under study today still have to be validated and standardized, and it remains to be seen whether they prove to be superior to established diagnostic procedures in terms of sensitivity, specificity, time, and cost (Baker 2007, 378f). The experience from genetic testing, for instance, indicates that even insufficiently validated tests may be prematurely introduced into practical application. That this could also be the case in neuroimaging is indicated by the fact that pioneer companies have already been founded in recent years, mainly in the United States, which offer a diverse assortment of such services (see table 5.1). However, they are few in number, they serve a very heterogeneous customer base, and the market is presently small and volatile, with many uncertainties (Baker 2007, 377).

Table 5.1

Overview of selected companies offering services in the field of neuroimaging of cognitive abilities

Company Name	Location	Products and Services
Advanced Brain Monitoring, Inc.	Carlsbad, CA , USA	Combination of EEG with vigilance, attention, and memory tests in an Alertness and Memory Profiling System to quantify impairment and measure fitness for duty
Applied Neuroscience Inc.	St. Petersburg, FL, USA	EEG-based support to type or diagnose cognitive functions and disorders, EEG-based biofeedback
Aspect Medical Systems	Norwood, MA, USA	EEG to monitor effects of anesthesia during surgery, EEG biomarkers for rapid identification of treatment efficacy
Biobehavioral Diagnostics	Cambridge, MA, USA	Improved diagnostic technique for assessing ADHD by clinicians

Table 5.1

(continued)

Company Name	Location	Products and Services
Brain Master Technologies, Inc.	Oakwood Village, OH, USA	EEG brainwave training, brain modification technology, neurofeedback
Brain Resource Company	Sydney, Australia	PC- and Internet-based test batteries, EEG, measures of brain function and cognition for pharmaceutical companies, clinicians, scientists, and so on. Database with results from cognitive performance tests, partly also with fMRI, EEG, and genetic data, as reference for clinical trials
Cephos	Pepperell, MA, USA	Detection of intent, prior knowledge, and deception by fMRI
Cyber Learning Technologies LLC	San Marcos, CA, USA	EEG neurofeedback technology and equipment
Human Bionics	Purcellville, VA, USA	Neurofeedback therapy for ADHD, with cognitive assessment and analytical service
Imagine NeuroSolutions	Flower Mound, TX, USA	EEG neurofeedback program for improvement of attention problems
Lexicor	Augusta, GA, USA	EEG tool to diagnose ADHD
Neurognostics	Milwaukee, WI, USA	fMRI for probing sensorimotor or cognitive functions (f)MRI-based support for mapping brain before tumor or seizure surgery
Neuronetrix	Louisville, KY, USA	EEG tool to diagnose Alzheimer's disease in early stages
Neurosense	Oxford, U.K.	Consultancy in neuromarketing, fMRI, MEG, and behavior testing in marketing research
No Lie MRI	Philadelphia, PA, USA	Detection of intent, prior knowledge, and deception by fMRI
Omneuron	Menlo Park, CA, USA	Reducing chronic pain by biofeedback using MRI
SalesBrain LLC	San Francisco, CA, USA	Neuromarketing
SleepMed	Kennesaw, GA, USA	Internet-based services to collect and analyze EEG data for clinicians for sleep disorders and epilepsy
Unique Logic and Technology	Asheville, NC, USA	EEG neurofeedback learning software for ADHD

Note: ADHD, attention-deficit/hyperactivity disorder; EEG, electroencephalography; fMRI, functional magnetic resonance imaging; MEG, magnetoencephalography; MRI, magnetic resonance imaging.

Sources: Baker 2007, 377–379; Hüsing, Jäncke, and Tag 2006, 149f; Pearson 2006, 918f.

Nevertheless, the following drivers make it likely that more diverse and more sophisticated applications will reach the marketplace in the years to come:

• Imaging technologies are increasingly being adopted by scientific disciplines not traditionally related to neurosciences, such as economics (Camerer 1999; see Ulshöfer, this volume), learning and instruction research (Stern et al. 2005), or different branches of psychology. The reputation-building effect of the required highly sophisticated instrumentation may play a role in this trend, and even more so, as access to the limited research resource of imaging equipment fulfills a gatekeeper function, giving persons with access a competitive advantage. Finally, the exploitation of synergies between the disciplines forms a fertile ground for the development of new, original research questions which are only addressable with interdisciplinary cooperation, which thus further broadens the scope of possible future applications (Hüsing, Jäncke, and Tag 2006, 145–147).

• Advanced neuroimaging devices such as MRI or PET scanners are expensive equipment with rather high fixed costs for the equipment, building, maintenance, and qualified staff for operation. Fixed costs must be shared based on the volume of examinations conducted annually. As a consequence, users of PET and MRI will aim to maximize the number of analyses performed. On the other hand, as most analyses are carried out for medical purposes, income significantly depends on the reimbursement conditions set by the relevant health insurances. Against this background, there are economic incentives for operators of neuroimaging devices to acquire additional sources of income beyond those services reimbursed by health insurance. Moreover, imaging device companies offer flexible and attractive financing and leasing options, including sales of refurbished and used systems, thus contributing to the expansion of imaging service providers. For reasons of qualification, quality assurance, the high number of patients, and versatile use of expensive imaging devices, equipment manufacturers also develop application-specific sequences which allow a "push button" use of the imaging devices for different diagnostic and analytical procedures (Hüsing, Jäncke, and Tag 2006, 181–186). This also supports the diffusion of neuroimaging beyond specialized centers with specifically qualified staff.

• Although the practically usable information that can be gleaned from neuroimaging in the analysis of cognition and emotion is in most cases not new or unique, and could also be obtained with conventional, established testing, there is a demand, albeit small, from a heterogeneous group of customers and stakeholders for such information and services (Baker 2007, 377). The extraordinary attractiveness of neuroimaging, the (often unjustified) perception of its superiority to conventional psychological tests, coupled with an overestimation of its performance and an underestimation of its limits and risks, contribute to this demand.

While it is likely that sufficiently validated and standardized neuroimaging procedures will eventually complement existing psychological and genetic tests for a broad variety of mental disorders and cognitive abilities, a key question is what the validity and explanatory power of brain imaging for potentially far-reaching judgments about a person's cognitive abilities and behavior presently is and could become in the future. The following methodological issues should be taken into account here.

Although the visual maps generated by neuroimaging seem convincing, it must be kept in mind that the method employed to measure an ability (in terms of experimental setup, paradigmatic, and protocol variables) may significantly affect the result and may, consequently, be misleading or used in a manipulative way, especially if presented to nonexperts. The complex traits under study must be transformed into highly controlled, highly artificial, and abstract test situations and therefore require a careful discussion about the extent to which inferences can be made from this test situation to human behavior in "normal life" outside experimental settings. Most neuroimaging methods require the comparison of one cognitive or emotional state (e.g., active, impaired function) to another (e.g., passive/baseline, normal function). This is often done by comparing data from the human subjects under study to data from a control group.

Brain imaging studies with fMRI are often performed with rather small study groups of 10 to 16 study subjects, which raises the question of how statistically significant the results really are (Thirion et al. 2007, 105). This is especially true if one considers, additionally, that behavioral sex differences may depend on age, stages of life, and/or the reproductive cycle, or these differences may only become apparent in certain environments (Institute of Medicine 2001, 79–116; Arnold et al. 2004, 1057; Becker et al. 2005, 1650). Moreover, data from individuals are also compared to databases, which for these reasons should be controlled with respect to possible sex and ethnicity bias. Moreover, data which have been obtained with a specific subset of the population (e.g., psychopaths) must not be applied to the general population. For that reason, there is a need for clarification about when a database, which is to serve as a standard, is sufficiently large, representative, and medically, psychologically, and culturally serviceable to deliver valid assessments of individual cognitive function for a given purpose (Eaton and Illes 2007, 395). Such a discussion will most likely challenge our understanding of what can be considered "normal" and what is "pathological deviation from normal ranges." At the present level of knowledge, there is not yet a scientific basis for applying neuroimaging for a "screening" of the general population.

All of the potential future applications mentioned above imply that knowledge about cognitive abilities and mental state gleaned from neuroimaging can be transformed into "appropriate action." This requires a closer look at the knowledge gathered and the possible actions. On the one hand, the information obtained from neuroimaging may deviate substantially from initial expectations (Hüsing, Jäncke, and Tag 2006, 76–78). According to recent estimations, in 2% to 8% of brain imaging studies in the context of nonmedical, cognitive experiments on mentally healthy people, unexpected brain anomalies were detected (Illes et al. 2004, 743). Incidental findings that appear to be outside the norm are therefore not quantitatively negligible. People informed of the unanticipated discovery of anomalies in their brain will find themselves, their partners, and their relatives exposed to significant psychic stress due to the possibly far-reaching consequences for the subject but perhaps also for third parties, such as relatives. Moreover, in many cases, it will not be known—or there will be considerable prognostic uncertainty concerning—what possible impact a "positive" finding might have for the individual. This situation requires careful counseling and support by specially qualified staff. Moreover, referral to specialists and additional diagnostic procedures and therapeutic interventions are often required, which may lead to additional costs and may pose health hazards to the person affected.

It is obvious that high professional standards and well-established procedures for the management of such cases are required. However, brain imaging studies in cognitive neuroscience are often performed by psychologists or other scientists who have not received formal training in interpreting brain scans with respect to abnormalities of clinical significance and with respect to disclosing sensitive personal information to patients and counseling them appropriately. This raises the question of whether the investigator is in a position to diagnose and interpret an abnormality reliably. There is also the risk that unanticipated findings may go unrecognized and thereby subjects are left without appropriate referral or counseling. Additionally, data may be inappropriately interpreted, confronting the subject with a false-positive result. It also raises the question of under which conditions an investigator or an institution can be held liable for a pathological condition which goes undetected. On the other hand, if scans of all study participants were subjected to routine clinical assessment by specially trained medical staff, this would substantially increase the workload, staff requirements, and costs for such studies and impede cognitive neuroscience research. In terms of both legal and ethical considerations, study participants also have the right not to know. As a consequence, informed consent procedures must be so designed that the person concerned is offered the opportunity to decide on his or her own whether he or she wishes to be informed (and, if so, to what degree) of possible incidental findings of treatable or nontreatable conditions. Unfortunately, there is evidence that established procedures in institutions conducting neuroimaging of healthy volunteers often do not fully take into account the above-mentioned concerns (Hüsing, Jäncke, and Tag 2006, 291–294).

"Appropriate action" especially raises the question of the type of intervention possible (e.g., selection vs. remedial action or even enhancement) and the availability of and access to appropriate interventions which can effectively influence the condition. Due to the widespread overrating of neuroimaging and the failure to take its limitations fully into account, the risk exists that conditions may be perceived as "determined" and therefore not amenable to interventions. However, recent findings of brain research emphasize the remarkable plasticity of the human brain, and the often conveyed notion of "closing windows" in cognitive development cannot be substantiated for the human brain.

Neuroimaging implies the acquisition, collection, processing, and storage of large amounts of data in digitized form. Data processing, analysis, and interpretation can, therefore, be separated, both spatially and temporally, from the physical neuroimaging investigation and direct involvement of the patient or research subject. The data can also be interlinked with other data. As brain functions are closely related to personality and individuality, with quality of life, the ability to lead an autonomous and fulfilled life, and with social interaction, neuroimaging and brain data derived from neuroimaging can potentially yield very sensitive information about the individual, requiring special protection. As social stigma is attributed to the impairment of brain functions, a deviation of a subject's brain scan from "normal" findings might lead to negative conclusions about the person's personality and behavior, with subsequent discrimination toward the person concerned (see the Introduction to this volume). This points to the need to continuously assess whether existing data protection legislation and established privacy practices are keeping pace with progress in neuroimaging, in order to adequately address the data protection risks inherent in neuroimaging (Hüsing, Jäncke, and Tag 2006, 294–297).

5.5 Summary and Conclusions

Brain imaging in cognitive neuroscience is a dynamically developing research field. Presently, its application in psychological research has mainly confirmed what was already known before, from a different analytical perspective, and the diagnostic specificity and sensitivity of neuroimaging of cognitive abilities does not go beyond established psychological and psychiatric diagnostic tests. However, it has the potential to provide additional and complementary tools for the diagnosis of cognitive impairments and the monitoring of therapeutic interventions. Nevertheless, intensive efforts in validation and standardization are still required, and its usefulness and/or superiority to established procedures in terms of sensitivity, specificity, validity, costs, and applicability in practice remains to be demonstrated. A broad variety of potential applications outside the research context can be anticipated in the medium to long term, and significant scientific, economic, and social drivers have been identified which support this development.

In order to prevent a premature application of insufficiently substantiated findings in "everyday life," there is a clear need for safeguards against "unscientific" applications. In research, the enforcement of rigorous peer-review processes, a high level of awareness of and transparency with regard to the limitations of neuroimaging methods and experimental approaches, and a critical discussion of what can be inferred from experimental or diagnostic procedures to far-reaching assessments about cognitive abilities and likely future behavior of affected persons are important elements of these safeguards. With respect to sex and gender issues, the perceived "objectivity" of neuroimaging bears the risk that results will be interpreted as the "biological basis" of the traits under study and that cultural aspects, sex stereotypes, and environmental influences will not be sufficiently and appropriately taken into account. Against this background, an interdisciplinary reflection about the (uncritical) reception of neuro-imaging findings by target audiences and about the possible instrumentalization of neuroimaging findings is desirable.

Given the sensitivity of the personal information that could one day be gleaned from neuroimaging of cognitive abilities, the possibly significant impact on the individual's self-image, behavior, and future way of living, and the potential for misuse and discrimination, applications of these techniques on a broader scale require a prior social debate and clarification about which tests should be permissible on whom, by whom, for which purposes, and under which conditions, and which consequences must not or should follow from these tests.

6 Emotional Intelligence, Professional Qualifications, and Psychologists' Need for Gender Research

Myriam N. Bechtoldt

6.1 Introduction

In 1995, Daniel Goleman, a former editor of *Psychology Today* and at that time working for *The New York Times*, published *Emotional Intelligence: Why It Can Matter More than IQ*. In this book he asserted that people's life success would be more dependent on their emotional quotient (EQ) than on their intelligence quotient (IQ). The public reaction was tremendous: Goleman's book became a best-seller, and in 1995 the American Dialect Society declared EQ to be the "most useful word of the year."[1]

What makes Emotional Intelligence (EI) a best-selling topic among laypeople and a fascinating yet at the same time controversial issue among psychological scientists? Though not a researcher himself, did Goleman detect a psychological characteristic that had been overlooked by experts in the field? What does psychology actually know about EI and its impact on people's lives? This chapter focuses upon these central questions. First, it relates EI to the older concept of social intelligence, which had been of considerable interest to psychologists for decades before the term EI was invented. The chapter then proceeds with a discussion of different approaches to measuring EI. It follows with a review of findings concerning the impact of EI on job performance, as it is particularly in the work context that EI has achieved great popularity. It concludes, finally, with a brief review of findings on gender differences in EI.

6.2 Historical Development of EI

Although the term EI had been generally unknown before the publication of Goleman's best-seller, it is not Goleman but doctoral student Wayne Payne who is said to have coined it: In 1986, Payne completed his unpublished thesis entitled "A Study of Emotion: Developing Emotional Intelligence." Four years later, in 1990, Peter Salovey and John Mayer published the first paper on EI in a scientific psychological journal. The paper received little recognition from the scientific community, however, until Goleman's best-seller in 1995. Since then, the number of publications about EI has increased to more than 650. Moreover, Mayer and Salovey's conception of EI has become influential in the field of psychology. In their 1990 paper, they define EI as "a subset of social intelligence that involves the ability to monitor one's own and others' emotions, to discriminate among them, and to use this information to guide one's own thinking and actions" (Salovey and Mayer 1990, 189). They explicitly describe EI as a subcomponent of social intelligence. Given that Mayer and Salovey clearly relate EI to social intelligence, why did they not employ this traditional term?

6.2.1 Social Intelligence

In 1920, Edward Thorndike defined social intelligence as "the ability to understand and manage men and women, boys and girls—to act wisely in human relations" (Thorndike 1920, 228). Though narrative rather than scientific, the definition was seminal. It indicated two major components of social intelligence: the ability to analyze people (perceptual ability) and the necessary skills to act appropriately in social encounters (behavioral skills). Social intelligence was part of Thorndike's tripartite model of intelligence, which consisted of abstract intelligence (the ability to understand and effectively deal with ideas and concepts), mechanical intelligence (the ability to understand and effectively deal with objects), and social intelligence.

It is important to note that Thorndike's three-part model was not immediately influential in psychological intelligence research. The dominant intelligence model of that time had been published by Charles Spearman in 1904 and included just one general factor of intelligence (g). Using a new statistical method, factor analysis, he had shown that there was a strong positive correlation in the performance of all mental tasks requiring intellectual abilities, irrespective of their content.[2] Accordingly, he favored a unitary concept of intelligence. The g-factor model, which is still dominant today, subsumes social intelligence as a subcomponent of general intelligence and does not see it as an independent factor as the EI literature suggests.

Although Spearman's model did not devote any attention to the question of whether social intelligence existed independent of general intelligence, Thorndike's idea triggered much activity among scholars trying to develop tests for social intelligence. For example, the George Washington Social Intelligence Test (GWSIT; Moss and Hunt 1930), one of the oldest tests, measures recognition of others' moods via their verbal and facial expressions, memory of names and faces, and sense of humor. However, because there was a high correlation between GWSIT test results and tests for general intelligence, it was questioned from the beginning whether the GWSIT measured anything beyond the traditional concept of intelligence. The same arguments were made against other early tests of social intelligence like the Vineland Social Maturity Scale (Doll 1935) and the Social Insight Test (Chapin 1942, 1968). Typically, there was a high correlation between social intelligence tests and general intelligence, especially with subtests measuring verbal comprehension. Although Thorndike's definition had declared that perceptual and behavioral skills were essential elements of social intelligence, psychometric tests of social intelligence obviously failed to address these two components. The latter would have required confronting test takers with social interactions instead of paper-and-pencil tests. Thorndike himself had anticipated these assessment difficulties. To him, it seemed easier to define social intelligence than to measure it: "Convenient tests of social intelligence are hard to devise. . . . Social intelligence shows itself abundantly in the nursery, on the playground, in barracks and factories and salesrooms, but it eludes the formal standardized conditions of the testing laboratory" (1920, 231). Given the dissatisfying results of the first era of test development, he concluded that psychology still lacked adequate measurement tools for assessing social intelligence; therefore, it would remain to be seen whether social intelligence could be empirically differentiated from general intelligence.

However, further attempts to do so did not yield any breakthroughs. In 1960, Lee Cronbach, an educational psychologist who made significant contributions to the field of psychological testing and measurement, concluded that in spite of "50 years of intermittent investigation . . . social intelligence remains undefined and unmeasured." Moreover, he concluded that "enough attempts were made . . . to indicate that this line of approach is fruitless" (Cronbach 1960, 319). Thereafter, although some ambitious researchers still attempted to prove the contrary (e.g., Guilford 1967), psychologists' interest in research on social intelligence declined significantly over the following two decades.

6.2.2 Interpersonal and Intrapersonal Intelligence

In the early 1980s, Howard Gardner (1983) presented a theory of multiple intelligences, which included a social intelligence component that he called "interpersonal intelligence" and a more inwardly focused counterpart called "intrapersonal intelligence." Interpersonal intelligence, which denoted the ability to accurately perceive others' moods, feelings, and motivations, overlapped with Thorndike's perceptual component of social intelligence. Intrapersonal intelligence added a new component by emphasizing the ability to understand one's own emotions and motivations. Gardner's methodological approach deviated from the traditional procedure of psychological intelligence research established by Spearman, because it did not statistically assess the independence of interpersonal and intrapersonal intelligence from general intelligence. His nonstatistical approach was one reason the conception of social intelligence was, once again, ignored by mainstream psychology.

6.2.3 Social Intelligence as a Core Element of Laypeople's Implicit Theory of Intelligence

Even though Gardner's model did not gain academic favor, it became widely known and popular in the field of education. It even inspired schools to adapt their curricula to the idea of multiple intelligences. Social scientists outside of psychology and especially laypeople had far fewer problems with the idea of social intelligence than intelligence researchers themselves: One of the leading intelligence experts in psychology at the time, Robert Sternberg, asked 186 people waiting for trains or entering a supermarket to list examples of behaviors that they considered indicators of "intelligence" (Sternberg et al. 1981). Subsequently, the complete list was given to another sample of 122 laypeople who rated these behaviors in terms of prototypicality: Participants were asked to judge how characteristic of an "ideally intelligent person" they considered each of these behaviors to be. Sternberg and his colleagues statistically analyzed the relations between the characteristic ratings and identified those with the highest correlations. The findings were intriguing. One of the three dimensions that emerged reflected skills and behaviors the researchers referred to as "social competence." Behaviors comprising this factor were, for example, "is sensitive to other people's needs and desires," "has social conscience," "thinks before speaking and doing," "makes fair judgments," "is frank and honest with self and others," and "accepts others for what they are" (Sternberg et al. 1981, 45). The other two factors were "practical problem-solving ability" and "verbal ability." When the same behaviors were rated by experts in the field of intelligence, that is, by psychologists holding doctoral degrees, a strikingly different picture emerged: Analyses of their characteristic ratings also yielded two factors comprising "practical problem-solving ability" and "verbal ability" but not a factor of social competence.

Three points appear noteworthy about these results:

1. Laypeople have a clear implicit theory about intelligence.
2. Laypeople, in contrast to experts, consider social abilities as central to their understanding of intelligence.
3. Although not explicitly discussed by Sternberg et al. (1981), social abilities also seem to imply moral values in laypeople's view.
What consequences can be derived from these results?

Explicit theories of intelligence are scientific constructions, addressing the question of what intelligence really is. They are inferred from empirical data, for example, test results of people performing various mental tasks. In contrast, implicit theories reflect peoples' genuine understandings of intelligence, which, although not necessarily based on scientific findings, significantly influence their everyday behavior. In many situations, people try to assess one another's intelligence without having intelligence test results at hand, for example, in job interviews. As the outcome of such everyday assessments may have considerable consequences for the individual being evaluated (such as being offered a new job), it is important to know what characteristics and behaviors people actually focus on when they judge an individual's mental abilities. Sternberg and colleagues' work demonstrates that when they judge, people take social skills into account.

While psychological scientists have been struggling with the concept of social intelligence for decades, laypeople seem to have a much clearer understanding of it. When social abilities are essential to people's conceptions of intelligence, one may expect a positive attitude among laypeople toward intelligence models including or even prioritizing this component, regardless of their scientific evidence. From the point of view of laypeople, intelligent people are not only capable, they are also considerate, fair, self-disciplined, and tolerant. Thus, laypeople seem to assume that intelligence results in high moral standards.

6.2.4 The Bell Curve

In 1994 the American public learned more about intelligence when psychologist Richard Herrnstein and political scientist Charles Murray published *The Bell Curve*, a book summarizing empirical findings on the impact of general intelligence on people's lives. They presented analyses of a large longitudinal data set, the National Longitudinal Survey of Youth, compiled by the National Bureau of Labor and Statistics. The data contained the results of traditional intelligence tests from a nationally representative sample of Americans as well as data about their achievements and living conditions.

Based on this large data collection, the authors made several assertions. They argued that intelligence is one of the most, if not the most, important factors in both economic and social success in life. Furthermore, intelligence is distributed unequally among different ethnicities, with African-Americans scoring significantly lower on intelligence tests than white Americans. Moreover, intelligence is largely (40%–80%) genetically determined. The heritability factor assigns a subordinate influence to differences in upbringing conditions. Accordingly, attempts to significantly raise individuals' IQ levels by means of schooling or training programs yield rather disappointing results.

The Bell Curve became both a best-seller and a highly contentious issue at the same time. Critics reproached Herrnstein and Murray for promoting an elitist model of society and racial discrimination. For example, based on their assertions, it could be argued that African-Americans had lower incomes, jobs of lower status, and a disproportionately high share in statistics on delinquency not because they were discriminated against but because they were genetically less intelligent than white (Caucasian) Americans. This conclusion was rejected by the American Psychological Association (1996) because of a lack of scientific evidence supporting the hypothesis of genetic differences in intelligence between ethnic groups.

6.2.5 Goleman's Conception of EI

Just one year after the publication of *The Bell Curve,* Daniel Goleman published his best-seller. Combining findings from neuroscience and cognitive psychology, he explicitly derogated the primacy of general intelligence in favor of EI. He defined EI as "abilities such as being able to motivate oneself and persist in the face of frustrations; to control impulse and delay gratification; to regulate one's moods and keep distress from swamping the ability to think; to empathize and to hope" (Goleman 1995, 34).

Two aspects seem particularly interesting about this definition. First, Goleman equates cognitive abilities—intelligence—with personality variables that are not typically considered indicators of intelligence. An individual's self-control, persistence, mood, and hope do not enable logical reasoning or verbal comprehension—two mental capacities which psychologists since Spearman and laypeople alike (see Sternberg et al. 1981) consider prototypical indicators of intelligence. Goleman himself seems to be aware of the inconsistencies in his definition when he summarizes the essentials of EI as follows: "There is an old-fashioned word for the body of skills that emotional intelligence represents: character" (Goleman 1995, 34). Still, he insists that emotional intelligence is a purely cognitive ability.

Second, the series of personality variables he subsumes under the heading of EI create a picture of committed, considerate, sociable, and emotionally stable individuals who are able to pursue their goals against all odds. Thus, Goleman's emotionally intelligent individuals possess a series of traits that define a psychologically healthy, socially valuable member of society. He is, therefore, in line with laypeople's conceptions of intelligence (see Sternberg et al. 1981).

This definition of EI was heavily criticized by intelligence researchers from the very beginning. Definitions of intelligence in psychology all agree on the fact that intelligence enables individuals to learn from experience and thereby to adapt to their environment. Personality, by definition, refers to an individual's habitual style of acting toward and reacting to his or her environment (Pervin 1980). These styles are neither clearly adaptive nor maladaptive—it is the situational context that determines their usefulness (see Illouz, this volume). Neuroticism, for example, an individual's tendency to react anxiously, to experience depression, and to ruminate, conflicts with the variables in Goleman's catalogue of EI. However, it may be highly adaptive for a child to develop neurotic tendencies, like trait anxiety and hypervigilance, if these make him or her alert to sudden mood changes in an alcohol-addicted and abusive father. Neurotic tendencies in this case might help the child to avoid the father in these moments. As a grown-up, however, the same reactive patterns might be rather dysfunctional if displayed toward colleagues or supervisors because now individuals should have more assertive conflict management strategies at their disposal. Therefore, selecting a series of personality variables and calling them "intelligent" without taking into consideration the situational context appears to be a questionable approach.

Second, the relationship between intelligence and adaptability seems to be linear, that is, the higher the intelligence, the higher an individual's ability to learn and adapt. With regard to personality variables, however, curvilinear relationships seem more realistic. For example, a very low level of optimism could be just as dysfunctional as a very high level. The latter might result in a distorted view of reality and even prevent the individual from successfully coping because he or she refuses to take potential risks and dangers into account.

While there are complications involved in using a personality-based model of EI like Goleman's, the intuitive appeal is clear. If intelligence is crucial to success in life, then it is highly desirable to be intelligent. Herrnstein and Murray (1994) asserted that intelligence is genetically determined and thus hardly modifiable by environmental factors. Goleman (1995) instead suggested that everyone who wished to be (emotionally) intelligent could be. One had only to work on self-discipline, confidence, and optimism. This made EI an appealing concept to the public. Similarly, Salovey and Mayer's decision to speak of "emotional" instead of "social" intelligence might have expressed their desire to evoke more openness and less negative emotions among scientists toward what had previously been a rather contentious subject.

6.3 Measuring EI

If EI is supposed to have a considerable impact on people's success in life, the question arises of how to assess an individual's EI. Companies, for example, might be interested in including the measurement of job applicants' EI in their personnel selection procedures. A series of EI tests have been developed in psychology since the mid-1990s (e.g., Bar-On 1997; Mayer, Salovey, and Caruso 2002a and b; Salovey et al. 1995; Schutte et al. 1998), including commercially available tests that have received little scientific attention. The tests can be grouped into two categories: questionnaires and performance tests. The first group follows Goleman's understanding of EI as a collection of personality traits. They consist of questionnaires asking people for their habits and attitudes (self-reports). The second group of tests comprises performance tests. Test takers are presented with tasks akin to those on general intelligence tests, implying that their answers can be judged as either right or wrong. Both approaches will be reviewed below.

6.3.1 Self-Reports

To prove that EI is a kind of intelligence that can be separated from general intelligence, tests of EI need to fulfill certain criteria, for example, their results must correlate with intelligence but not too highly; otherwise, the independence of EI from general intelligence will remain questionable (as was the case for social intelligence). Their results should not correlate too highly with traditional personality measures either; otherwise, it will be impossible to differentiate EI from known personality traits. The latter, in fact, is true of the self-report questionnaires on EI.

For example, the Emotional Quotient Inventory (EQ-i) by Bar-On (1997) aims to measure five different components of EI: (1) intrapersonal intelligence, (2) interpersonal intelligence, (3) adaptivity, (4) stress management, and (5) general mood. Conspicuously, one of these components, general mood, openly addresses personality instead of intelligence: It clearly asks for an individual's dispositional level of happiness and optimism. Similarly, a close examination of the other four components' subscales reveals considerable overlap with traditional personality measures. As to intrapersonal intelligence, the questionnaire assesses self-regard, assertiveness, and independence. These aspects, in turn, are also part of the California Psychological Inventory (CPI; Gough 1957), an established and well-known personality questionnaire. Similar findings pertain to the aspects of interpersonal intelligence and adaptability component, which are also covered by the CPI. Not surprisingly, correlations between the EQ-i total value and basic personality dimensions are so high that "these data suggest that the EQ-i is nothing but a proxy (and likely crude) measure of . . . personality" (Matthews, Zeidner, and Roberts 2002, 212). More specifically, it seems to be a measure of psychological health, because it has a high negative correlation with neuroticism, obsessive–compulsive behavior, and anxiety (all correlations between $r = -60$ and $-.70$; Newsome, Day, and Catano 2000; Dawda and Hart 2000). Moreover, there is absolutely no correlation between EQ-i and intelligence ($r = .01$; Newsome, Day, and Catano 2000). To sum up, there is no empirical evidence whatsoever to confirm the assertion that EQ-i measures a kind of intelligence. Instead it assesses personality components indicating psychological health. These findings are representative of other questionnaires on EI (Davies, Stankov, and Roberts 1998): They seem to endorse known concepts rather than to add substantially to the assessment of human abilities. Moreover, they are prone to "self-deceptive enhancement and deliberate faking" (Lopes, Côté, and Salovey 2006, 58), which is true for personality tests in general. Job applicants, for example, know exactly which answers will leave the best impression on their potential employer: A person applying for a job as an insurance agent and facing one of the items of the Schutte Self-Report Inventory on EI (Schutte et al. 1998), like "I find it hard to understand the nonverbal messages of other people," will know which answer meets the demands of the job.

Generally, if EI is supposed to indicate an ability, self-report instruments like questionnaires are not an appropriate assessment tool. This argument is further strengthened by the failure of people to accurately judge their own abilities; correlations between self-estimated intelligence and intelligence test scores do not exceed $r = .30$, that is, they are of moderate size only (Paulhus, Lysy, and Yik 1998). The assessment of cognitive abilities requires performance tests which confront people with problem-solving tasks.

6.3.2 Performance Tests

Mayer and Salovey were among those who chose to design performance tests for EI. They first published the Multifactor Emotional Intelligence Scale (Mayer, Caruso, and Salovey 1999), which was later succeeded by the Mayer–Salovey–Caruso Emotional Intelligence Test (MSCEIT V2.0; Mayer, Salovey, and Caruso 2002a and b). It consists of 141 items measuring four components, (1) emotional perception, (2) assimilation of emotions, (3) understanding emotions, and (4) managing emotions:

1. To measure *emotional perception*, test takers are confronted with photographs of faces, abstract designs, or landscapes and must judge the degree of certain emotions (anger, sadness, happiness, disgust, fear, surprise, and excitement) present in these pictures.
2. The second component, *assimilation of emotions*, demands that test takers "translate" emotions into cognitions. For example, they are asked to evoke a certain emotion in themselves (e.g., envy) and must rate how hot or cold it is.
3. The third component, *understanding emotions*, asks test takers to identify emotions that can be combined to form other emotions, for example, envy and aggression form malice.
4. The last component, *managing emotions*, asks test takers to judge how likely it is certain actions would affect either their own feelings or those of other people, for example, what could be done to reduce an individual's anger or to prolong joy (Mayer, Salovey, Caruso, and Sitarenios 2003).

Among other things, critics scrutinized the problem of scoring respondents' answers. While a proposed solution to an arithmetic problem is either right or wrong, the question of how to most effectively prolong a person's joy or reduce his or her anger is more open to debate. The three scoring alternatives proposed, consensus scoring, expert scoring, and target scoring, will be briefly reviewed below.

Consensus scoring If the majority of an audience watching a movie reacts with terror, it is not an important question whether the movie is really shocking in nature. EI would not seek to prove the majority of people wrong if the movie was in fact harmless, because people's emotions are neither right nor wrong. EI would, rather, consist in perceiving the audience's reaction and dealing with it appropriately. Thus, concerning the perception of emotions, one might say that the majority is always right. One way to score respondents' answers in an EI test is therefore to apply a consensus scoring method. In the case of the MSCEIT it was a normative sample consisting of 5,000 individuals. If the majority of these people perceived an abstract design as aggressive, this would be the correct answer—a fact that clearly differentiates

EI from traditional measures of intelligence which apply objective evaluation criteria. The problem inherent in consensus scoring, however, is the inability to identify highly gifted individuals. By definition, highly gifted people are more skilled than the majority. If, however, the majority's opinion is the benchmark to compare their answers with, highly gifted people will receive lower scores and remain undetected.

Expert scoring   To establish a more objective measurement of performance, expert scoring was developed. In this method, EI experts decide which answer to a given item is right. The problem inherent in this approach is the identification of EI experts before having a valid test on hand. In the case of the MSCEIT, the group of experts consisted of 21 members of the International Society of Research on Emotions (10 men and 11 women) who volunteered for this task. They came from eight different but exclusively Western nations and were on average 39 years old. The question is whether or not researchers on emotions are necessarily emotionally intelligent themselves. This applies less to the more analytical components of EI like emotional perception: Across cultures people interpret expressions of emotions very similarly, and emotion researchers have developed a rich understanding of how to code emotional expressions. Emotion management, however, is different. Research in this field is more recent and has resulted in fewer consensual findings (Mayer, Salovey, Caruso, and Sitarenios 2003; see also Reddy, this volume). Different cultures vary considerably as to their advice about how to regulate emotions; therefore, research on emotion management is more context dependent. Thus, even if there is a satisfying degree of consensus among experts regarding the "best" strategy of emotion management, this agreement will probably not be universally valid. So far, empirical results on this issue are lacking.

Target scoring   The third alternative for scoring respondents' answers is the target approach: Individuals are asked to evoke a certain emotion in themselves and to express it nonverbally. Test takers score highly if they perceive the emotion the person is feeling. Again, the pitfalls of this strategy result from the impossibility of assessing truth: If the target insists on feeling an emotion, which, however, is interpreted differently by the observers, then who is right—given the impossibility of checking the target's emotions and given the fact that people sometimes have problems recognizing their own emotions, especially when they are low in emotion perception?

The MSCEIT applies both consensus and expert scoring. There is a very high correlation between both scoring methods, which suggests that experts share the majority's beliefs. Despite the complexity of scoring, findings on the validity of EI are encouraging: The subtests are reliable, something which was not true of earlier versions of the test. Statistical analyses indicate that the subtests form four different but interrelated components which can be subsumed under a general factor of EI (Mayer, Salovey, Caruso, and Sitarenios 2003). Test results reveal a moderate correlation with general intelligence, which is to be expected because EI is a type of intelligence, but they do not correlate too highly as was the case in the previous tests of social intelligence. Additionally, the MSCEIT does not correlate considerably with mood or personality (Lopes, Côté, and Salovey 2006). The highest correlation with a fundamental personality dimension refers to agreeableness and is moderate (Lopes, Côté, and Salovey 2006). Thus, people with high scores in the MSCEIT tend to be more social and less hostile.

Most important, the MSCEIT seems to predict a variety of positive work-related outcomes, like overall job performance, teamwork, stress tolerance, and leadership qualities.

6.4   EI and Job Performance

From a theoretical point of view, the ability to perceive, use, understand, and manage emotions should impact job performance in several different ways:

Direct effects on performance   For example, employees working in service lines of business may directly benefit from these abilities because they might be better equipped to analyze and manage their customers' emotions, which could result in better job performance.

Moderating effects on performance   Similarly, employees skilled at managing their own emotions might have valuable strategies on hand to cope with negative emotions resulting from stress, thereby moderating the negative effects of stress on well-being and job satisfaction, which in turn affect job performance.

Indirect effects on performance.   Supervisors who are able to manage their employees' emotions might be better at motivating them and maintaining their enthusiasm, which in turn should result in better team performance.

Indirect effects of EI on job performance might also result from higher quality interpersonal relationships between coworkers that people with emotional abilities might be expected to establish. Thus, they would probably receive more support, when necessary, which should decrease their workload and their perceived level of stress. Similarly, people high in EI might contribute to a positive atmosphere within teams and appear to act more socially. As supervisors consider not only task performance in their performance ratings but also employees' general behavior, that is, their engagement in behaviors which are not explicitly part of their job, people high in EI should receive better job performance ratings.

Research findings in this field are new and rather tentative but point in the directions hypothesized. For example, service workers rated high in emotional competence experienced less strain in customer interactions. Moreover, they were better at managing the stress resulting from customer interactions. Consequently, their general well-being and job satisfaction exceeded that of lower ranking coworkers (Giardini and Frese 2006). Similarly, in teams at a large insurance company involving 164 team members, the higher the performance ratings they received, the higher they scored on the ability to manage emotions.

Empirical results which suggest that the influence of EI on job performance becomes stronger with lower individual scores on traditional intelligence scales are of particular interest (Côté and Miners 2006). This suggests a compensatory model of intelligences: If employees are rather low in traditional intelligence, they can compensate for this disadvantage with high EI. Because there is ample room for performance improvement in people with low traditional intelligence, the ability to decode coworkers' and supervisors' emotions may facilitate coordination and interpersonal relationships. Additionally, EI will help to establish good interpersonal relationships with colleagues, thereby increasing the chance of receiving social support with difficult tasks. These findings also suggest that abstract and emotional abilities can indeed be separated.

6.5 Negative Effects of EI

However, there have also been hints of some negative effects of EI on stress. Whereas the ability to manage emotions seems to provide a buffer against stress, findings on perceiving emotions suggest the opposite. In a sample of Australian students, those who were highly perceptive of others' emotions coped less easily with daily hassles that could range from minor annoyances to major problems (e.g., financial insecurity). Their well-being was more strongly impaired, that is, they reported higher levels of depression, hopelessness, and more suicide ideation than people low in emotional perception (Ciarrochi, Deane, and Anderson 2002). To explain this finding, the authors offered both an "insensitivity hypothesis" and a "confusion hypothesis." The insensitivity hypothesis suggests that people low in emotion perception acknowledge the existence of hassles in their life but tend to ignore them. The confusion hypothesis, on the other hand, asserts that people low in emotion perception are sensitive to stress but are not aware of it. Since they should be less clear about their own emotions, due to the fact that they are low in emotion perception, the association between their levels of stress and negative emotions should be weaker. Further research is necessary to clarify these assumptions.

6.6 Gender Differences in EI

Do men and women differ with regard to EI? Goleman (1995) claims that women are at an advantage when compared to men because their socialization places more emphasis on emotions in general: For example, parents use more emotion words when they tell stories to their daughters than to their sons, and mothers display a wider range of emotions when they interact with their daughters than with their sons. Thus, girls seem to receive more training with regard to emotions, which might predispose them to become more competent in dealing with them. However, as research on EI is still in the early stages, results on gender differences in EI are still sparse. The results that do exist vary depending on the kind of assessment which was applied. In self-report questionnaires on EI, there is no sex difference with regard to total values, but women describe themselves as more empathetic and socially responsible, and they report they have better interpersonal relationships, whereas men ascribe to themselves higher self-regard, stress tolerance, and optimism (Bar-On 1997, 2000). Since self-reports are not an appropriate method of assessing abilities, these results reveal more about the different self-images of men and women than real differences in their abilities. These different self-images also reflect typical stereotypes about women and men. A "typical" man is described by laypeople as aggressive, tough, courageous, strong, forceful, arrogant, egotistic, boastful, hard-headed, and dominant. A "typical" woman, in turn, is affectionate, sensitive, sympathetic, nagging, and emotional (Hosoda and Stone 2000).

To obtain insights into sex-related ability differences rather than into stereotypes about men and women, performance tests are more informative. Indeed, on the MSCEIT, women seem to score slightly higher than men (Lopes, Côté, and Salovey 2006). It remains unclear whether these differences result from different innate abilities or from socialization effects. Probably both factors will be causal, as is the case for gender differences in general intelligence (American Psychological Association 1996). For example, it would be too rash to interpret the above-mentioned findings of different parental styles toward sons and daughters as reflecting parents' motivation to educate "typical" men and women. Parents also react to their children, and boys and girls differ regarding their interactional style from birth on. Female babies not more than a day old are more interested in looking at faces than are male babies of the same age (Connellan et al. 2001). At the same time, they are more emotionally stable than male babies, who are more irritable and are more difficult to comfort. Thus, that female babies seem to be more interested in social contact and apparently cope better with emotions might explain why mothers display a wider variety of emotions toward their daughters than toward their sons, which in turn might help them to further develop their emotional skills.

Before addressing the question of gender differences, however, it is necessary to establish the validity of EI and to make sure that EI can indeed be differentiated from general intelligence or known personality traits. As psychological research on EI was and is still concerned with this question, statements about gender differences in EI are rather preliminary at this stage.

Notes

1. American Dialect Society. "1995 words of the year." http://www.americandialect.org/index. php/amerdial/1995_words_of_the_year/ (accessed May 26, 2007).

2. A correlation (r) indicates the strength and direction of a linear relationship between two random variables. It can range between −1 and +1. A value of $r = +1$ describes a perfect positive interrelationship, that is, a high value on variable X goes along with a high value on variable Y. A correlation of $r = -1$ describes a perfect negative interrelationship, that is, a high value on variable X goes along with a high negative value on variable Y. A correlation of $r = 0$ denotes that the two variables are independent. In general, a correlation refers to the departure of two variables from independence, although correlation does not imply causality. If two variables are highly positively correlated, they can be conceived of as indicators of a common underlying factor that causes their high empirical overlap. The analysis of intelligence tests typically yields high positive correlations between tasks that seem to measure different abilities—mathematical or verbal skills, for example. Thus, people who are good at one of these tasks very often also succeed with the other type of task. Therefore, it is justified to summarize these seemingly two different types of tasks as indicators of a common underlying factor called "general intelligence."

7 Emotional Intelligence as Pop Science, Misled Science, and Sound Science: A Review and Critical Synthesis of Perspectives from the Field of Psychology

Carolyn MacCann, Ralf Schulze, Gerald Matthews, Moshe Zeidner, and Richard D. Roberts

7.1 Introduction

Emotional Intelligence (EI) refers to a set of abilities in perceiving one's own and others' emotions, in regulating emotions, and in coping effectively with emotive situations (e.g., Matthews, Zeidner, and Roberts 2007). Bounded by this and other potential, definitional frameworks, EI seems to be everywhere. Educators, executives, and life-style gurus all claim that what people need the most is emotional awareness and sensitivity, largely because the vast majority of us fail to manage emotions successfully. Indeed, individuals appear blind to their own emotional reactions, or fail to control their emotional outbursts, or act inappropriately in pressure situations. In fact, EI is commonly offered as a panacea for many of modern society's ills. Training EI in schools, workplaces, and psychiatric clinics may offer a solution to many of the maladies afflicting contemporary society.

Despite considerable enthusiasm, some caution and skepticism are needed. Perhaps EI is nothing other than a popular fad along the lines of crystal healing or other New Age excesses. Our primary goal in this chapter is to offer a state-of-the-art overview for the reader, evaluating different approaches to EI according to the principles of psychological science. In this chapter, we set out the case for developing a rigorous science of EI. A central part of such a science is accurate, fair, and valid measurement, and we will survey some of the techniques used for measuring EI. We argue that three approaches to EI can be distinguished: (1) *a popular-science approach* that first drew both public and scientific attention to the importance of emotions for intelligent functioning but never fully attained the status of a science, (2) *a misled science approach* where the study of emotional aspects of personality was mislabeled as the study of Emotional *Intelligence*, and (3) *a sound scientific approach* to the study of Emotional Intelligence. In evaluating the various accounts of EI, we outline why we believe these three phases are distinct, and how the third approach may be useful for applied psychology. We conclude the chapter with some concerns and possible future directions that theoreticians, scientists, and practitioners alike might collectively explore.

7.2 Emotional Intelligence as an *Intelligence*

It is important to acknowledge that EI, as the second word in the phrase suggests, is a form of *intelligence*. That is, individuals differ in some objective ability for dealing with emotion. What psychological processes might make a person especially capable in this regard? Some suggested processes include detecting a person's emotions by facial cues, voice pitch and rhythm, or body posture. Other processes suggested in the literature are understanding the antecedents and consequences of emotions, facilitating thought by evoking particular emotions, or expressing emotions to improve interactions with others. As we may encounter emotional geniuses and elites, we also may come across the emotionally challenged and the typical person of moderate EI.

There is a contrasting, alternate position that how people typically deal with emotion is a qualitative style of behavior, which is neither intrinsically good nor bad. For example, some people may tend to be calm whereas others are more excitable, but calmness is not necessarily better than excitability. The notion of EI implies a strict hierarchy of emotional abilities. Thus, to understand what is meant by EI, we need fairly early on in this chapter to look at how it might be different from standard forms of intelligence.

7.2.1 General Intelligence and Its Critics

The concept of EI is firmly rooted in past psychological thinking and research. The concept has come to prominence against a background of dissatisfaction with conventional theories of intelligence, and the sense that a narrow range of academic abilities does not do justice to all the potential that an individual may possess. To understand the historical underpinnings of EI, we briefly discuss the concept of human intelligence and how it is currently viewed among experts.

Most people believe they know what intelligence is. The term typically refers to intellectual and academic aptitudes for abstract reasoning, analysis, and problem solving. Indeed, with over a century of cumulative expertise, psychologists have become especially adept at devising ever more sophisticated tests of these qualities. These efforts have borne fruit to the extent that standardized cognitive tests are able to predict an individual's future academic and occupational success (Roberts et al. 2005). College professors and NASA scientists do indeed typically obtain higher scores than most people on a variety of IQ tests. At the genesis of intelligence research, Charles Spearman (1927) argued for the idea of a unitary *general intelligence* (which he called *g*), based on research showing that all IQ tests measured one common entity to some extent. That is, although people differ somewhat in their aptitudes for particular kinds of thinking (e.g., had *specific abilities* such as verbal or mathematical reasoning), there was one overarching general ability that determined a wide range of intelligent behaviors.

This historic *g* model of intelligence undoubtedly captures something of what it means to be intelligent. However, in the following decades, many psychologists proposed models that emphasized the *specific abilities* over *general intelligence*. Some of these models included specific abilities in processing or understanding social or emotional phenomena. Indeed, the idea that general intelligence might not be the only factor important for social functioning harks back to the pioneers of IQ testing such as Alfred Binet and David Wechsler (Kaufman and Kaufman 2001; Landy 2005; Matthews, Zeidner, and Roberts 2002).

EI may be viewed as a subset of the "social intelligence" domain. Landy (2006) traces the term "social intelligence" to the philosopher and educator John Dewey, whom he quotes as follows, from 1909 (p. 43): "Ultimate moral motives and forces are nothing more or less than social *intelligence*—the power of observing and comprehending social situations—and *social power*—trained capacities of control—at work in the service of social interests and aims" (italics in the original).

One of Dewey's concerns was school curriculum. Dewey's general philosophical position is commonly known as "instrumentalism," which means that any kind of knowledge is regarded as instrument. Subsequently, the psychologist Edward L. Thorndike (1920, 228) described social intelligence as an ability distinct from abstract intelligence, defining it as "the ability to manage and understand men and women, boys and girls, to act wisely in human relations." Thorndike never attempted to develop a paper-and-pencil test for social intelligence, believing that it should be observed in real-life behavior. This again corresponds with Dewey's philosophy, which was widely influenced by the phenomenological approach of William James and his basic work *The Principles of Psychology* (1890). According to James, psychological observation is dependent on the ("real") life world.

In the decades that followed, researchers sporadically tried to develop and validate standardized tests for social intelligence. These included tests designed to capture the respondent's ability to recognize emotive gestures and facial expressions (see Matthews, Zeidner, and Roberts 2002 for a review; Fahlenbrach and Bartsch, this volume, analyze how facial expressions are used in media culture to evoke meta-emotions). However, these efforts never led to especially important scientific principles. The measures proved to be unstable over time, yielded inconsistent and sometimes conflicting results, and/or measured abilities that could not be distinguished from verbal or reasoning abilities already assessed in standard IQ tests. There was also little evidence accrued that social intelligence tests predict real-life behavior (other than through their overlap with intelligence). Frank J. Landy (2006) cautioned that current work on EI may revisit these generic problems of social intelligence.

One model of intelligence to include social abilities was put forward by Howard Gardner (1999). He proposed that there are multiple intelligences such as musical and mathematical intelligence that are important to human functioning. Gardner refers to two types of ability that resemble EI and most likely were a major factor in its development—interpersonal intelligence (understanding the feelings and intentions of others) and intrapersonal intelligence (awareness and discrimination of one's own feelings). If theories of multiple intelligences are correct, we can no longer refer to people as being more or less intelligent in some general sense. Instead, people typically show more complex patterns of higher aptitude for some activities and lower for others. At the extreme, Gardner describes cases of so-called "savants," who may be *subnormal* in terms of intelligence test score but capable of remarkable artistic accomplishments.

The specific term "Emotional Intelligence" has been attributed originally to the German psychologist Barbara Leuner. Writing in 1966, she suggested that the hallucinogenic drug LSD, in concert with psychoanalysis, might help women with emotional problems (low EI) deal with early separation from their mothers. Wayne Payne (1985) was the first author to use the term in English, as part of an unpublished doctoral dissertation discussing the development of emotional awareness in children. The first systematic research on EI was performed by two psychologists: John ("Jack") D. Mayer and Peter Salovey (e.g., Mayer and Salovey 1993). In any case, the popularity of EI appears to reflect the impact of a single book, Daniel Goleman's (1995) *Emotional Intelligence*. In addition to being an international best-seller, it turned out to be the stimulus for a feature article in *Time* magazine (Gibbs 1995).

7.2.2   How Daniel Goleman Created a New Type of Intelligence

Goleman (1995) set out a comprehensive account of "EQ" (emotional quotient) and its relevance to society. His central thesis was that emotional illiteracy is responsible for many social problems including mental illness, crime, and educational failure. Furthermore, people at work often fall short of their potential by failing to manage their emotions appropriately. Job satisfaction and productivity are threatened by unnecessary conflicts with coworkers, failure to assert one's legitimate needs, and failure to communicate one's feelings to others. Goleman pushed the intelligence envelope in various ways. Notably, this thesis conflicts with conventional psychological theory as follows:

1. *Definition of intelligence.* Goleman included qualities such as optimism, self-control, and moral character as part of this proposed new intelligence. In standard psychological research, such qualities are considered aspects of *personality* rather than intelligence.

2. *Stability of intelligence.* Typically, intelligence has been viewed as fairly stable over time, but Goleman emphasizes that EI can be learned and increased at any time during one's life.

3. *Intelligence in everyday life*. Goleman (1995, 1998) has claimed that EQ is a more important factor than IQ in enjoying a successful life, for example, in being promoted at work and in maintaining secure and fruitful relationships with others. Indeed, a subtext of his 1995 book is that IQ is much overrated; as one of the chapter headings succinctly puts it, "Smart is Dumb." Empirical evidence so far indicates that EI is probably no more important than IQ in predicting success.

4. *Intelligence has a moral dimension*. Conventionally, "intelligence" refers to a set of aptitudes and skills that are equally at the service of the philanthropist and the evil genius. Goleman (1995, 286), however, relates EI to moral character: "emotional literacy goes hand in hand with education for character, for moral development and for citizenship."

So, what exactly did Goleman (1995) mean by "Emotional Intelligence" or "EQ"? In fact, his first book set out a laundry list of desirable qualities, including self-confidence, sensitivity, self-awareness, self-control, empathy, optimism, and social skills. Indeed, Goleman has been criticized for listing almost every positive quality that was not actually considered part of intelligence (e.g., Matthews, Zeidner, and Roberts 2002). Subsequently, Goleman sought to put the traits that focally define EI on a more systematic basis (Cherniss and Goleman 2001).

Goleman's revised model of EI separates two different aspects of EI. First, he distinguishes between those elements of EI that refer to *personal competencies*, such as self-awareness, from those that relate to *social competencies*, such as empathy. This distinction parallels Gardner's (1999) intrapersonal and interpersonal intelligences. Second, he distinguishes between facets of EI that relate to *awareness* from those that concern the *regulation* of emotion. For example, recognizing that someone is unhappy is different from being able to cheer the person up, but both "reading" emotions and constructively changing emotions relate to the overall facility of EI. Putting together the two divisions of "self versus others" and "recognition versus regulation" yields the four major dimensions of EI listed below. Each of the various attributes of EI can be classified as belonging to one of these four dimensions:

Dimension 1: Recognition Applied to the Self (Personal Competence)   Attributes included are Self-Awareness, Emotional Self-Awareness, Accurate Self-Assessment, and Self-Confidence.

Dimension 2: Recognition Applied to Others (Social Competence)   Attributes included are Social Awareness, Empathy, Service Orientation, and Organizational Awareness.

Dimension 3: Regulation Applied to the Self (Self Management)   Attributes included are Emotional Self-Control, Trustworthiness, Conscientiousness, Adaptability, Achievement Drive, and Initiative.

Dimension 4: Regulation Applied to Others (Relationship Management)   Attributes included are Developing Others, Influence, Communication, Conflict Management,

Leadership, Change Catalyst, Building Bonds, as well as Teamwork and Collaboration.

Goleman (1998) further argued that EI is a set of learned skills that may translate directly into success in the workplace. For example, "the empathy competence" helps team leaders to understand the feelings of team members, leading to greater team effectiveness. It also helps those lower in the organizational chain. For instance, such a competency should help sales personnel to close more sales by being better able to "read" the customer's emotional reactions to the product and the sales pitch. Conversely, emotionally unintelligent behaviors may be highly damaging to organizations. As Hogan and Stokes (2006, 269) note, "the primary reason employees leave a company is poor management—people don't quit organizations, they quit managers." Goleman's ideas concerning why EI may be valuable and how specific competencies may apply to the workplace environment are no doubt important. However, to move from the realm of pop psychology to the status of science, these ideas need to be informed both by existing theories within psychological science and by data showing that such ideas hold true.

7.3   Toward a Science of Emotional Intelligence

In contrast to the preceding, a scientific account needs a clear definition of what EI is and is not. Even if we have a definition, EI may be hard to measure. Social-emotional abilities may not be expressed in conventional psychological tests, even those that purport to measure emotional abilities. Finally, even if it transpires that we can measure EI reliably, "all that glistens is not gold." Perhaps EI will turn out to be no more than the superficial slickness of the salesperson, or an inflated ego, or even the dark art of manipulating others emotionally. Evidence is needed that people who obtain high scores on EI actually function better in their social and emotional lives.

There are several reasons why a scientific understanding of EI would be useful. These include the following:

1. *Mapping the "ecology" of EI.* It is unlikely that EI is distributed at random across human social groups. For example, both popular stereotypes and personality research suggest that women are more likely to possess agreeable characteristics thought by some to be central to EI (e.g., Costa, Terracciano, and McCrae 2001). These include empathy, awareness of the feelings of others, and coping with stress through "tending and befriending." Valid measurement of EI is necessary to test whether there are in fact meaningful *gender* differences. Measures are also required in order to identify other possible group differences including those related to age, social class, and culture. For example, it is often believed that emotional wisdom increases with age and life experience (sometimes referred to as "personal growth"). It also is important to look

at how EI might be distributed across different occupational groups (see Illouz, this volume): Are social workers really more emotionally intelligent than computer programmers?

2. *Discovering the sources of EI: genes, brains, and the social environment.* Assuming EI exists, what determines whether it is high, low, or intermediate in a given individual? If EI is like most other human characteristics, we may assume that it reflects both genes and the social environment in which the child grows up. The individual's DNA interacts with external stimulation in building the brain, including those brain structures that influence emotion. Perhaps EI may be linked to the neurology of structures in the frontal lobes of the brain that are known to be important for regulating and controlling emotion (e.g., Bechara, Tranel, and Damasio 2000). In addition, the quality of interactions that the child experiences with caregivers and peers is known to affect emotional development. For example, maltreatment and deprivation are known to have various adverse effects (e.g., Zeidner et al. 2003). Perhaps EI in part reflects the extent to which the child is exposed to good role models for expressing and managing emotion (see Fahlenbrach and Bartsch, this volume).

3. *Understanding EI as a process.* It is often said that intelligence as a construct is incomplete. Simply enumerating a person's IQ fails to suggest how intelligence plays out as an ongoing process as the person performs meaningful actions in some real-life context (Sternberg 1985). Similarly, we need a scientific account of how EI is expressed in handling the problems and challenges of life. For example, one pivotal question to ask might be this one: How does EI help the person to *adapt* to threats and opportunities? In fact, a process view of EI is especially important if it is indeed correct that EI is more easily changed than IQ. We may only be able to understand EI in relation to dynamic interaction between person and environment.

4. *Targeting the exceptional.* If we want to foster EI and brilliance in order to profit from the wisdom of the emotionally gifted as well as to intervene to help the emotionally impoverished, we need to know who they are. Just as good IQ tests are needed to identify cognitively gifted as well as challenged individuals, standardized EI tests are required to identify individuals who may need enrichment, support, and/or training in dealing with emotive situations. Thus, valid measures and assessment techniques are needed to discover emotional geniuses as well as the emotionally challenged.

5. *Understanding abnormality.* One of Goleman's themes is that low EI leads to various mental problems, including emotional disorders and antisocial behaviors. However, is this opinion actually true? We need a scientific account of the role of EI in abnormality to inform us of a high profile issue EI research might profitably impact.

6. *Debunking myths.* Some of the claims made about EI, a subset of which we have covered, are grandiose. Moreover, popular culture is vulnerable to new ideas in proportion to their media coverage and sense of importance (rather than their actual importance and factual basis). A sound science of EI is needed to sift out the unimportant

and the unsound so that widely adopted ideas and applications are useful and helpful rather than misleading or harmful.

7.4   The Three Pillars of a Science of Emotional Intelligence

In this section, a brief purview of the state of the art in scientific research on EI is given. The aim is to summarize different approaches researchers have taken in their search for the essence of EI. Matthews, Zeidner, and Roberts (2002) list three essential pillars for a scientific treatment of EI: (1) measurement (that EI exists), (2) theory (that EI makes sense), and (3) applications (that EI is useful). We evaluate different approaches to EI in light of these three pillars.

7.4.1   Pillar 1: Measurement of EI

The case for EI measurement is pivotal because of uncertainties over what EI actually is. Some prominent theories of EI include long lists of many desirable personal qualities from the psychological fields of emotion and intelligence (and, in some cases, also from the field of personality). Combining elements from two fields (emotion and intelligence) is not sufficient to posit a third field (EI) that spans between them. It is also necessary to demonstrate that the selected elements meaningfully cohere to form a single entity and that this entity is logically labeled as "emotional intelligence." Such a demonstration requires both empirical data and theory showing this new EI entity is an *intelligence* requiring some processing or transformation of *emotions*. For this reason, if models of EI are to mature into full-blown theories, the construct must be *measured* as a distinct personal attribute reflecting the interplay between an individual's intelligence and emotions. Without measurement, from a scientific psychological perspective at least, accounts of EI are little more than verbiage, the truth of which cannot be determined.

Thus, an empirical approach is needed to investigate the speculations surrounding EI. Measurement places the study of this concept in the field of *individual differences*, or differential psychology. Standard differential psychology recognizes that *intelligence* (or superior performance in some domain) is fundamentally distinct from *personality* (referring to styles of behavior that differ from one another qualitatively, but are not correct or incorrect). Thus, an important goal for research is to show how tests of EI fit into this larger scheme of individual differences: Theoretically, EI should relate to conventional measures of intelligence but be relatively distinct from personality (as EI is itself a type of intelligence and *not* an aspect of personality). If we cannot measure EI accurately enough to evaluate these theoretical claims, the concept is unfalsifiable and, therefore, outside the domain of science.

Quite a large number of psychology research teams have attempted to measure EI in various ways, and these attempts may be divided into two types of measurement:

maximum performance and typical performance. Maximum-performance measures assess how close test takers' responses are to the correct or best answer. An example item for this approach might be "Which emotion is expressed most strongly in this facial expression?" Within the EI field, such maximum-performance tests are referred to as *ability measures, information-processing measures,* or *performance-based measures* (Mayer, Caruso, and Salovey 2000; Petrides and Furnham 2001). In contrast, typical-performance measures ask test takers whether they generally behave in certain ways, or have a certain set of beliefs. An example item might be: "I often talk to other people about their problems," rated on a scale with categories labeled *Strongly Agree, Agree, Neither Agree nor Disagree, Disagree,* and *Strongly Disagree.* In the parlance of EI research, roughly overlapping terms for typical performance include *mixed measures, self-report measures, trait emotional intelligence,* and *personality emotional intelligence* (Mayer, Caruso, and Salovey 2000; Petrides and Furnham 2001; Barchard and Christiansen 2007).

In the paragraphs below, we evaluate the validity of maximum-performance and typical-performance measures separately, ascertaining whether these two measurement traditions really measure EI, rather than some other related entity or entities. For instance, since emotional *intelligence* should clearly be an intelligence, EI test scores should relate more strongly to IQ than to personality. The relatedness of test scores can be judged with the correlation coefficient (r), where 0 indicates no relationship and 1.00 indicates identity. Heuristics for small, medium, and large degrees of relationship are values above .10, .30, and .50 respectively (Cohen 1988). Bechtoldt's chapter in this volume gives further details on the correlation coefficient.

Evaluating Typical-Performance Measures of EI   Vastly more EI measures use a typical-performance approach than a maximum-performance approach. In fact, the number of typical-performance measures is increasing exponentially, particularly in areas outside of the peer-reviewed psychology journals. The major problem with such tests is that what they measure has virtually no relationship to intelligence but instead overlaps to a large extent with established personality traits, particularly the dimensions of Emotional Stability/Neuroticism and Extraversion/Introversion.

The personality traits Extraversion and Emotional Stability relate to typical ways people interact with others and the depth and frequency with which they experience emotions. People with low Emotional Stability are generally more anxious, hostile, easily depressed, self-conscious, impulsive, and easily stressed out than those with high Emotional Stability. Extraverted people are generally more warm, gregarious, assertive, active, excitement seeking, and cheerful than introverted people (Costa and McCrae 1992). Table 7.1 shows the degree of overlap between three typical-performance measures of EI with extraversion, stability, and intelligence, respectively.

These typical-performance EI measures generally show large correlations with both personality dimensions but generally show small to zero correlations with

Table 7.1
Correlations for three typical performance measures of Emotional Intelligence with Extraversion, Emotional Stability, and Intelligence

Instrument	Correlations with Extraversion	Correlations with Emotional Stability	Correlations with Intelligence
AES	.43 to .54	.21 to .64	.01
EQ-i	.46 to .53	.62 to .72	−.21 to .13
TEIQue	.68	.70	—

Note: AES, Assessing Emotions Scale (Schutte et al. 1998); EQ-i, Emotional Quotient Inventory (Bar-On 1997); TEIQue, Trait Emotional Intelligence Questionnaire (Petrides and Furnham 2003).
Adapted from Roberts, Schulze, and MacCann, in press.

intelligence, indicating that these measures are personality traits (typical ways of behaving) rather than intelligence (knowledge, skills, or abilities). The label "emotional *intelligence*" is thus not an accurate characterization of typical-performance measures. In addition, the *very* high relationship between the Trait Emotional Intelligence Questionnaire (TEIQue) and the two personality traits suggests that the TEIQue may be assessing a subset of these existing personality traits. After statistically correcting for measurement error, these correlations reach $r = .84$ for Extraversion and $r = .87$ for Emotional Stability. All three typical-performance measures are part of the personality domain, but the TEIQue particularly seems to be located within the research tradition of Extraversion and Emotional Stability specifically. The assessment of Extraversion and Emotional Stability has been researched extensively since at least the 1940s (e.g., Hathaway and McKinley 1942, Fiske 1949), and the theoretical bases for these two personality traits arguably stretch back over 2,000 years to Hippocrates and Galen's humorism. Thus some measures of EI (such as the TEIQue) appear part of this long tradition of describing and assessing emotional temperaments and should properly be studied within this domain rather than under the banner of "emotional intelligence."

Evaluating Maximum-Performance Measures of EI   In contrast to typical-performance measures of EI, there is really only one group of tests that measures EI as maximum performance: the Mayer–Salovey–Caruso Emotional Intelligence Test Battery (MSCEIT; Mayer, Salovey, and Caruso 2002a and b). Sometimes an earlier version of the MSCEIT is also used for research purposes: the Multifactor Emotional Intelligence Scale (MEIS; Mayer, Caruso, and Salovey 1999). Since the MSCEIT tests are the only comprehensive and commercially available maximum-performance tests of EI, we outline the distinctive features of these tests. There are eight tasks in the MSCEIT, two for each of the four *branches* of EI. The four branches are (1) Perception of Emotion, (2) Emotional Facilitation of Thought, (3) Understanding Emotions, and (4) Managing Emotions. The four-branch theory of EI is described in more detail in the Pillar 2 section of this chapter, but we describe the tests here, to illustrate how they measure EI.

1. *Faces*. For each of four photographs of faces, test takers rate the presence of five emotions on a scale ranging from 1 (no emotion) to 5 (extreme emotion).

2. *Pictures*. For each of six pictures, test takers rate the presence of five emotions from 1 to 5.

3. *Sensations*. For each of five statements, test takers make three judgments about the similarity of an emotion to a physical sensation on a scale ranging from 1 (not alike) to 5 (alike).

4. *Facilitation*. For each of five scenarios, test takers rate the helpfulness of three different moods on a scale ranging from 1 (not useful) to 5 (useful).

5. *Blends*. Test takers answer 12 multiple-choice questions assessing which combinations of emotions form complex emotions.

6. *Changes*. Test takers answer 20 multiple-choice questions assessing which emotions are related to particular situations.

7. *Management*. For each of five scenarios, test takers rate the mood management of actions on a 5-point scale ranging from "very ineffective" to "very effective."

8. *Relations*. For each of five scenarios, test takers rate the effectiveness of three responses on a 5-point scale ranging from "very ineffective" to "very effective."

Scoring of the MSCEIT   In standard intelligence tests, the correctness of an answer can be obtained from trusted sources of knowledge (e.g., arithmetic tests are scored according to mathematical rules, vocabulary items with thesauri or dictionaries). The MSCEIT does not use equivalent formal systems for determining the correct answer on EI test items (Roberts, Zeidner, and Matthews 2001). Instead, correctness is determined using social consensus—whatever the majority independently agree on constitutes the best answer. This approach to scoring is undertaken in three different ways: (1) expert scoring, (2) consensus scoring, and (3) target scoring. Bechtoldt (this volume) describes these three approaches in some detail.

Using consensus to score test items might be conceptually problematic for a maximum-performance test, particularly for ratings. As an example, people who are exceptionally good at facial expression recognition might perceive nuances of expression that the ordinary person would miss, and so they might rate faces as showing some slight level of emotion where most people see no emotion. These exceptionally sensitive people would receive low scores with consensus scoring, despite a high level of skill. This relates to another important issue: whether EI can be said to exist as an entity. If we cannot specify *why* some emotional reactions, perceptions, or insights

Table 7.2

Correlations between Mayer–Salovey–Caruso Emotional Intelligence Test Scale scores and personality–intelligence constructs

| Branch | Five-Factor Model Personality Constructs | | | | | Intelligence |
	E	A	C	ES	O	
1. Perception	−.06 to .06	.02 to .14	−.05 to .07	.03 to .14	−.02 to .10	.00 to .17
2. Assimilation	−.04 to .07	.08 to .19	.01 to .12	.04 to .15	.02 to .14	.01 to .21
3. Understanding	−.04 to .08	.05 to .16	.00 to .11	.00 to .12	.08 to .20	.10 to .43
4. Management	.04 to .15	.22 to .32	.07 to .18	.03 to .14	.13 to .24	.05 to .23

Note: E = Extraversion, A = Agreeableness, C = Conscientiousness, ES = Emotional Stability, O = Openness to Experience.
Adapted from Roberts, Schulze and MacCann, in press.

are better than others, except that experts or large groups of people agree that this is so, it is hard to argue convincingly that such an entity actually exists.

The MSCEIT's Relationship to Personality and Intelligence   Maximum-performance tests of EI must meet the same criteria as typical-performance tests, correlating more highly with intelligence than personality. Table 7.2 summarizes the range of correlations that the four MSCEIT branch test scores share with personality and intelligence (Roberts, Schulze, and MacCann, in press, provide a more detailed version of this table).

With one exception, correlations with intelligence were higher than correlations with the five major personality traits for all four components of the MSCEIT. The one exception was the Management branch, where correlations of .24 with Openness to Experience and .32 with Agreeableness were higher than the maximum observed correlation of Management with intelligence ($r = .23$). Agreeable people are trusting, truthful, kind, cooperative, modest, and sympathetic. Open people are imaginative, artistic, and open to a variety of feelings, thoughts, values, and different experiences. Traditional intelligence tests also typically show a small degree of relationship with Openness to Experience. The highest relationship to intelligence was found for the Understanding branch. Thus, the Understanding Emotions branch best meets the criteria for a valid test of EI, with the Management branch involving personality to some extent (but notably, to a much smaller extent than for the typical-performance measures of EI).

In any case, the patterns of correlations among EI and personality are quite unlike the patterns found for self-reports of EI. For the latter, the strongest relationships were with Extraversion and Emotional Stability, whereas for maximum-performance measures of EI, Extraversion and Emotional Stability show the weakest correlations. Note, too, that the significant correlations with Agreeableness and Openness to Experience are of no more than small to moderate magnitude. Clearly, variables assessed with the MEIS and MSCEIT are distinctive enough from personality factors to suggest they are outside of this domain.

7.4.2 Pillar 2: Theory and Definition of EI

The second pillar needed to support a science of EI is no less important. A theory of what it means to be emotionally intelligent is needed, a theory that identifies the key psychological processes involved. Suppose there is a test that succeeds in selecting people who have a talent for understanding and dealing with emotions. What is special about the way that these emotionally gifted individuals input emotion-laden stimuli, process emotional information, and respond to emotive situations? Conversely, features of emotional processing that may contribute to emotional illiteracy also must be understood.

Definition of EI   The four-branch hierarchical definition of EI offers some suggestions as to what differentiates high-EI and low-EI individuals. This definition forms the theoretical basis for the MSCEIT tests. In this model, there are three levels at which EI can be conceptualized, as shown in the paragraphs below.

Level III: General EI

Level II: Broad Areas of EI

- *Area 1: Experiential EI.* The ability to perceive, respond, and manipulate emotional information without necessarily understanding its meaning.
- *Area 2: Strategic EI.* The ability to understand and manage emotions without necessarily experiencing the feelings of emotion.

Level I: Narrow branches of EI

- *Branch 1 (from Area 1).* The ability to "Perceive Emotions" in faces and pictures.
- *Branch 2 (from Area 1).* "Facilitating Thought" by cognitive processing of emotions.
- *Branch 3 (from Area 2).* "Understanding Emotions" and how they blend and change over time.
- *Branch 4 (from Area 2).* "Managing Emotions" by using feelings to create better outcomes.

At the broadest level, EI can be considered one entity: the skilled performance on emotion-related tasks. At a narrower level, this performance can be differentiated into two areas: the immediate processing of emotional stimuli (the experiential area) versus the more thoughtful, cognitive, or strategic processing of emotional information (the strategic area). At the narrowest level, four different branches of EI are separable. These four branches increase in complexity from the first to the fourth branch, with component abilities in the higher branches depending or building on abilities in the lower branches. At the simplest level, EI is the perception and expression of emotions (Branch 1—*Perceiving and Expressing Emotion*). Branch 2 consists of the productive integration of emotions in thought processes (*Assimilating Emotions in Thought*). Branch 3 includes the understanding of the use of emotion terms in language, relations between emotions, between emotions and circumstances, and transitions among emotions (*Understanding Emotions*). Finally, the fourth and highest branch involves managing emotions in order to moderate negative and enhance positive emotions (*Reflectively Regulating Emotions*). The first two branches collectively form the *Experiential EI* area, whereas the higher two form the *Strategic EI* area.

Mechanism for EI   One possibility explaining the mechanism for emotional abilities is that EI is engrained in the neurons of the brain. Neuroscientists have been especially interested in areas of the frontal lobes of the brain that seem to control the infusion of emotion into decision making. Damage to these areas causes emotionally unintelligent behaviors such as violent mood swings, reckless impulsivity, and poor real-life decision making. Alternatively, we may look to the software rather than the hardware of the brain for the mental models that people build to establish their place in the social world around them. There is an important cognitive-psychological tradition of linking emotion to personal beliefs and evaluations. This tradition also traces emotional dysfunction to excessively negative cognitions. Perhaps EI resides in building mental models that promote productive social engagement with others. A related issue is whether the attributes of EI are truly adaptive in the sense of promoting success in real life.

7.4.3   Pillar 3: Possible Utility of EI

The final pillar rests on demonstrating the practical value of EI in fields such as education, organizational psychology, and mental health. We are not painting on a blank canvas here. Applied psychologists have already contributed much toward the development of practical interventions that improve the human condition. In many cases, interventions are based on theory and supported by evidence. Thus, it needs to be shown that EI offers something altogether new or, at the least, adds something to current practice. In fact, applied research has tended to proceed on a path separate from laboratory-based research that is more focused on measurement issues; it may indeed be seen as its own strand of research, although both basic and applied research would benefit from greater integration (Roberts, Schulze, and MacCann, in press).

Practical Implications of Gender Differences in EI   One important difference that EI shows from traditional tests of intelligence is a marked female superiority, observed largely in the *management* or *regulation* of emotional situations, rather than the processing, recognition, or understanding of emotional phenomena (Ciarrochi, Chan, and Caputi 2000; Day and Carroll 2004; Kafetsios 2004; Mayer, Caruso, and Salovey 1999). Previous psychological research has found that women outperform men on memory tasks that are episodic or autobiographical (i.e., memory of real-life situations; Herlitz, Nilsson, and Backman 1997; Seidlitz and Diener 1998). Compared to men, women accurately recall more of their own emotional life events, recall them in more vivid detail, and are faster at accessing these memories (Davis 1999, Ross and Holmberg 1992, Seidlitz and Diener 1998). Davis found that this difference was only the case for *emotional* memories. In contrast to this female superiority on test items with emotional or situational content, men generally outperform women on intelligence test items in most domains of "general knowledge" (Lynn, Irwing, and Cammock 2001; Lynn and Irwing 2004) or when items involve spatial content (Ackerman et al. 2001; Colom, Escorial, and Rebollo 2004). The various methodological problems and inconsistencies (e.g., merging different definitions and tests of intelligence, using different social contexts and groups for volunteer recruiting and interview, etc.) involved in comparing women's and men's intelligences elucidates the comparative study of Ali A. Loori (2005).

In applied settings (e.g., job selection) the IQ tests most frequently used resemble these traditional test items more than the context-rich test items used to assess emotion regulation. The possibility of using EI tests as an alternative or adjunct in such applied settings might usefully reduce adverse impact (at least in terms of gender). Naturally, this argument rests on the assumption that EI should predict criteria just as well as existing measures of intelligence do. Section 4.3.3 (Relationships of EI with Real-World Outcomes) assesses whether this assumption holds true.

Self-Insight, Faking, and Operational Use   One of the primary barriers to using EI in the real world is that the identification of someone's EI level may depend on their self-knowledge and truthfulness, particularly if self-ratings are used (as they often are in typical-performance tests). It is not entirely clear whether or not an individual can have rational insights into his or her emotional life, as indeed is evidenced, most dramatically, by various forms of psychopathology. In addition to lack of self-knowledge, the desire to fake, lie, or cheat on such tests also presents an obstacle to their use in applied settings. Self-report measures of EI appear vulnerable both to faking bad (i.e., giving a poorer impression of your "self" than is warranted by the objective facts) and faking good (i.e., giving a better impression of your "self" than is actually the case), rendering the use of such instruments in anything but low-stakes applications highly problematic.

Relationships of EI with Real-World Outcomes One of the possible advantages associated with EI is the prediction of valued criteria in formal academic and workplace environments, as well as areas of life where understanding emotions and their management may be more important than reasoning or knowledge.

Space precludes a detailed discussion of all such relations, though they have been the topic of a recent review (Mayer, Roberts, and Barsade 2008). Some representative relations between EI and criteria covered by these commentators include the following:

1. Higher levels of EI in male college students relates to lower consumption of alcohol and illegal drugs (Brackett, Mayer, and Warner 2004). This relationship between EI and alcohol and drug use was not found for female college students. EI scores also related to less reported use and intention to use tobacco and alcohol among adolescents (Trinidad and Johnson 2002, Trinidad et al. 2004). Gender differences in this relationship were not reported in these studies.

2. Veneta A. Bastian, Nicholas R. Burns, and Ted Nettelbeck (2005) found small to moderate relationships between anxiety and the Perception and Understanding aspects of EI. They also found some evidence that EI related to lower anxiety above and beyond the effects of intelligence and personality. When other forms of intelligence and personality factors were controlled, MSCEIT scores predicted an additional 6% of the variance in anxiety. Separate effects for men and women were not reported in this study.

3. Carol L. Gohm, Grant C. Corser, and David J. Dalsky (2005) found significant relationships between MSCEIT subscale scores and coping styles. Understanding and Management were related to behavioral disengagement ($r = -.25$ and $r = -.21$) and denial ($r = -.30$ and $r = -.21$), while Management also related to seeking emotional support ($r = .25$), and seeking instrumental social support ($r = .23$).

4. Marc A. Brackett et al. (2006) found that MSCEIT total scores significantly predicted constructive/destructive responses after controlling for the Big Five personality factors, psychological well-being, empathy, life satisfaction, and Verbal Scholastic Aptitude Test results (partial correlations ranged from $-.22$ to $-.33$; negative correlations are expected because of the nature of the criteria). Notably, these relations were found only for the male participants.

5. Mark A. Brackett, Rebecca M. Warner, and Jennifer S. Bosco (2005) found that heterosexual couples where both partners were low on EI reported (1) lower relationship depth, (2) lower support and positive relationship quality, and (3) higher conflict and negative relationship quality. Similarly, Brackett et al. (2006) found that MSCEIT scores predicted confederate and judge ratings of social behaviors after a social interaction, but only among men.

6. Paulo N. Lopes et al. (2004) found that the Management subscale of the MSCEIT predicted self-reports of positive interactions with friends ($r = .31$). MSCEIT Manage-

ment also predicted reports by friends of positive and negative interactions and emotional support ($r = .33$, $-.30$, and $.26$). After controlling for the Big Five personality factors and gender, almost all relationships remained significant.

7.5 Summary and Concluding Comments

The editors of this book charged our team with a difficult mission: to provide an evaluation of the scientific merits of the burgeoning literature on EI and, furthermore, its relevance and need for gender research. We have touched on certain issues in this chapter; for more extensive treatments the reader may refer to Matthews, Zeidner, and Roberts (2007), who assembled a panel of international experts charged explicitly to deal with such issues. Based on the arguments presented in this chapter, and those embellished in this source, we believe that three separate approaches have emerged:

1. *A popular-science approach.* Our review of Goleman's account points to several points of disjuncture for empirical evidence. Popular accounts often gloss over contradictions and caveats in arriving at a digestible set of conclusions. Moreover they often reinforce stereotypes and popular heuristics without empirical evidence (e.g., the innate nurturance of women). It is necessary to realize their limitations in informing scientific theories; the cart should not, and cannot, lead the horse.

2. *A misdirected science approach.* Our review of the correlates of self-report measures shows that such measures do *not* assess an intelligence and, therefore, should not be used to assess EI. Our conceptual arguments for a constrained definition of EI support this conclusion (more detailed descriptions of the underlying logic of such arguments are given in Schulze, Wilhelm, and Kyllonen 2007). Nevertheless, the study of emotionality within the personality field is an interesting and potentially fruitful undertaking. Richard D. Roberts, Ralf Schulze, and Carolyn MacCann (in press) describe how such research may be continued with self-reports, more correctly treating these measures as a detailed and focused expansion of research within the personality domain.

3. *A reputable science approach.* By contrast with self-report measures, maximum-performance assessments show better qualities as measures of EI, although there remains much work to be done. First, the very fact that only two measures (the MEIS and the MSCEIT) have a research background that goes beyond initial stages of test development is a suboptimal state of affairs.

We started this chapter by noting that EI seems to be everywhere, from preschool to the boardroom, and close by pointing out that it is only *one* of the three varieties of EI that truly seems to be all around us. Not surprisingly, this is the popular science of EI. While this approach has been the catalyst for much discussion about the importance of social skills, character, and morality, programs and conclusions based on pop-science approaches are of negligible value at best. Such approaches are best viewed as a social barometer or zeitgeist, highlighting the cultural premium placed on soft skills and "people smarts" rather than technical proficiency alone. Scientific approaches are far less prevalent, and the maximum-performance-based approach the least prevalent of all, in part because there is really only one single test commercially available for applied use (i.e., the MSCEIT). The *idea* of EI is everywhere, but the popular demand for scientifically rigorous applications currently far outstrips their real availability. Although the pace of academic science is slow compared to the escalating fascination for promising new ideas, we are optimistic that science may yet catch up, such that exciting innovations within the EI field may narrow the bridge between what is known and what is hoped for.

Acknowledgments

We thank Matthew Ventura, Devendra Banhart, and Lydia Lunch for supporting the preparation of this chapter. We would also like to thank the editors for their comments and feedback on an earlier version of this chapter, as well as Walter Emmerich and Lydia Liu for their internal Educational Testing Service reviews. The views expressed here are those of the authors and do not reflect on the Educational Testing Service. Correspondence concerning this chapter should be directed to Carolyn MacCann.

III Socioeconomic Contexts: Emotional Brains at Work

8 Emotional Capital, Therapeutic Language, and the Habitus of "The New Man"

Eva Illouz

8.1 Freud, Emotions, and Social Stratification

In this chapter,[1] I examine in a somewhat preliminary and tentative way some of the effects of psychological knowledge on social structure. If culture is central to the sociological project, it is not only because it bestows meaning onto action but also because it shapes the very structure of economic and symbolic resources. As Friedland and Mohr put it, "Materiality is a way of producing meaning; meaning is a way of producing materiality" (Friedland and Mohr 2004, 9).

In 1883, before the birth of psychoanalysis, writing a letter to his future wife Martha Bernays, Sigmund Freud commented on the differences between the pleasures of "the masses" and those of the middle and propertied classes:

The mob gives vent to its appetites, and we deprive ourselves. We deprive ourselves in order to maintain our integrity, we economize in our health, our capacity for enjoyment, and our emotions. We save ourselves for something, not knowing for what. And this habit of constant suppression of natural instincts gives us the quality of refinement.... Why don't we get drunk? Because the discomfort and disgrace of the after-effects gives us more unpleasure than the pleasure we derived from getting drunk. Why don't we fall in love with a different person every month? Because at each separation a part of our heart would be torn away.... Our whole conduct of life presupposes that we are protected from the direst poverty.... The poor people, the masses, could not survive without their thick skins and their easygoing ways.... Why should they scorn the pleasure of the moment when no other awaits them? (Freud 1975, 50f)

In these surprisingly sociological remarks on the emotional and instinctual structure that separates the working classes from the middle classes, Freud anticipates what would become a cliché in the 1960s, namely, that the middle and propertied classes achieve economic security at the price of constraining and constricting their emotions, impulses, and desires. Using such metaphors as "economizing," "saving," and "deprivation," Freud suggests that his middle-class contemporaries treat their emotions as an economic asset; they "invest" emotions in objects that do not threaten their stability and security; they make their emotions yield social benefits such as "refinement" and a genteel demeanor. Conversely and symmetrically, Freud suggests that the working classes are less stifled by emotional constraints. The middle-class emotional ethos would be of no use to the working classes, Freud tells us, because it would weaken them (they need their "thick skins" in order to survive) and because emotional deprivation serves no purpose when one may not expect future reward such as respectability and social standing. The working classes have no choice but to enjoy ordinary pleasures when they can.

Freud succinctly describes a relationship between a psychic economy of emotions and social class or, more precisely, between emotions and what Pierre Bourdieu would later call "economic necessity" (Bourdieu 1979/1984). The more pressing one's economic necessity, the less restrained one's emotions are likely to be: This is clearly what we can read between the lines in Freud.

In a later text, Freud brings a new twist to these evocative statements. Freud imagines a house divided between "basement" and "first floor." The caretaker's daughter lives in the basement and the landlord's daughter on the first floor (Freud 1963, 352f). Freud imagines that early in their lives, the two girls engage in sexual play. However, Freud tells us, they will develop quite differently: The caretaker's daughter, who does not think much of playing with genitals, will remain unharmed and may perhaps become a successful actress, marry above her condition, and even eventually become an aristocrat. By contrast, the landlord's daughter, who at a young age has learned the ideals of feminine purity and abstinence, will view her childhood sexual activity as incompatible with such ideals. She will be haunted by guilt, will take refuge in neurosis, and will not marry. Given the prejudices of Freud and his contemporaries, we are led to presume that the landlord's daughter will lead the lonely and dull life of a spinster. Thus, Freud suggests that the social destiny of these two girls is intertwined with their psychic development and that their neurosis (or lack thereof) will determine their social trajectory. However, the idea proposed herein by Freud differs from what he had expressed in his letter to Martha. That is, Freud suggests that members of different classes have access to unequal emotional resources, but here, the lower classes are, so to speak, better equipped emotionally. It is precisely their lack of sexual inhibition that will prevent the birth of neurosis and will, in turn, help the caretaker's daughter achieve upward social mobility.

In these two texts, Freud makes a complex claim about the relations between social and psychic trajectories: He points to reciprocal connections between emotions and social position, for he argues that if class determines emotions, emotions may play an invisible but powerful role in social mobility. By suggesting that the economic ethos of emotions, engendered within the capitalist work sphere, is incompatible with successful personal and emotional development, Freud implicitly relies on a model in which psychic development *may disturb and invert* the traditional hierarchical supremacy of money and social prestige.

Freud's observations have important consequences for our understanding of the relationship between culture, emotions, and social class. First, Freud suggests that the middle-class private sphere is not sealed from the economic marketplace, nor is it a zone of free-flowing, spontaneous, and disinterested emotions. On the contrary, Freud clearly suggests that even within the confines of their private lives, members of the middle class continue to treat their emotions as *capital*—as something to be properly amassed with a view toward the acquisition of a respectable social identity and "distinction." Second, he suggests that by using the economic ethos to manage one's emotions and libido, members of the middle class deprive themselves of emotional fulfillment and happiness. Economic success and "distinction" come at the price of "true" intimacy and stand in the way of happiness. Conversely, emotional development and happiness may ultimately curb and disturb conventional class hierarchies. In the few sentences quoted above, Freud tentatively sketches out some interesting ideas, namely, that there are some significant points of connection between social stratification and emotions and that emotional life can shape one's social destiny and success. Freud offers here a supremely sociological idea, namely, that emotional life is not only stratified but stratifying as well.

However, in order for emotional life to play this role in social structure, a mechanism must exist which enables the conversion of emotional action into social resources. In fact, Freud's remarks are strangely premonitory of the ways in which psychological ideas have contributed greatly to making emotions play an increasingly crucial role in social mobility. In other words, the mechanism mediating between social structure and emotions is the vast cultural apparatus deployed by psychological persuasion. Karin Knorr-Cetina puts it as follows: "With the current understanding of the society, we tend to see knowledge as a component of economic, social, and political life. But we can also turn the argument around and consider social, political, and economic life as part and parcel of a particular knowledge culture. . . . *Knowledge cultures have real political, economic, and social effects that are not neutral with respect to social structures and interests and with respect to economic growth*" (emphasis added; Knorr-Cetina 2005, 74).

8.2 The Rise of Emotional Competence and Emotional Intelligence

Freud's ideas, quoted at the beginning of this chapter, have nowhere been more thoroughly applied than in the personality tests that were established during the first decade of the twentieth century.[2] "Psychological tests, both intelligence tests and personality tests, have been a central part of organizational America since the 1920s" (Abbott 1988, 149).

Personality tests were aimed at selecting the most suitable candidates for work in organizations and thus were premised on the assumption that there was a close connection between personality traits, emotional makeup, and job performance. "Psychoanalytic concepts and psychoanalysis itself have had a rather profound impact on the assessment process" (Walsh and Betz 1985, 110).

Psychoanalysis played an important role in making emotions and personality an aspect of social mobility by providing the tools with which to recruit people and to evaluate their performance in corporations.

In the 1940s, the field of personality screening went through an important phase of development with the use of Jungian "archetypes." On the basis of their interpretation of Jung's archetypes, Katherine C. Briggs and Isabel Myers developed the famous Myers–Briggs Type-Indicator, which included such categories as "sensate" or "intuitive," subsequently used widely for personality evaluation and job placement (Briggs and Myers 1976).

Through psychologically inspired categorization and classification, emotional behavior imposed itself as a central criterion for the evaluation and prediction of economic behavior. Personality tests have become so widespread that they can be said to be to emotions what scholastic tests are to cultural capital: a way to sanction, legitimize, and authorize a specific way of handling feeling. In her *Cult of Personality*, Ann Murphy Paul argues that today there are 2,500 kinds of personality tests and that testing has become a $400 million industry. No less than 89 of the *Fortune* 100 largest corporations make use of personality tests for hiring and training employees (Paul 2004).

Personality tests are predicated on a few core assumptions: that individuals' actions and reactions can be captured under the category of personality; that personalities are stable and therefore predictable; that personalities can be measured; and, finally, that certain personalities—the patterned cluster of attitudes and emotions with which we respond to situations—are more suited to certain professions than others. Expanding upon this core notion, some personalities came to be viewed as more competent than others.

The practice of measuring personality included two components, *attitudinal* and *emotional*. It is the emotional component, however, which has over time become the most decisively developed. The idea that emotions point to (professional and social) competence has nowhere been more apparent than in the now widespread notion of "Emotional Intelligence" (EI), a notion which, more than others, makes an explicit connection between emotional management and social success. According to such notion, one's emotional makeup, however subjective, can be objectively evaluated, thus enabling comparisons between people with regard to their *emotional capacities*.

When the notion of EI emerged in the 1990s, it swept through the American corporations and even American culture at large and quickly became a new instrument for the evaluation of work performance. With it, psychologists could now "discover" characteristics in the world they had helped shape, namely, the fact that emotional demeanor had become a marker of social identity. The notion of EI claimed that the way we handle our emotions points to essential aspects of who we are and that emotions can, in turn, be currencies to be exchanged for a variety of social goods, most noticeably that of *leadership*.

"Emotional intelligence" marks the culmination of a century in which the presence and hegemony of the therapeutic loomed large. Even before the concept was coined, the following quote from the article "Is it OK to Sob on the Job?" by Ann Curran (published in *Redbook* 1985) is one example of the many ways in which psychologists had promoted the tenets of EI *avant la lettre*:

At your job you can take advantage of your greater ease with emotion if you start using it strategically. You can begin by thinking about what you're feeling, trying to understand why you feel the way you do. Consider your emotions an early warning system, to alert yourself that an office situation needs to be adjusted. "If you are angry or upset," Dr. Potter says, "something's wrong. That's what your emotions can tell you. Then use your intelligence to decide what to do. Analyze the degree of risk you face, and decide whether it's in your best interests to express your emotions. If you think before you speak, revealing your feelings might actually turn out to be savvy office politics"

Indeed, this article, written in 1985, puts forward the central idea behind the later notion of "emotional intelligence," namely, that emotions should be at the service of one's intelligence, always equated with the capacity to understand and further one's self-interest. To be emotionally intelligent is tautologically defined as one's ability to manage one's emotions in such a way that they are disciplined by the cognitive and practical understanding of one's interests. A second illustration raises the idea that emotional literacy is the key to a happy life lived without *emotional mistakes*. What is required in a variety of situations, such as a street riot, wife beating, or a magistrate lying under oath, is nothing less than the skills of emotional literacy. As Claude Steiner suggests in his recounting of numerous anecdotes, "emotions like anger, fear, or shame makes smart people behave stupidly, rendering them powerless" (Steiner 1997, 13).

If Daniel Goleman, a journalist with training in clinical psychology, was able to turn his book *Emotional Intelligence* (Goleman 1995) into a worldwide best-seller and a new standard with which to evaluate conduct, it was because American popular culture had already been saturated with an almost century-long psychological culture in which emotions were increasingly central to the evaluation of the self and others. Psychological culture had long been advocating the central tenet behind the notion of EI, namely, that emotions ought to be informed and guided by rational judgments.

EI is, among other things, an offshoot of Howard Gardner's pioneering notion of multiple intelligence (Gardner 1983) and, more specifically, of his notion of "personal intelligence."[3] Peter Salovey, David Caruso, and John D. Mayer, three prominent researchers in EI, define the concept as the ability to perceive and express emotion, cognitively understand and relate to emotion, and control emotion in the self and others, leading to better problem solving in an individual's life (Mayer, Salovey, and Caruso 2000).

According to this definition, EI is the cognitive ability to process one's own feelings mentally and verbally, such rational processing being, in turn, important for the reflexive management of situations.[4] When emotions are used adaptively to solve a situation, then one might be said to have displayed "emotional intelligence."

Given that sociology has been very preoccupied with mechanisms of social reproduction and exclusion (Bourdieu 1979/1984), the concept of EI should be a welcome guest: At face value, it should help us build more complex models of social stratification—helping us to introduce another variable that may or may not explain and predict social mobility. In addition, the notion of EI might offer an alternative to the much criticized concept of IQ. Indeed, the standard measurements of intelligence have been sharply criticized by sociologists on the ground that they reflect the cognitive competence and the social environment of the middle and upper middle classes, thus subtly discriminating against those whose socialization excludes the cognitive skills that are tapped into by IQ tests. Oprah Winfrey's 1998 show on EI, in which she enthusiastically endorsed the concept, provides an example of the ways in which the notion of EI has been seized in popular culture as a welcome alternative to standard notions of intelligence. In the context of the show, these notions have been addressed as follows: "Unlike your IQ score which is pretty much set in stone, you can actually raise your EQ score and become emotionally smarter."[5]

It is also easy to understand why the notion of EI would be enthusiastically endorsed by feminists who hold that women are more attuned to interpersonal relations than men and that they base their moral decisions on empathic thinking. If it is indeed frequently the case that women develop the skill of tuning into the emotional needs of others, of managing social relations in a nonconfrontational fashion, and of monitoring their verbal and emotional behavior, they should thus score high on EI tests. Consequently, making our institutions sensitive and responsive to EI could be an important tool in the rehabilitation of the emotional competence of minorities who were disadvantaged when competing with others on the basis of formal intellectual skills. In light of this, it would seem that the concept of EI is analytically useful, as it complicates our picture of social stratification, and normatively important, as it could help us to positively define skills other than those traditionally used to rank children and adults. Hence, at face value, the concept of EI should be welcome as it confirms the repeated claims that forms of intelligence are multiple, that intelligence does not necessarily demand formal cognitive skills, and that our institutions (schools or corporations) should be more attuned to identifying and rewarding this new form of competence.

And yet, despite the promise of EI to enable a more pluralistic and democratic distribution of resources, I argue that in fact it represents a new axis of social classification, which creates new forms of social competence (and incompetence).

8.3   Emotional Intelligence and Therapeutic Ideology

Let me refer to a vignette presented in a seminal article by two most prominent academic researchers in the field of EI, Mayer and Geher, who define EI by its opposite, namely, through the lack of EI:

A patient (a woman) was having an affair with a married man. One day she asked the married man to promise her that he would not come from his home when he visited her and that he would not return home when he left her. She formulated what she expected from him more clearly the next day: "You must not come from her or go to her when you see me." She spoke of it as if it were an indifferent thought that had occurred to her, a convenient arrangement, yes, even a kind of amusing idea. But the analyst could put himself into the place of his patient . . . he got an inkling . . . of the emotions of his patient: her jealousy, her suffering from the thought that her lover left her to go home to his wife (Mayer and Geher 1996, 90f).

The authors suggest that this woman's request is formulated in such a way that it renders her own interest unintelligible; unable to tell to herself and to her lover what her "real" feelings are, she runs the risk of seeming capricious, irrational, and demanding—thus one must conclude that her coping strategies are inadequate to help her achieve her goals.

The authors' analysis of the vignette is interesting precisely because it helps expose the assumptions contained in the notion of "emotional intelligence," assumptions derived mostly from the ideology of the psychological persuasion.

Their first and perhaps most obvious assumption concerns the fact that the authors assume that there are "real" feelings *trapped* inside the self, only waiting to be appropriately named and known by a conscious and knowing subject. Such an "ontological" view of emotion is central to clinical psychology and stands in opposition to the view that feeling an emotion is a labile process, a result of interpretation and labeling which, in turn, depend on symbolic cues provided by the environment. As numerous anthropologists and even social psychologists have argued (Lutz and Abu-Lughod 1990b), there is no emotional "substance" waiting to be known, named, and revealed. Rather: Far from being blocks of experience or consciousness waiting to be discovered and appropriately named, names of emotions and the experience of emotions are fluidly and contextually generated. The view that emotions are blocks of experience, repressed, stored, and only waiting to be named and freed, feeds directly into the interests of psychologists whose profession consists in defining their work as that of exposing, adequately naming, and transforming emotions.

Furthermore, the authors assume that grounding one's claims on "what one feels" is socially more competent. It should be clarified that this claim is never made explicit in the text but only axiomatically assumed and is, once again, a central tenet of the therapeutic persuasion. I would, however, argue that a competent emotional response depends on the constraints embedded in situations and not on a context-free rational processing, understanding, and labeling of emotions. In other words, a competent emotional response does not necessarily entail a self-conscious awareness of one's emotional responses. For example, in the above vignette, the woman's request was, in all likelihood, perfectly comprehensible to her lover, who would have had to be singularly ignorant of contemporary codes of love not to understand that her request was an attempt to claim the uniqueness of their relationship and to isolate their relations from his married life. As it was formulated, this woman's request *was not only reasonable, but highly competent* precisely because she did not verbalize her motivations. She was able to make a clear demand on this man's movements without expressing anxiety, jealousy, or possessiveness, all emotions likely to have weakened her position and status within the relationship. This suggests an important theoretical point: Social actors attend to situations and function in them with *stored cultural knowledge, or cultural codes*, which make them finely attuned to the constraints embedded in a situation without going through the elaborate operation of identifying, naming, and explicitly expressing the emotions produced by these constraints. In other words, what guarantees that social interactions "flow" is the fact that so much of these interactions rely on tacit and stored knowledge. Echoing the psychological persuasion at large, Mayer and Geher's suggestion that emotional "intelligence" involves the reflexive and explicit naming of emotions for oneself and for others is oblivious to the fact that people attend to the meaning of the emotions felt by others without having recourse to a reflexive foregrounding and manipulation of emotions. EI, as defined by the scholars, would in fact make most social interactions cumbersome, as it would hamper interactional flow and fluency. Reflecting the rational views of actors and action that have engulfed and colonized the social sciences (Smelser 1998), the notion of "emotional intelligence" equates intelligence with the harnessing of emotions to problem solving. In contrast, for cultural sociologists, situations are construed and dealt with through the tacit knowledge we bring to them; it is this tacit knowledge that makes us opt for *roundabout* emotional responses grounded in practical and habitual knowledge. Like pianists playing difficult sonatas, we attend to situations by using rules we have perfectly internalized, not by mentally reflecting on and contemplating different courses of action. Pianists or social actors who become too intensely aware of themselves and of the rules they use, of their bodily and emotional movements, play their score in a cumbersome fashion and lack the flow and fluency that distinguish virtuosity from rote learning.

In short, mental awareness of one's emotions is not always possible, nor is it always desirable. This leads to another crucial point: In this particular social situation—a situation in which a married man has control over a single woman—making her claim in a roundabout fashion rather than clarifying her emotions in an outright fashion is the *most* competent emotional response, as it is precisely this approach which enables this woman to retain control of the situation. Indeed, as this example suggests, control of situations is often maintained precisely by veiling emotions, both to ourselves and to others, not by disclosing them. Given that power and control are such fundamental dimensions of social interactions, and given that they crucially depend on *hiding* emotions (from oneself and from others), this implies that the reflexivity and verbal disclosure of emotions advocated by psychologists and by experts in EI may ultimately disturb a subtle and more efficient manipulation of social relations and situations. To be more precise: The aforementioned woman is caught in a double bind, which she had been placed in by her lover. Her roundabout request elegantly reconciled two contradictory requirements—one was to retain control by seeming detached from the difficulties inherent in the situation, and the second was to ascertain her amorous territory. Therefore, this example does not illustrate the woman's incompetence but rather the fact that actors often operate in situations that have *contradictory demands* by *unreflexively* navigating in them and improvising responses. Emotional ambiguity, ambivalence, and lack of clarity are highly *competent* because they are ways of coping with contradiction-ridden social situations. Had this woman been "emotionally intelligent"—by becoming conscious of her feelings and by voicing such feelings to ground her claims—she might have lost her control over the situation or over her lover.

The rationalist assumptions guiding the notion of EI curiously contradict a line of research in cognitive psychology about some of the processes involved in decision making. This research paradigm shows that many intelligent decisions are based on intuitive thinking, or what cognitive psychologists call "thin slicing," the ability to make accurate snap judgments about people, problems, and situations without going through a formal process of labeling and cognitively rehearsing the dimensions of the situation, emotional or otherwise. Such snap judgments derive from unconscious thought processes, the capacity to mobilize past experiences and to zero in and focus on only a few elements of the object judged. Additionally, in groundbreaking experiments, cognitive psychologists Timothy Wilson and Jonathan Schooler have shown that introspection can in fact be an obstacle to problem solving based on insight. When introspecting about such tasks as tasting a jam or choosing an interesting university course, people are not as good at recognizing the good from the bad jam, the interesting from the boring course (Wilson and Schooler 1991). To translate their findings into the vocabulary of sociologists, introspection interferes with action moved by the logic of practice, such as taste and social tact (Wilson and Schooler 1991; see also Schooler, Ohlsson, and Brooks 1993).

Let me thus make the following suggestion: The competence to meet the emotional requirements of specific organizational and social contexts has more to do with the mechanism of habitus than with the self-aware introspection of one's emotional makeup or with the rational capacity to process one's emotions in thought. Emotional competence does not necessarily depend on the reflexive and verbal foregrounding of emotions. We should then ask ourselves whose social and emotional skills such a notion naturalizes and legitimizes.

8.4 Emotional and Social Competence

It is not by chance that in the vignette offered by Mayer and Geher, the therapist is presented as the one who is emotionally intelligent. This is so because to define emotional incompetence is, simultaneously, to define competence and the social bearers of that competence. This is not surprising in light of the fact that the notion of EI is the outcome of the worldview of a particular class of professionals—the psychologists—who have historically been extraordinarily successful in claiming a monopoly on the definition and the rules of emotional life in the private and public spheres and have redefined professional success in terms of emotional demeanor and management. To be emotionally intelligent has become the prerogative of a *professional* class responsible for the management of emotions, and being emotionally competent would seem to consist in acquiring the cognitive and emotional skills of which clinical psychologists claim to be the virtuosos. In the same way that IQ served to classify people in the army and in the workplace so as to increase their productivity, EI has become a way to classify productive and less productive workers, this time along the lines of emotional rather than cognitive skills. In claiming to describe different forms of emotional competencies, the notion of EI in fact helps to organize social groups around a new axis of social classification. Emotions have come to be increasingly defined as a form of competence, which, in turn, can be "played" within social fields of struggle.

Emotional fields work by constructing and expanding the criteria for evaluating health and pathology. These emotional fields construct and regulate access to new forms of social competence, which I will dub "emotional competence." In the same way that cultural fields are structured by cultural competence—the capacity to relate to cultural artifacts in a way that signals familiarity with high or legitimate culture sanctioned by the upper classes—emotional fields are regulated by emotional competence—the capacity to display an emotional style defined and legitimized by the main actors in that field, namely, psychologists and mental health workers.

Like cultural competence, emotional competence may be translated into a social benefit such as professional advancement or social capital. Indeed, for a particular form of cultural behavior to become a capital, it must be convertible into something that agents can play with in a field, such as an economic and social benefit which will, in turn, give them a right of entry, that will help them seize what is at stake in that field (Bourdieu 1979/1984). In that sense, we may speak of a concept of *emotional capital*, similar in function to that of cultural capital.

Browsing the Internet on EI yielded several examples of the uses of the construct in modern corporations. An article reviewing the various uses of EI in industry deserves to be quoted at length because it (unwittingly) provides an illustration of the way in which EI is used as a new form of classification that can be converted into real economic capital:[6]

1. The U.S. Air Force used the EQ-i to select recruiters (the Air Force's front-line human resources personnel) and found that the most successful recruiters scored significantly higher in the EI competencies of Assertiveness, Empathy, Happiness, and Emotional Self Awareness. The Air Force also found that by using EI to select recruiters, they increased their ability to predict successful recruiters by nearly three-fold. The immediate gain was a savings of $3 million annually. These gains resulted in the Government Accounting Office submitting a report to Congress, which led to a request that the Secretary of Defense order all branches of the armed forces to adopt this procedure in recruitment and selection.[7]

2. Experienced partners in a multinational consulting firm were assessed on the EI competencies and three other tests. Partners who scored above the median on 9 or more of the 20 competencies delivered $1.2 million more profit from their accounts than did other partners—a 139 percent incremental gain.[8]

3. In jobs of medium complexity (sales clerks, mechanics), a top performer is 12 times more productive than those at the bottom and 85 percent more productive than an average performer. In the most complex jobs (insurance salespeople, account managers), a top performer is 127 percent more productive than an average performer (Hunter, Schmidt, and Judiesch 1990). Competency research in over 200 companies and organizations worldwide suggests that about one-third of this difference is due to technical skill and cognitive ability while two-thirds is due to emotional competence (Goleman 1998). In top leadership positions, over four-fifths of the difference is due to emotional competence.[9]

EI is used as a way to predict and control economic productivity and to classify the people in charge of production in a new way. It employs what Espeland and Stevens call "commensuration," a common metric to standardize and compare different objects in order to build (symbolic and/or material) equivalence between them (Espeland and Stevens 1998). Here, the equivalence they are trying to build is between jobs and people. As Joan Acker puts it: "[A job] is an empty slot, a reification that must continually be reconstructed, for positions exist only as scraps of paper until people fill them. . . . Human beings are to be motivated, managed, and chosen to fit the job. The job exists as a thing apart" (Acker 1990, 148).

The system of equivalence enabled by the notion of "emotional intelligence" suggests that the self is becoming commodified in a way that is unprecedented in the cultural history of capitalism: "EI" essentially translates one's emotional makeup into monetary terms.[10] Moreover, following the logic of capital described by Pierre Bourdieu, emotional forms of capital can be converted into monetary ones. The emergence of the corporate field has given rise to what Bourdieu terms new forms of symbolic capital, which are used in fields of struggle (Bourdieu 2000, 166). If, as Bourdieu suggests, fields maintain themselves through the mechanism of habitus or "the structuring mechanism that operates from within agents" (Bourdieu and Wacquant 1992, 18), then we may suggest that in an increasing number of fields, emotional habitus is a prerequisite to enter and play in them. Surpassing traditional forms of cultural capital—such as wine tasting or familiarity with high culture—emotional capital seems to mobilize the least reflexive aspects of habitus. This capital exists in the form of "long-lasting dispositions of mind and body" and is the most "embodied" part of cultural capital (Bourdieu 1986, 243).

Although Randall Collins' approach differs substantially from that of Bourdieu, some of his insights may perhaps help explain the formation of emotional habitus. Collins has famously discussed the notion of emotional energy to account for what holds interaction rituals together (Collins 2004). I would argue that while emotional energy is not equivalent to EI or competence, it is a precondition for it. Collins argues that emotional energy is the type of energy we accumulate from a series of successful interactions with others (Collins 1990). Emotional energy—undoubtedly an important component of sociability—is the self-confidence we gain from having repeatedly gained a sense of belonging in a status group. Collins depicts here a kind of Durkheimian synergism and enthusiasm we derive from feeling that we are a member of a group and that we are able, in turn, to feed back to the group. People with such emotional energy, Collins claims, are likely to assume a position of leadership because they have the energy that derives from the group which can, in turn, embody the group. If, as he argues, emotional energy is accumulated through past membership in a status group and successful interactions, then displaying emotional energy becomes a way of signaling one's previous successful interactions—*a sort of positive emotional capital that can be converted into candidacy for leadership*. Emotional demeanor may thus be the accumulation of the frequency of interactions and of one's status in these interactions.

Emotions function as a capital not only because they are derived from one's social bonds and one's position within those bonds but also because emotional habitus, like one's taste, is defined by one's social position and social identity. To the extent, however, that cultural capital, at least in the Bourdieusian sense, means access to an established corpus of artistic creations identified as "high culture," EI does not qualify as a subspecies of cultural capital. Emotional habitus lies thus at the intersection of three domains of social experience: the interactional, the bodily, and the linguistic.

By claiming that personality and emotions were leadership assets and that these assets could be acquired through a self-reflexive work of introspection and self-observation, psychologists contributed to the conversion of emotional style (see Reddy, this volume) into a social currency, or capital, and articulated a new language of self-hood with which to seize that capital. While in Freud's descriptions, the economic self exacted a high price from private life—that peculiar flavor of morose repressiveness that leads to repression and neurosis—the psychic economy of people working in the contemporary service industry (especially the lower- and middle-rank managers) demands a subtle and complex emotional work that includes rather than excludes others, that is both assertive and other oriented, attuned to the emotional aspects of interaction yet also in full cognitive control of them. EI is thus fundamentally connected to *class dynamics* and this in a few different but related respects: Because contemporary capitalism demands both speed and mobility, it tends to loosen the fit between the structure of social fields and the inner structure—the habitus—of the subject. That is, contemporary capitalism demands—symbolic and emotional—skills, which will help one cope with a wide variety of social situations and persons, in complex and uncertain markets. For this reason, EI is a *procedural "empty" form of habitus*, that is, a habitus that has been emptied of its cultural weight and content. In its capacity to detach itself from one's concrete cultural soil, EI reflects the emotional style and models of the middle classes: Their work in the contemporary capitalist economy demands a careful management of the self, they are highly dependent on collaborative work, they constantly evaluate others and are, in turn, evaluated by them, they move in long interactional chains, and they must meet a wide variety of persons in a wide variety of contexts. EI is a form of capital which is central to social capital because emotions are the nuts and bolts of how people acquire networks, both strong and weak. Emotions are essential components of the mechanism of social capital in the two senses identified by Alejandro Portes: One designates the ability to form positive social networks, that is, a positive form of sociability in which solidarity and emotional energy are produced; the second refers to the ways in which personal relationships are converted into forms of capital, such as career advancement or increased wealth (Portes 1998).

Emotional capital has become particularly prominent in a form of capitalism which can be characterized, following Luc Boltanski's expression, as "connexionist." As he puts it, in connexionist capitalism, the "class *habitus of the dominant classes* can no longer rely on its own intuition. This habitus needs to know how to establish relationships between people who are geographically and socially distant from oneself."[11]

In connexionist capitalism, status is established by one's capacity to know many people and to establish connections between them. Adding a new layer to our conceptualization of emotional capital, here, emotions have become capital because establishing social relationships is central to connexionist capitalism.

8.5   The Global Therapeutic Habitus and "The New Man"

Let me take this analysis one step further. I am going to argue now that the therapeutic habitus marks the emergence of new forms of masculinities, which, through processes of cultural globalization, have come to interlock with local class dynamics.

In a series of articles, John Meyer and his associates have argued that globalization is the process by which an increasing number of states worldwide adopt the same cultural models (of the economy, the polity, the individual), which thus penetrate social life (see, e.g., Meyer et al. 1997). In the modern globalized polity, individuals constitute themselves by using standard rules in order to establish the essence of modern actorhood such as being rational and purposeful. Psychology is one of the main cores of cultural globalization, generating worldwide models for the organization of individuality. This model is diffused globally through university curricula and training programs and through the regulated practice of professional therapy.

I would add that it also circulates through the lighter, faster, and more informal structure of the market. An illustration of this process can be found in a workshop on EI I attended in Israel in 1998. The purpose of the workshop was to teach and spread the insights of the then newly discovered concept of EI.[12] Approximately 200 participants attended the workshop. The translator of the Hebrew version of Goleman's book (Goleman 1997a) made the introductory remarks and was followed by a variety of speakers, most of whom were in the field of organizational consulting, claiming expertise in leadership training. In response to one of the organizers' question as to "who had read" the book, everyone, as far as I could tell, had read Goleman's book. Yet, although the book and its insights were the main topic of the day, there was very little coherence in the different approaches to EI offered by the speakers. One speaker claimed that EI consisted of knowing how to be determined and stubborn, while another claimed that the failure to understand when to stop trying signified a lack of EI. One speaker argued how important it is to plan and think ahead about what we do and what we say, while another claimed that spontaneity was of paramount importance. One advised attendees to "look at what people do, not what they say," while another argued that "what people do may have so many meanings that we don't know for sure what it means. We can only know from their intentions, and thus we must always ask them."

None of these contradictions seemed to disturb or to be perceptible to the audience because they are in fact in line with the therapeutic persuasion which "works" by seizing upon a wide variety of mutually contradictory narrative pegs, all of which can retrospectively organize the proper management of the self. EI is one such narrative peg that also functions as a classification scheme around which various consultants and psychologists, in turn, organize their professional practices.

The second part of the day entailed a workshop delivered by David Ryback, PhD, author of *Putting Emotional Intelligence to Work* (Ryback 1998). He claimed that EI skills are essential to both the private and public spheres, and the skills required for a good marriage are equivalent to the skills required to conduct business or even international negotiations between nations. For the most part, these skills are gender neutral, but if they were to be gendered, they would undoubtedly be female. Ryback, like all psychologists, distinguishes between appropriate and inappropriate emotions and posits that emotional life should be conducted in accordance with objective rules. A competent emotional life contains skills which mix neutrality with spontaneity, sincerity and lack of judgmentality, self-assertion and listening skills, and flexibility and firmness. In short, EI, as advocated by this psychologist, contains a "mix" of conflicting attributes, precisely the "mix" that has made the therapeutic persuasion so effective, because it creates a permanent uncertainty and desire to reconcile conflicting attributes.

It is very doubtful whether this workshop can single-handedly transform the emotional makeup of its participants. However, such workshops should nonetheless interest the sociologist because they point to the formation of what I would like to call a "global emotional habitus." The formation of such habitus takes place in the usual sites of socialization (family, school, media), but, as the plethora of psychological workshops which have flourished in Israel for the last two decades attests to, the acquisition of such habitus also takes place in the voluntarist cultural framework of the didactic workshop such as the one analyzed above. The primary goal of these workshops, I argue, is instilling new emotional dispositions or skills required to navigate the conditions of late modernity, to move along long chains of social networks, and to meet the demands of global connexionist capitalism.

Such habitus is related to globalization, understood as a process, which *gets* deployed within local class structures (even if it often ends up disturbing that class structure). In this vein, John Meyer's ambitious and highly persuasive analyses have remained curiously oblivious to the class dynamic through which the process of globalization occurs. Indeed, not only have psychological models of selfhood given rise to a new habitus—which could be characterized as a "global" therapeutic habitus—but I would also argue that this habitus is characteristic of the social group of managers and cultural specialists most involved in the process of globalization.

A 1998 interview with an Israeli man, who had earned a graduate degree from Tel
Aviv University and worked as a cultural specialist in an association with a global orientation, provides an example of this "global therapeutic habitus." During the interview, he distinguished between two types of men. One he called "the hero type," who
had served in the army, ate national foods (e.g., hummus), and did not express his
feelings under any circumstances. The second type is the "new man," as he called it
in Hebrew (*Ha Guever Hachadasch*), who is able to "get in touch with his feelings,"
with what he called "the feminine side of things." The interviewee claimed that all
his male friends were "like that," like the new man, and that he could not have other
kinds of friends. The following excerpts of the interview further outline the profile of
the "new man":[13]

Interviewer: Do you think you are typical in that? Or rather do you think that your
views of men and emotions are strange in Israeli society?
Respondent: No. I am quite typical of a certain social group, a certain social milieu.
Interviewer: What do you mean?
Respondent: I mean that to be able to enter a certain social territory, to belong to
certain groups, emotional complexity is a must.
Interviewer: Can you point to a character known or unknown which would embody
for you that kind of emotional complexity?
Respondent: That would have to be the movie *Annie Hall*. I saw that movie perhaps
30 times. That was a very formative movie for me and for many others.
Interviewer: Let me go back to something you said just before, with regard to belonging to a certain social group, men, or at least the men you know, have to have a certain
way of expressing their emotions. Did I understand you correctly?
Respondent: Absolutely. Definitely. It is a part of the "entry exams." Let me give you
an example. My wife, Liora, is a clinical psychologist. She has a sister who lives in
[Jerusalem]. Her husband is some kind of redneck. He comes from a *Moshav* [agricul-
tural settlement]. He is a stereotypical *moshavnik*. He lacks in any kind of emotional
expressivity. He has no emotions. And we make fun of him, all three of us, me, my
wife, and my wife's sister precisely on that, on the fact that he does not have feelings.
He never longs for anything, or never misses anything, or never feels depressed. He
does not know the concept of "being depressed." Where have you seen anything like
that? So that's the criteria. When I used to date women, if she did not know what
"being depressed" meant—I don't mean a big clinical depression but just regular ordinary depression—then she would not qualify. She would not be a possible candidate.
No way (Eyal, 29, graduate degree in social sciences).

Cultural globalization is largely at work in the above excerpt: Woody Allen's movies
have been a powerful instrument for the diffusion of a certain therapeutic style and
for new forms of masculinities. This style of masculinity is strongly associated with a

specific emotional style (anxious, nervous, self-conscious, verbal, reflexive) and has become diffused mostly among the new middle classes. Emotional style functions here as a token of membership to certain social groups, educated, Western, secular, and, perhaps, most importantly, it is not defined by the nation, that is, global. That style is associated with regular markers of taste, that is, how one dresses and what one eats. The "new man" here does not express membership in an economic or social group but rather a distinction in emotional competence, itself a marker of social status. Two men might technically be members of the same socioeconomic group yet have a very different emotional habitus. If globalization creates new forms of inequalities, dividing the mobile from the stationary, it also requires a kind of habitus that is closely connected to therapeutic cultural practices. We may thus suggest that therapy is a cultural structure mediating between globalization and class structure through the formation of new masculinities. I will now turn to an examination of how the formation of new masculinities creates new hierarchies.

8.6   Intimacy as a Social Good

If it is indeed the case that therapy mediates between class structure and new masculinities, how are we to understand its effect on the shape and distribution of resources?

Much of the Marxian or Weberian sociology of capitalism has implicitly held the same view offered by Freud at the beginning of this chapter: The Bourgeois may exploit others in the realm of production, but he or she finds himself or herself, after all, the victim of poetic justice that disposes him or her of the poor man's emotional riches. While transforming the world into a place where the dispassionate pursuit of gain is central, the Bourgeois sacrifices his or her well-being and his or her capacity to forge long-lasting meaningful bonds on the altar of Mammon. This cliché—at the heart of which lies the dichotomies of "market" and "gift," and "interest" and "sentiment,"—has prevented sociologists from understanding the ways in which the new middle and upper middle classes may in fact have better chances of achieving well-being and intimacy through access to therapy. What if the Bourgeois, or his or her postindustrial version, had turned out to be the best candidate for love and well-being precisely because of his or her access to the language of therapy?

In the context of contemporary American society, definitions of intimacy are intimately linked to the language of therapy, which has naturalized and legitimated the emotional and verbal style of the new middle class. In the period following World War II, the language of therapy, at once making sense of objective transformations of the workplace and shaping a new language of selfhood, became the privileged cultural repertoire within which members of the new service class, in the United States, constructed and understood their self, *both at work and in the family*. Such a transformation was made possible by the fact, as documented in my book (Illouz 2008), that psychologists straddled the work sphere and the family and codified intimacy, in the very same categories they were using in parallel to prescribe a new type of corporate selfhood. Because most critiques of therapy oppose the therapeutic ethos to a model of civic virtue or political engagement, they have usually ignored the question of its *social uses*, its pragmatics, thus failing to grasp that the therapeutic discourse orients perceptions, classifications, and modes of social interactions toward the pursuit of symbolic goods that still remain to be specified. The most interesting social effect of the cultural domination of therapy has been the creation of new forms of social goods and new forms of social competence with which to attain such goods as intimacy. If there is one single contribution of feminist scholarship from which there is no possible return, it is its central insight that the public sphere cannot be our only way to evaluate the "good society"; rather, intimate relations, friendship, and parenthood, are no less—and perhaps even more so—the arenas with which to evaluate how good and how just a society is (Moller-Okin 1989). Andrew Sayer expresses it as follows: "Class inequalities involve not merely differences in wealth, income and economic security, but differences in access to valued circumstances, practices and ways of life—'goods' in a broad sense and in the recognition or valuation of those goods and their holders" (Sayer 2005, 95).

This, in turn, implies that in order to critically examine the therapeutic discourse, we cannot rely on an Aristotelian model of social relations based on *public participation*. Intimate relations ought to figure no less in our accounts of the connection between culture and just social arrangements. If we examine the language of therapy in order to isolate what actors claim makes it perform in their lives, then we may be able to illuminate the new forms of goods and hierarchies it reifies. If we take intimacy to be *a sphere of meaning in its own right*, the therapeutic ethos appears to be a cultural resource that helps certain actors implement standards of well-being *as they are socially and historically constructed*. In other words, if we view intimacy as a good of a special kind, we may inquire about the cultural and symbolic forms that grant access to such spheres of well-being.

This proposition runs counter to the dominant paradigm of the sociology of domination which typically addresses various forms of capital in the context of competitive arenas and finds it disconcerting to approach the family and intimacy as goods in their own right. Bourdieu's theory of social reproduction, for example, approaches the family as an institution that is ultimately subordinate to social structure (Bourdieu 1979/1984). In the theory of symbolic reproduction, the family is the institution that instills the early and invisible dispositions that will later be converted into practical choices in competitive fields of social struggle. However, as Michael Walzer (1983) has so persuasively suggested, a theory of justice ought to account for (and respect) the values of each sphere of life. Michael Rustin (1991) works with the same premise when he suggests that we include "well-being" as a category of social right. According to Rustin, with the increasing complexity and variety of human values, there is a parallel increase in the need for personal development which becomes "one of the goals which people seek through relationships of kinship or friendship, through education, through work and culture" (Rustin 1991, 45).

Rustin suggests that psychoanalysis should be accorded status as a "sphere of justice," with its own criteria of value, helping one to achieve one's definition of the good life, and that psychic development and satisfaction can and should matter to public institutions. In this respect, we may inquire about intimacy, not only as a sphere subservient to socioeconomic structure at large but also as a sphere of meaning and well-being in its own right. It would then make sense to ask whether intimacy is "justly" distributed.

If we approach the family and intimacy as autonomous spheres of meaning and action, we may then analyze them as institutions meant to provide *moral goods* in which the content of *selfhood and well-being are at stake*.[14] That is, if we reverse the Bourdieusian model and inquire into the ways in which one's professional habitus helps one reach particular forms of *eudaimonia* (happiness and well-being), *then we may inquire about the ways in which intimacy, like other forms of goods*, is socially distributed and allocated. This is, what Anthony Giddens has in mind, I think, when he suggests that "life politics" restructures older social divisions—life politics includes such issues as self-realization, intimacy, and the good life in general: ". . . [C]lass divisions and other fundamental lines of inequality, such as those connected with gender or ethnicity, can be partly *defined* in terms of differential access to forms of self-actualization and empowerment. . . . Modernity, one should not forget, produces *difference, exclusion* and *marginalization*" (Giddens 1991, 6).

If Giddens is correct, then we must inquire into the "mechanics" of inclusion and exclusion from such spheres of well-being as intimacy. How is exclusion from such (moral) goods as well-being and intimacy produced? I would argue that the language of therapy plays an important role in relaying such exclusions. The following example may help us begin to illustrate what I mean here.

A 32-year-old female interviewee is a professional editor and holds a PhD in English Literature from a top American university. For four years, she has been married to a university lecturer in philosophy. She has been in therapy off and on for the past 11 years.[15]

Interviewer: Do you have negative emotions?
Silence.
Interviewer: You don't have to answer if you don't want to.
Respondent: Well, I am not sure if I should say.
Interviewer: It is completely up to you.

Respondent: Well . . . I am jealous. I am very jealous. And I know where it comes from. It basically comes from my father leaving my mother for another woman, and growing up with a mother who told me over and over again not to trust men.

Interviewer: Does it have any impact on your relationship with your husband?

Respondent: Yes, oh yes, I can become very jealous, very possessive, and feel really threatened by other women. Like the other day, we were having dinner with friends of ours, and one of my friends asked Larry [her husband] if he had been to India. And he said he did but he did not want to talk about it, because he had been there with a girl-friend, and he knew it would upset me to talk about it. So he didn't want to talk about it, but she kept asking him questions, until I told her: "Look he does not want to talk about it. He was there with a girl-friend, and that's making me upset." Larry and I we had some rough times over this issue . . .

Interviewer: Did you do something about it?

Respondent: Yeah. . . . Just talking, we talked for a long long time about it. Both of us are sort of very aware of ourselves; both of us have a strong interest in psychoanalysis and therapy; so we talked and talked about it, and analyzed it. So it was just talking about it, understanding it, and having him tell me over and over again that he loved me, and that he would not leave me for another woman. And I think that the fact we could talk about our feelings and really understand them is what got us through.

This highly educated couple displays "emotional competence" (dubbed "intelligence" in the psychological persuasion), namely, self-awareness, the ability to identify their feelings, name them, talk about them, empathize with each other's position, and find solutions to a problem. It is not a coincidence that this man and woman display such emotional and linguistic practices: Both have earned PhDs in fields where language is crucial to their professional performance and where self-awareness can be converted into a symbolic capital. These skills are closely intertwined with their cultural capital. Both hold PhDs in fields in which self-expression is important and in which the cultivation of self and authenticity are rewarded. The therapeutic language and this couple's EI are "real" cultural resources, not because they understand the "real" nature of their emotional problems but because the couple can deploy a common cultural habitus—in which language is viewed as a tool for solving problems and for expressing the inner self. They can, in turn, use this tool to make sense of difficult emotions and put them "to work," by eliciting a narrative of verbal intimacy and self-help, which they can both share and capitalize on to further their intimacy. Clearly, they are both using a single habitus transposable from the workplace to the sphere of intimacy and vice-versa. What is perhaps most conspicuous is the fact that, as previously discussed, this habitus destructures *gender identities*. As is obvious from the interview, both this woman and her husband display similar linguistic and emotional competence; they share common emotional models; the man is no less able than this woman, presumably, is to show empathy and care.

EI may thus have real effects (in the same way that IQ does), because it reflects the kind of competence most readily available to the new middle classes. Moreover, it is a form of competence that is, in fact, a cultural resource adapted to the social conditions of selfhood in late capitalist modernity: the collapse of normative frames presiding over marriage, the individualization of intimacy, and the burdening of the self with the injunction to improvise the rules for coping with normative plurality and uncertainty. All of this places new demands on the self to live within and meet the requirements of marriage.

The therapeutic language and model of "communication" is a habitus, which directs feelings, thoughts, and action in both the private and public spheres and is transferable from one sphere to the other. As a self-help book puts it: "It is only recently that organizations have begun to value employees who can deal effectively with people. The best place to learn that skill is in your intimate relationship" (Sellner and Sellner 1991, 14).

By the same token, corporate skills may contribute to intimate relationships: "Because conversation control [i.e., communication] is central to everything we do, we will see the benefits not only in our work life but in our home with our family and with our friends in social relations" (Margerison 1987, 7).

Bargaining and consensus building through verbal communication have become the cultural models underlying both corporate and domestic bonds. Thus the therapeutic ethos has contributed to a blurring of the cultural boundaries between the spheres of work and intimacy and has transformed the dialogical and emotional skills central to intimacy into skills that can be capitalized on in the work sphere. The middle-class domestic sphere and work sphere, far from being opposed to each other, are contiguously connected to each other through the cultivation of a common *reflexive and communicative selfhood, which, in turn, tends to blur distinctions of gender roles and identities*.[16] The reflexive and communicative selfhood codified, made visible, and legitimated by psychologists has thus contributed to articulate male and female identities in a common and convergent *androgynous* model of selfhood.

In their use of therapeutic cultural frames, middle- and upper-middle-class men may have access to new forms of masculinities, more compatible with "feminine" models of selfhood. As Frank Furedi argues, hegemonic masculinity—silent, strong, self-reliant, unemotional—is now pathologized, and feminine masculinity is clearly preferred (i.e., thought to be healthier) by mental health workers (Furedi 2004). "According to the emotionally correct hierarchy of virtuous behavior, feminine women come on top. Feminine men beat masculine women for second place. And of course, masculine, macho men come last. This hierarchy informs the attitude of many health professionals" (Furedi 2004, 35).

This hierarchy indeed also reflects a social hierarchy of forms of masculinity, for the nonmacho men are significantly more likely to have a college education and to be involved in types of work oriented toward the manipulation of knowledge and cultural symbols. This becomes clearer when we compare the interviews discussed earlier with that of a 56-year-old African-American working-class man, who works as a janitor in the Chicago area:[17]

Respondent: I was married a few years ago and had a stepson who was knowing that he was an only child and his mother was a whole entire different breed compared to what my mother—compared to what my first wife was in the way she raised kids. I mean she let him do a lot of different things that I didn't approve of like—to telephone all night long and so after eight years of her I wouldn't give a damn about the telephone line, you know, because the phone would ring all night long. I don't believe in that.

Interviewer: Did the phone bother you?

Respondent: Yeah, oh yeah.

Interviewer: Did you tell him?

Respondent: Oh yes. Oh yes. I told him and her.

Interviewer: What did you tell her?

Respondent: Well, I don't know. Well I have a . . . I have a . . . a . . . I can be foul at times. I told her more than once. So in the eight years we were together we've always had problems with the phone ringing all night long and then as he got older, 'cause he was fifteen years old when I met him, we broke up two years ago—he was a full grown man.

Interviewer: You broke up with your wife?

Respondent: Well we broke up. I'm I'm I'm the one . . . so—in the process of that—that was one the big reasons why we broke up. And she, of course, was someone who thought he couldn't do any wrong and uh so therefore he got away with a lot of stuff being an only child. I mean it's halfway dangerous about kids when you meet women out there nowadays who have teenage kids and they run 'em in. You know what I mean? I mean I have several buddies of mine who have relationships with women who have teenage kids and it's a misfit.

Interviewer: Did your marriage fall apart because of that?

Respondent: Well well well well it wasn't all his fault. It was part of the problem.

Interviewer: Did you have arguments?

Respondent: Oh yes. Sure I shouted at him. I shouted at her. There's only so much you can take but but also like I said I can do my shouting but in the end I've got it all out of my system and I'm going on with my business. I don't hold grudges to anybody, you know what I mean? I hate to go to bed—I hate to wake up in the morning—I hate to wake up in the morning mad at your woman. I like to settle all the stuff before going to bed, you know what I mean? We may be fighting all day long but holding a grudge and being angry at each other is something I try to avoid. It's also nice to make up you know, after you've had your fight you know to make it up.

Interviewer: How do you make up?

Respondent: On different ways. Well it's always nice when you have a good sex partner. That's always nice. I most enjoy it after a fight. . . .

[later in the interview] and the second [wife] she left me—I didn't leave her. I mentioned that I left her but I didn't leave her. She left me. I came home one morning from work at two o'clock in the morning and she had took a lot of stuff that she shouldn't have took and didn't tell me anything about it. See so I would've told her—

Interviewer: And she did not tell you anything before hand that indicated that she might leave?

Respondent: No. No.

Interviewer: How do you explain she left?

Respondent: She left. And she didn't tell me anything about it. That's the only thing I can think. . . . [later in the interview] After she left—after I got the initial shock and it wasn't so much the shock about her going it—it was the shock over what she done you know. That's the thing that upset me more than anything else.

Interviewer: What is this that she had done?

Respondent: Well uh uh you know, uh I mean the way she didn't sit down and talk to me. She could've told me about. I would've felt much better if she would've told me—if she says, "George, uh uh I am not satisfied with the situation and I'm going to move." I would've loved her to come straightforward and told me. 'Cause that's the way I—I told her on several occasions that I wasn't satisfied and uh you know—

Interviewer: And how did she tell you?

Respondent: I don't know. I don't know.

Interviewer: And what is the thing that is difficult in having her move without telling you?

Respondent: It makes me feel like I can trust very few women or for that percentage trust anybody because once you sleep with somebody every night and all of a sudden then you come home one day that's a horrible feeling. It's like "I let you break into my house and then you devastate my sixty years on earth." It's like leaving like she did—I come home from work and somebody has broken the house and taken a lot of stuff out of it. It's something that I worked hard for, you know what I mean? That's a devastating feeling. You know. When I picked up the wreaths at the hospital and they told me that my [first] wife was deceased in an automobile accident—those were the biggest shocks in my entire life.

This working-class man exemplifies in a dramatic fashion the fact that working-class marriage contains potential for havoc, not merely because of the objective difficulties to which working-class lives are incessantly subject but also because working-class men and women lack a clear common language for the articulation of needs and goals, to articulate a common project for two different biographies. Notice that this man mentions they frequently screamed at each other and that they resolved their conflicts by having sex, two modes of actions opposed to the therapeutic persuasion's gospel of verbal communication. That is, they lacked a common cultural resource, which they could use in the framework of daily life in order to manage their relationship and their conflicts. This working-class man was left with the experience of suffering all the more intolerable as it remained meaningless, that is, he had no interpretative frame to account for it. He did not have readily available a narrative which could provide this event, nor could he put himself to "work" toward a psychological goal to process, integrate, or overcome it.

Working-class people whom I (and other researchers) interviewed, complain, much more than their middle-class counterparts, of silence, of difficulties in communication and in having a satisfying relationship. As women have entered the workforce, and as norms of equality have progressively penetrated marriage, the need for functional cooperation and communication between partners has increased. In the context of an increasingly complex family, in which partners have to verbally coordinate their actions and tasks, the potential for conflict (and the attendant negative emotions such as anger or resentment) increases. The skills to "communicate" successfully become crucial assets in achieving intimacy, not because they refer to invariant psychological properties of the psyche but because they refer to *sociological skills* for navigation in conditions of late modernity, conditions which disorganize relationships, disorganize the self, and burden it with the demands to improvise the rules of action and interaction. Those (therapeutic) emotional and linguistic skills are less present in working-class intimate lives because they have less currency in the working-class man's workplace. As the British sociologist Paul Willis has shown in his ethnographic study of the shop floor, blue-collar work mobilizes an ethos of bravery, strength, and distrust of words (Willis 1980). Skills in human relations, that is, the ability to attend to one's emotions and to negotiate with others, have little relevance in the working-class man's work sphere. Contrary to middle-class men, whose emotional makeup plays an important role in their work performance, working-class men are more likely to conform to models of hegemonic masculinity. More broadly, these differences reflect disparities between working-class individualism and middle-class individualism, in that the former can be described as "rugged" or "tough" and the latter as "soft" and "psychological" (Jusserow 1999, 169). The individualism of working-class men and women is interwoven with narratives of struggles with adversity and displays the properties of rugged individualism, which contains distrust, toughness, and an emphasis on physical strength. In contrast, middle- and upper-middle-class individualism can be characterized as "soft psychologized individualism," emphasizing a sense of uniqueness, individuality, and self-confidence as well as the emotions, needs, and desires of the psychological self. These differences represent unequal opportunities to access ordinary forms of well-being.

8.7 Conclusion

Let me now conclude by considering an example that provides a good summary of the preceding discussion. In an article attempting to explain why black males and females marry each other in much lower proportions than their white counterparts, the author—a sociologist specializing in the African-American family (Dickson 1993)—offers the following explanation. She locates one of the possible sources of the problem in what she calls "the cool pose of the Black male." In her own words: "This term refers to the ability to present oneself as emotionless, fearless, and aloof, and functions both to preserve the Black male's pride, dignity, and respect, and to express bitterness, anger, and distrust toward the broader society. Although this behavior may be functional in protecting Black males from the pain of living in an oppressive society, . . . it may be dysfunctional in relationships with not only Black women but other Black men and White men" (Dickson 1993, 481).

The cool pose illustrates the point raised earlier, namely, that our emotional responses are, more often than not, roundabout responses to situations which involve conflicting demands—in this case, the contradiction between self-dignity and the need to express rage. It also illustrates that what is adaptive in protecting oneself from an unjust society might be maladaptive for finding a mate and that one of the social sites in which inequality might be visible is precisely in the realm of intimacy, or in the capacity to form long-lasting bonds based on trust. Finally, were we to measure these men according to scales of EI, we would introduce yet another dimension along which they would, no doubt, fare poorly. Using EI as a classificatory device would, again, categorize black men with the "cool pose" as being emotionally unintelligent and inept. Hence the notion of EI may in fact deepen the exclusion of working-class men by offering yet another measurement of their social incompetence. The notion of EI imposes the emotional style, through the back door so to speak, of those who have had the time, leisure, money, and the cultural predispositions to dwell on their emotions, to cultivate the art of having social relations, and to strategically plan their lives and their interactions. In using and adopting the notion of EI, we must be alerted to the possibility that we are tautologically defining as "competence" what our institutions have already in fact defined as competence, and that we are in fact reaffirming the social privileges of those who are already privileged.

However, the social identity of the privileged may have changed: In the new emotional economy, women may indeed play a far more significant role than has been traditionally assigned to them. In connexionist capitalism women are equipped with skills and forms of capital which enable them to play new and different games in the social field. The point here is not to deny current hierarchies and distributions of power but rather to suggest that, increasingly, the cultural category of emotions is making our traditional models of social hierarchy increasingly untenable. It is possible not only that women compete in social markets with specifically women's emotional skills but also that they might have access to forms of goods that have been imperfectly accounted for by the (male) sociology of stratification. Indeed, people have been traditionally classified and stratified according to their access to goods such as money or prestige. Yet, from the standpoint of the sociology of emotion, we could also say that people have unequal access to eudaimonic goods, intangible goods which constitute the good life, the capacity to give and receive what Axel Honneth calls "recognition," which according to him, is the keystone of successful membership in social communities. One of the urgent tasks which lies ahead for the sociology of gender and emotion is to explore the differential position of men and women vis-à-vis eudaimonic goods in order to unravel new forms of inequality (Honneth 1996).

Notes

1. This is a shortened and slightly modified version of chapter 6 in my book Eva Illouz. 2008. *Saving the Modern Soul: Therapy, Emotions, and the Culture of Self-Help.* © The Regents of the University of California. Published by the University of California Press.

2. Hugo Münsterberg was the first in a long series of psychologists to devise personality tests for workers (see his 1913 *Psychology and Industrial Efficiency*) and started almost single-handedly the field of vocational guidance counseling.

3. This is according to Salovey and Mayer (1997). For a further analysis of personal intelligence and the psychological definitions and understanding of emotional, social, and personal intelligence, see Myriam N. Bechtoldt's chapter (this volume), as well as Salovey et al. (1995, 126) and Mayer and Salovey (1993, 433).

4. EI subsumes Gardner's inter- and intrapersonal intelligences and involves abilities that may be categorized into five domains: *self-awareness*, or recognizing in oneself a feeling as it happens; *managing emotions*, or handling feelings so that they are appropriate, realizing what is behind a feeling, and finding ways to handle such negative emotions as fear and anxiety, anger, and sadness; *motivating oneself*, or channeling emotions in the service of a goal, delaying gratification and stifling impulses, and being able to exercise self-control; *empathy*, or sensitivity to others' feelings and concerns and taking their perspective and appreciating the differences in how people feel about things; *handling relationships*, or managing emotions in others and social competence and social skills.

5. The Oprah Winfrey Show. 1998. Emotional Intelligence, October 6, broadcast, Harpo Studios, Chicago.

6. The Business Case for Emotional Intelligence, by Cary Cherniss: http://www.eiconsortium.org/research/business_case_for_ei.htm (accessed April 12, 2007).

7. The GAO report is entitled "Military Recruiting: The Department of Defense Could Improve Its Recruiter Selection and Incentive Systems," and it was submitted to Congress January 30, 1998. Richard Handley and Reuven Bar-On provided this information.

8. Boyatzis, Richard E. 1999. From a presentation to the Linkage Conference on Emotional Intelligence, September 27, in Chicago, IL.

9. See Boyatzis (1999 presentation to the Linkage Conference on Emotional Intelligence, September 27, Chicago); Goleman (1998); Hunter, Schmidt and Judiesch (1990); Spencer and Spencer (1993); and Spencer, McClelland, and Spencer (1992). This research was provided to Daniel Goleman and is reported in Goleman (1998); Clarke Associates (1996).

10. Notice that this argument differs from Arlie R. Hochschild's important work on the commodification of the self (Hochschild 1983). In her work, it is emotional performance, not emotional makeup, which is commoditized.

11. " 'Dans un monde en réseau, ou les connexions ont d'autant plus de chances d'être profitables qu'elles sont plus imprévisibles et plus lointaines, l'habitus de classe, sur lequel repose la convergence spontanée des goûts (Bourdieu, 1979/1984) dans les ordres sociaux a dominante domestique, n'est plus un support suffisant de l'intuition, du flair. Le grand est au contraire celui qui établit des liens entre des êtres, non seulement éloignes les uns des autres, situes dans des univers différents, mais aussi distants de son milieu d'origine et du cercle de ses relations immédiates.' C'est la raison pour laquelle un capitalisme connexioniste, contrairement a l'ancienne société bourgeoise, accepte bien un capital d'expériences et une connaissance de plusieurs mondes leur conférant une adaptabilité importante" (Boltanski and Chiapello 1999, 176, in text quote, transl. Eva Illouz).

12. The program was organized by an Israeli company called "Anashim ve Machchevim"; translation: "People and Computers." See a detailed description and analysis in Illouz (2008).

13. The following text is a transcribed interview. The personal data has been changed.

14. See for a somewhat similar approach Sayer (2005).

15. The following text is a transcribed interview. The personal data has been changed.

16. This is not to say that there are not many important differences between the corporate and the domestic self, most notably the fact that the corporate self wears many more masks than its domestic counterpart. However, the fact that the corporate self is self-consciously masked is the cultural analogue to the ideal of self-disclosure in the private sphere, for "self-revelation" and "disguise" belong to the same binary code of selfhood conceived in terms of "authenticity." Furthermore, whether masked or disclosed, this self must cope in the same way with the question of how to live with another.

17. The following text is a transcribed interview. The personal data has been changed.

9   Technologies of the Emotional Self: Affective Computing and the "Enhanced Second Skin" for Flexible Employees

Carmen Baumeler

9.1   Introduction

Daniel Goleman, psychologist and author of several best-sellers about Emotional Intelligence (EI), argues, "[t]he rules for work are changing. We're being judged by a new yardstick: not just how smart we are, or by our training or expertise, but also by how well we handle ourselves and each other. This yardstick is increasingly applied in choosing who will be hired and who will not, who will be let go and who retained, who passed over and who promoted" (Goleman 1998, 3). As his statement *how well we handle ourselves and each other* indicates, not only education and work experience but, above all, the management of emotions promises professional success. EI, as a result, has become prominent in human resource management and is currently a popular topic in managerial discourse.

This chapter argues that the concept of EI can be interpreted as a Foucaultian technology of the self which aims at the development of flexible employees. First of all, I will discuss the conception of the flexible worker as a historically contingent ideal of the productive subject which is closely linked to the rise of flexible capitalism. Second, the psychological agenda of EI, as developed by Goleman (1995, 1998), will be presented. This program of self-transformation constitutes a guide to successful behavior in the workplace and reflects the contemporary conception of the flexible employee. While EI is often regarded as a mere psychological skill, acquired through mental training, it is not well-known that the concept has also spread to the computer sciences. Here, contemporary research in the fields of wearable and affective computing is trying to develop a "technologically enhanced second skin" (Andrejevic 2005, 113) in order to create the ideal productive subject. In exploring suggested workplace applications, this chapter will reveal the normative assumptions about the user as a completely informed and emotionally controlled individual. The article concludes with a summary of the main points and a discussion of gender issues which have largely escaped notice.

9.2   Changing Conceptions of the Subject at Work

Conceptions of the productive subject have changed over time. Accordingly, different management strategies have been developed to contend with these new ideas (Miller and Rose 1990, 1995). Whereas in the first two decades of the last century the well-known management program *Taylorism* viewed the productive subject as a physiological apparatus to be managed with the tools of scientific management, the *human relations movement* which followed had a different point of view. From this perspective, workers were first and foremost social people. They were not merely passive human machines but active participants in the work process. Employees, consequently, were perceived as individuals seeking comfort, communication, and reassurance. Therefore, management developed certain techniques to guide social groups toward efficiency, harmony, and work satisfaction.

In the 1960s, workers were again reconceptualized as *rational economic actors* seeking to maximize income in order to satisfy their needs in private life. However, this conception only lasted for a decade. In the 1970s, the productive subject was updated once more to an "active and motivated individual, seeking autonomy, control, variety, and a sense of worth" (Miller and Rose 1995, 441f). For this kind of individual, flexible hours, job enrichment, self-managed work teams, and so on were supposed to turn work into something democratic, creative, innovative, and productive.

The refashioning of the productive subject has continued. Since the 1990s, the emerging spirit of *flexible capitalism* has called for a new kind of employee (Sennett 1998; see also Ulshöfer, this volume). On the one hand, this kind of economic regime has been characterized by forced globalization, swift technological change, intensified competition, and the reorganization of production systems. On the other hand, alongside the economic transformation has come an increase in unemployment rates, job obsolescence, and the political agenda of neoliberalism.

In the age of flexible capitalism, bureaucratic organizations have faced widespread criticism regarding their lack of enterprise. To adapt to the new business environment, plants have had to increase flexibility and innovation. Managerial solutions to the problem have been sought in the decentralization of organizational structures, wholesale restructuring on a massive scale, and the reduction of hierarchy. Because the post-Fordist workplace demanded a new kind of workforce, the new economic regime has also affected the micropractices of everyday working life. Gideon Kunda and John van Maanen (1999, 65) claim that "Change, on all fronts, personal, social, and institutional, is the mantra of our times; we are reminded—endlessly and relentlessly—that the only constant is change. To survive, we must come to terms with turbulent environments, thrive on rampant chaos, welcome rapidly changing markets, adjust to high degrees of uncertainty, and celebrate seemingly perpetual technological revolutions."

As a result of this economic transformation, companies have promoted the enterprising capacities of all employees in order to achieve excellence, competitiveness, efficiency, and productivity (Rose 1997, 154). Consequently, the contemporary conception of the worker is the enterprising subject or the *flexible employee*. The current idea is that enterprises should neither rationalize management, so as to increase efficiency, nor manage social groups, in order to maximize contentment, but release the individual's autonomy and creativity and direct them toward organizational excellence and success (Miller and Rose 1990, 26). Thus, all employees are supposed to be transformed into entrepreneurial selves who are personally responsible for innovation, economic growth, and—because of the concomitant reduction in welfare state services—the safeguarding of their own employability.

Luc Boltanski and Ève Chiapello's (2003, 112ff) content analysis of French management literature supports these claims. They identified several features of the flexible employee, specifically, middle managers. According to their analysis, ideal workers are multitaskers, innovative, mobile, venturesome, and able to cooperate with people of various backgrounds and cultures. They are autonomous, informed, spontaneous, creative, and able to adapt to different work tasks. Additionally, they have a talent for communication and are capable of relating to others. Moreover, ideal productive subjects are active in continuing education and enthusiastic. Because of rising job insecurity, they accumulate social capital and cultivate expanding contact networks, which guarantee permanent employment in changing fields of work.

What is striking is the fact that the flexible employee is based upon a completely individualized concept of a disembodied, universal worker, which implies that every person has equal opportunity to adapt to this idealized image. Social attributes such as gender, ethnicity, or social background are generally not discussed. However, as is well-known, these are categories that structure social inequalities at the workplace and provide unequal resources for on-the-job success.

Before discussing these issues, I will first address the question of how the transformation to the universal flexible employee is accomplished. As section 3 shows, EI's psychological program is one of the key concepts in the self-government of individualized productive subjects directing them to become idealized workers.

9.3   Educating the Star Performer

Various experts have sought to understand people at work in an attempt to manage them more successfully. Hence, management has concentrated not only on the technical features of production but also on the psychological traits of the worker, for example, in recruitment, performance evaluation, and training (see Illouz, this volume). Therefore, psychological expertise has been in demand: "All sorts of problems of work—labor turnover, unrest, accidents, inefficiency, boredom, and much more—have been problematized in psychological terms, and attempts have been made to ameliorate these problems by acting upon the psychological dimensions of the workplace—at the level of the individual and the group" (Miller and Rose 1995, 429). Today, one of the most popular and widely used psychological concepts is EI.

This psychological program adopts an evolutionary perspective and draws on research results in the neurosciences in order to gain credibility. The emotional centers in the brain are held responsible for emotion regulation such as self-control under stress or the ability to adapt to change (Goleman 1998, 78), two of the core requirements of the flexible employee. Correct brain practice is said to prevent the hijacking by negative emotions. Additionally, brain functioning can be altered by mental training: "As a competence such as self-control strengthens, so do the corresponding circuits in the brain" (Goleman 1998, 239). If the brain is trained accordingly, people will be able to choose the emotions which are appropriate to and most useful in specific situations.

Whereas Goleman's 1995 book discussed the general concept of EI, his subsequent publications have dealt with the workplace in particular. According to Goleman (1998, 3), EI is especially important for on-the-job success (for an overview of the topic, see Bechtoldt, this volume). Emotional competence in dealing with ourselves and others is a crucial factor in becoming a star performer and can be learned with the help of mental training. Furthermore, as Goleman (1998, 4) declares, "In a time with no guarantees of job security, when the very concept of a 'job' is rapidly being replaced by 'portable skills,' these are prime qualities that make and keep us employable."

Though at first sight EI seems to be a value-free mental training technique, Goleman's transformation of the concept into emotional competencies in the workplace sheds light on the normative construction of the psychological agenda. Emotional competence is defined as a learned capability derived from EI resulting in outstanding work performance (Goleman 1998, 24ff). It includes traits such as innovation (being open to new ideas, approaches, and information), commitment (readily making sacrifices to meet a larger organizational goal), adaptability (flexibility in handling change), and achievement drive (striving to meet or improve a standard of excellence)—just to name a few. In particular, Goleman related the aptitude for leadership directly to the emotion management of others. In his view, the leader should act as an emotional guide: "Quite simply, in any human group the leader has maximal power to sway everyone's emotions. If people's emotions are pushed toward the range of enthusiasm, performance can soar; if people are driven toward rancor and anxiety, they will be thrown off stride" (Goleman, Boyatzis, and McKee 2002, 5).

The success of EI, with its emphasis on emotion management, reflects a shift in attitudes toward the display of emotions at work. Nowadays, emotions are no longer seen as a barrier to rational decision making. The management of emotions has become a symbol of a new rationality in the workplace (Fineman 2004). However, expressions of fear, anger, anxiety, and other disruptive emotions are still unacceptable in the occupational environment. In fact, personal needs, desires, and emotions have to be controlled in the service of organizational needs. The regulation of emotions in the self includes the channeling of negative emotions and the intentional activation of pleasant (e.g., enthusiasm) and unpleasant (e.g., anger) feelings (Matthews, Zeidner, and Roberts 2002, 472).

A negative emotion that is rapidly becoming one of the most serious economic concerns is occupational stress, frequently described as the Black Plague of the postindustrial era (Matthews et al. 2002, 489). The consequences of flexible capitalism—an increased workload combined with job uncertainty—have resulted in the widespread pressure of rising job performance expectations. Stress threatens not only the individual's health but also organizational success and, furthermore, places a burden on national health services. Again, emotionally intelligent individuals are said to be especially effective in responding to stress (Goleman 1998, 82ff).

In a nutshell, EI recommends certain self-regulatory practices which reflect some of the requirements of flexible capitalism and correspond to the conception of the flexible employee. With the benefit of the appropriate brain training, the productive subject is able to evoke positive emotions such as enthusiasm and self-motivation and to manage negative feelings such as frustration or stress. As Jason Hughes (2005, 609) accurately comments, "EI constitutes a reinvention of character such that it is better aligned to a new organization of work: character which encompasses a broad range of skills to be developed as a lifetime project, but character which, by definition, is flexible, adaptable, open to individual nuance, and to the ever-present change of the global market place." Drawing on Michel Foucault's (1988) concept of the technology of the self, the following section sheds another light on this reinvention of character.

9.4   Technologies of the Emotional Self

On the one hand, enterprising employees who readily adapt to changing circumstances promise rising productivity. On the other hand, they pose a managerial control problem. If direct hierarchical supervision is reduced to promote creativity and individual entrepreneurship, how can management be sure that the worker is completely devoted to the entrepreneurial goal? The solution lies in the worker's internalization of control.

Considering this, EI can be characterized as a *technology of the self* (Foucault 1988; Lemke 2000, 2001), as a technique for governing the subject. The concept developed by Foucault (1988, 18) permits "individuals to effect by their own means or with the help of others a certain number of operations on their own bodies and souls, thoughts, conduct, and way of being, so as to transform themselves in order to attain a certain state of happiness, purity, wisdom, perfection, or immortality." Workers, as a result, are actively and voluntarily involved in their own emotional refashioning.

Self-management is economically desirable, too. From the Foucaultian perspective, EI can be understood as a subjectification technique. The microtechnology of everyday life allows individuals to modify their lifestyle and live in accordance with the requirements of flexible capitalism. The technologies of the self are closely linked to entrepreneurs' aim of maximizing profit and dealing with political concerns about regulating the productive life of nations. The disciplining of the body and the optimization of its (emotional) capabilities ease its integration into the economic system undergoing transformation.

While individuals perform this transformation themselves in order to facilitate success at work, this does not indicate that the autonomous person is acting freely. On the contrary, processes of subjectification have always enjoyed a close relationship to political rationalities. The government of individuals, as a mentality that defines the logic of action and thought, leads groups of people toward certain aims that are supposed to be achieved with the help of programs, strategies, and tactics (Foucault 1979).

In democracies, psychology as a language of expertise plays an important role in the subjectification processes. In contrast to autocracies, domination and coercion of subjects cannot be legitimately exercised to achieve the desired practices in individuals. On the contrary, "government is achieved through educating citizens, in their professional roles and in their personal lives—in the language by which they interpret their experiences, the norms by which they should evaluate them, the techniques by which they should seek to improve them" (Rose 1997, 75–76). Governing practices such as EI seek to endow subjects with a certain shape and with a certain psychological state, which results in personal aspirations and desires appropriate to the contemporary political rationality.

The rise of flexible capitalism is also closely tied to neoliberalism as a political rationality, a governing mentality that subordinates the social domain to an economic logic. Moreover, the call for personal responsibility and self-care is accompanied by a reduction in welfare state services (Lemke 2001, 203). Where the regulatory competence of the state decreases, the individual should establish self-regulating practices in order to avoid social risks such as illness, unemployment, poverty, and so forth. Responsibility is assigned to individuals and not to state agencies, which had hitherto been charged with the administration of risks generated by the economic system. Emotional problems such as anger or stress are therefore not interpreted as outcomes of problematic events or inadequate organizational structures. On the contrary, managing negative emotions is regarded as a task of the individual's emotional work which thus places the responsibility for the prevention of bad feelings on the productive subject.

Nevertheless, EI is not simply a psychological program of self-transformation. The successfully merchandized and popularized concept gained ground not only in psychology, neurobiology, and business administration but also in computer science. Here, researchers in the fields of affective and wearable computing are trying to create computers capable of supporting human beings in the development of EI.

9.5 Affective Computing

Rosalind W. Picard (1998, x), a leading researcher in affective computing, reports, "I have come to the conclusion that if we want computers to be genuinely intelligent, to adapt to us, and to interact naturally with us, then they will need the ability to recognize and express emotions, to have emotions, and to have what has come to be called 'emotional intelligence.' " In her work, she refers to the publications of Goleman (1995), saying that "emotional abilities are more important than traditional IQ for predicting success in life" (Picard 1998, 13).

Affective computing is just one example of the so-called third generation of computing, where—after the diffusion of bulky mainframes and smaller personal computers—*computational components* are supposed to recede into the background of our lives. Since the middle 1990s, the top-ranking engineering university, the Massachusetts Institute of Technology (MIT), has been working on the construction of a "technologically enhanced second skin" (Andrejevic 2005, 113), where the human body is supposed to intimately connect to computers. These research fields appeal not only to scientists but also to politicians, governments, military agencies, and the computer, media and health industries (Baumeler 2005). Consequently, the MIT Media Lab—the birthplace of the technological vision of "being digital" (Negroponte 2000)—receives heavy funding from a large and various collection of private sponsors as diverse as Microsoft and Wal-Mart (Hassan 2003, 93).

According to the vision of *wearable computing*, users are wearing computers as clothes or accessories in an intimate way. Nevertheless, the wearability of computational components is not the only requirement, because computers are supposed to become smart. The computer envisioned should know the situation the user is in (context sensitivity), should enhance the user's perception (augmented reality), and should act according to user's anticipated wishes without having to ask (proactive acting). Smart clothes, as Alex P. Pentland (2000, 35) claims, "provide personalized information about the surrounding environment, such as the names of people you meet or directions to your next meeting, and can replace most computer and consumer electronics. The key idea is that because the room or the clothing knows something about what is going on it can react intelligently."

The vision of affective computing is closely related to wearable computing and proposes the construction of a computer that directly supports the user in emotion management. Rosalind W. Picard, who coined the term in 1994, reports that "research at the MIT Media Laboratory [is] aimed at giving computers the ability to comfortably sense, recognize, and respond to the human communication of emotion, especially affective states such as frustration, confusion, interest, distress, anger, and joy" (Picard 2000, 705). Sensors worn in long-term physical contact are supposed to recognize the user's emotions via physiological parameters of the human body such as respiration, heart rate, pulse, temperature, electrodermal response, perspiration, and blood pressure.

In this field of emotional context sensitivity, the affective computer envisioned provides the user with an augmented reality. Bodily sensors will identify more than human beings ordinarily do and, therefore, will recognize emotions that humans normally do not. While detecting the human emotional expression, the affective computer will also be able to act proactively and "undo some of the negative feelings it causes by helping a user manage his or her emotional state" (Picard and Klein 2002, 141).

In addition to the formulation of technical research questions (such as how to accurately identify emotions via biometric data), computer scientists are creating a variety of future application scenarios in order to clarify the (economic) benefit of their project. Some of the user scenarios for workplace applications presented below reveal the normative assumptions about the flexible employee as a completely informed and emotionally controlled individual.

9.6 Workplace Scenarios of Emotion Regulation

The analysis of user scenarios indicates the normative assumptions of a research field. Whereas some applications are suggested for autistic people, shopping, teaching, and so forth, there are also some proposals for the workplace. A suggested computational device, called an "affective mirror," aids emotion management in the context of applying for a job and responds to the issue of self-responsible employability in the age of flexible capitalism:

Imagine the most important interview of your life, with the head of the company that you have always wanted to work for. He asks you tough questions about problems you have solved, challenges you have faced, and why you want to leave your present job. At the end of this grueling meeting, he tells you that you were too nervous-sounding, had unusually short pauses in your speech, were evasive with eye contact, and had cold clammy hands. This was not the real thing, fortunately, but a practice session in front of your trusted computer. Your computer interviewing agent, displaying the face of the CEO, asked you questions while listening to changes in your voice and discourse parameters. It watched your facial expressions and body language, sensing changes in physiological parameters such as your skin conductivity and temperature. It watched your affective responses to see where they differed from what it usually senses from you in day-to-day interaction (Picard 1998, 86).

Another field of investigation is occupational stress. Picard and Du (2002, 14) argue that "many people are unaware of their stress levels and the effects of their emotional states." The researchers then visualize a device that aids in the collection of data for the measurement of (positive) stress and the ability of computers to support the positive state of so-called "flow" by blocking out interruptions. This scenario focuses on emotion management in order to raise productivity:

Some people lead such busy lives that their most precious commodity is an hour or two of uninterrupted time. It may be planned time, with the phone unplugged and a "come back tomorrow" sign posted on the door, or it may be fortuitous, occurring while a person gets deeply engrossed in work and loses track of time, and nobody happens to interrupt. One potential application of affective computing is to help the latter situation happen more often. With suitable sensors, a computer has a good chance of discerning your engrossed state, measuring EEG [electroencephalogram], blood flow, and other factors known to correlate highly with cognitive load and with deep involvement in a problem. The pleasurable and highly productive mental state people experience when they are deeply engaged in a task has been called "flow". . . . Once in this state, people usually do not want to be interrupted, except, of course for emergencies. If your computer could recognize your flow state without ruining it by interrupting to ask if you are in the state, then you might consider it desirable to have it notify your email agent, phone controller, and other potential interruptions to not disturb you except for an emergency (Picard 1998, 104).

Affective computing is also intended to help humans "manage difficult events, thereby rendering day-to-day existence less stressful and perhaps, more productive and pleasurable" (Picard and Klein 2002, 157). Negative emotions caused by stress, such as anger, cynicism, mistrust, and aggression, are said to have a direct link to heart disease. The following scenario provides an example of self-regulation, self-care, and self-management. The affective computer is supposed to actively monitor physiological changes related to stress (here: heart rate variability) in order to prevent cardiovascular disease:

Morning: Mike showers and before he dresses, he snaps on his health monitor. He grabs a bagel, his briefcase, and his freshly recharged cell phone and runs to catch the train. On the train, he flips open the phone for a quick chat with his Health Expert—"Bud." Bud tells Mike that yesterday's heart stress levels were the best yet—nice and low—except for during the evening, between 5:00 and 10:00 PM. He congratulates Mike on his steadfastness with checking in, saying his heart patterns are typical for someone four years younger. He asks if Mike wants to tell about what happened yesterday. Mike says, "No time now; later."

Afternoon: After five hours of meetings, Mike pops open the phone again while he's standing in line to grab lunch, to see how he's doing. Bud says that the morning levels were unusually high—similar to last night. Mike asks to see the graphs, and Bud shows them on the phone's display. Mike says, "Oh, this morning was a meeting with unhappy clients; I just heard about it last night at 5:00 PM and had to prepare for the meetings." Bud says, "I will annotate last night and this morning as 'meetings with unhappy clients' unless you say 'no.'" Mike says "that's fine" and Bud annotates the graphs. Bud asks Mike if he'd like some 1-minute tips for lowering his stress. Mike says "sure" and Bud walks him through a simple exercise. Mike asks Bud to give him a ring later that night, and then practices this exercise as he walks slowly back to the office. A glance at his phone shows him that it's helping—his stress level has gone down. That afternoon, while dealing with the crisis, Mike remembers how good he felt doing the exercise, and gives it another try.

Evening: On the train home, Bud rings Mike to see if now is a good time to follow-up. Bud shows Mike that he's back down to his previous good level for that time of day. Mike asks Bud to compare today to his worst (most stressful) day. Bud displays a graph from a day labeled "crisis with boss" and juxtaposes this with today's graph. Mike recognizes that he is much more in control of his stress now; he smiles and thanks Bud for the help (Picard and Du 2002, 16).

As this application demonstrates, users are supposed to manage stress themselves and, therefore, stay healthy and productive. This device was assembled with commercially available products such as sensors from a company called FitSense and a cellular phone from Motorola, a sponsor of the MIT Media Lab. Besides the reinvention of the self as a completely informed individual with self-regulating emotion management, the scenario proposes further applications for already existing technical devices. These technical devices would include a wide range of other potential sponsors: "It is also technically possible for the system to be adapted to display data on other devices, such as a wristwatch, hand-held computer, pager, or even your local refrigerator door with its future electronic display" (Picard and Du 2002, 18).

Taking a closer look at the proposed user scenarios, it is interesting to see that affective computing transforms Goleman's concept of EI. While Goleman focused on the understanding and labeling of emotions as a task that the individual has to fulfill, affective computing delegates the recognition and identification of emotions to the computer. From this perspective, the original concept of EI is redefined and solely based upon a one-way flow of biometric data.

The development of affective computing can be interpreted as a technological packaging for the ideal flexible employee who fulfills the demands of flexible capitalism (emotion and health management combined with high productivity) and, consequently, as a transformation of the self resulting from the merging of a psychological program with a computational technology. As these scenarios illustrate, EI does not remain on the level of mental training but is going to be developed as a materialized technology of the self.

9.7   Hidden Gender Issues

As this chapter has shown, EI and its offspring, affective computing, act in concert with the political rationality of flexible capitalism. Each period gives rise to distinct notions of the qualities of the worker, and the age of flexible capitalism calls for flexible employees who can master emotion and health management, as well as maintain their employability. Therefore, drawing on Foucault's technology of the self, EI and affective computing can be interpreted as related techniques for governing the productive subject. Both EI and affective computing start from the notion of a universal worker, rendering social attributes such as gender and social class invisible. Eva Illouz (this volume) shows that EI can be interpreted as a concept that reaffirms the social privileges of the middle classes, which, in contrast to members of the working class, have learned to talk about their feelings. From this perspective, EI is likely to reproduce the existing social inequalities. However, it is an open question whether EI and its computational counterpart will exert any influence on the widespread gender inequality in occupational success.

Neither Goleman's work nor affective computing take into account the influences of structural factors such as inequality regimes in the workplace. Thus, with the appropriate brain training or smart device, every person can become a star performer. This applies to the gender dimension as well. Basically, EI is promoted as a gender-neutral concept. The conventional wisdom is that women are more aware of their emotions and better at showing empathy, while men are more self-confident, optimistic, and adaptive and are better at handling stress. However, regarding total EI, Goleman (1998, 7) claims that there are no sex differences.

Some authors present a different view and even speak of the "feminization of management" (Fondas 1997), in saying that qualities defined as feminine (and culturally ascribed to women), such as empathy, caring, interpersonal sensitivity, and orientation toward the collective interest, have spread to organizational work. The redrawing of the traditional masculine/feminine hierarchy of logic/emotion (Hatcher 2003) and the demand for more emotionality in the workplace seem first and foremost to favor female employees. However, if we conceive of EI as a technology of the self with a close connection to the political rationality of flexible capitalism, hidden gender issues can be revealed which do not appear to favor most women.

As a wide range of organization studies demonstrates, organizations are not gender-neutral entities but are constituted by gendered inequalities, gendered images, and gendered interactions (Acker 1998, 196f). Representing an organization, a concept of a productive subject, or a form of intelligence as gender neutral obscures the fact that a gender substructure of organization exists, which reproduces gender inequality and provides unequal access to resources. This also applies to the concept of the "job" (Acker 1990) which generally is formulated for a disembodied, universal worker and implies that ordinary employees are people who have few obligations outside work, are devoid of daily family responsibilities, and immerse themselves completely in their work tasks. Based on the current separation of production and procreation, the worker is, effectively, masculine. This conception is also reflected in the contemporary productive subject, because—as I have shown—EI is just one element in the cluster of qualities expected in flexible employees and goes hand in hand with other requirements, such as the capacity for constant change, mobility, entrepreneurship, increased competition, self-responsibility for employability, increasing demands for overtime and higher productivity, and the decline in welfare state services. Considering the fact that most women in the industrial countries of the North still face the complex reality of raising children and earning money in part-time arrangements, flexible capitalism does not seem to favor women's careers in particular. As a consequence, it seems highly unlikely that increasing demands for EI in the workplace will change the persistent gender inequality regime and shatter the glass ceiling in the workplace.

10   The Economic Brain: Neuroeconomics and "Post-Autistic Economics" through the Lens of Gender

Gotlind Ulshöfer

10.1   Neuroeconomics and Its Challenges

A new discipline has emerged which brings together neurobiology, economics, and psychology: neuroeconomics. Economists and neuroscientists cooperate in focusing on the effects of products and economic behaviors on the human brain and on the brain's activities during economic decision making. Economic theory and marketing are affected by this research, which takes into view especially the emotional aspects of decision making.

In Germany, for example, the boom in neuroeconomics started in 2001 with one of the first public presentations of a marketing study which used neuroscientific results conducted at the University of Magdeburg, Germany. Institutes of neuroeconomics have been established at universities worldwide. However, for-profit imaging institutes have also been founded—for example, in the United States there were more than 88 for-profit imaging marketing institutes in the year 2004 (Hüsing, Jäncke, and Tag 2006, 149f).

In this chapter I want to look at neuroeconomic research from a gender perspective and analyze what brain research is doing in the area of economics, and how this research interest is connected to a broader view of economy and society. I will interpret neuroeconomic research as a reaction of capitalism to the critique that capitalism lacks emotions—in the sense of Luc Boltanski and Ève Chiapello (2006), who assume in their study *Le nouvel Ésprit du Capitalisme* (The New Spirit of Capitalism; French original 1999) that this economic system responds to these critiques. I will also try to explain where I see the deficiencies and problems of neuroeconomics, concerning present-day Western economic systems. My focus will be on scientific research in neuroeconomics, which does not exclude neuromarketing (e.g., Zimmermann 2006), but I will not place marketing and its problematic sides in the center of my analysis.

My analysis will take into account the following challenges of the self-understanding of human beings which emerge through neuroeconomics. First, how does neuroeconomics question the assumptions of economic theory with respect to its image of the model human being, *homo oeconomicus*, and the theory's individualistic methodology? This leads to a second point where the conventional "economic brain" is examined: The role of emotions has become a challenge for the economic rationality relevant in economic science (Priddat 2007, 215). What are the emotional aspects of economic decision making (e.g., Sanfey, Loewenstein, McClure, and Cohen 2006)? Third, neuroeconomics challenges the idea of power and influence over the self, especially in the field of neuromarketing: Can big companies—by knowing how the brain works emotionally—manipulate human behaviors? This is a fear expressed by Sandra Blakeslee in her article, "If Your Brain Has a 'Buy Button,' What Pushes It?" in *The New York Times* (October 19, 2004), referring to arguments from the U.S. nongovernmental organization Consumer Alert with respect to neuromarketing research. Fourth, neuroeconomics also challenges the self in the way it deals with society: Which underlying concepts of economy and society are used in neuroeconomics? What is the role of the individual from this perspective? Do individuals have to optimize themselves and adapt to the economic sphere? How are outstanding individuals, such as leaders, perceived? All four challenges are related to the question of how gender and sexual stereotyping influence the findings of neuroeconomics and vice versa.

10.2   The "Economic Brain" and Its Critiques

For mainstream economics, "the economic brain" has a clear characteristic: It is rational in the sense that the utility of the individual is maximized (Blaug 1993, 229ff), independent of any social influence. These assumptions are aggregated and labeled as *homo oeconomicus*, being central to the leading paradigm in economics, that is, neoclassical economics with its methodological individualism (Persky 1995). Economic rationality in general has been located in the human brain—and therefore we can also refer to *homo oeconomicus* as "the economic brain." In its traditional form, economic rationality is based on the idea of full information, which is processed in the brain to make rational decisions. *Homo oeconomicus* is a theoretical construct, enabling the "science" of economics to describe economic processes as processes of decision making which tend toward equilibrium. Emotions have not been considered important within economic theory. This might also be due to the fact that the bodily localization of emotions has been unclear for the last few centuries, and the finding of valid data concerning the influence of emotions and other factors on economic behavior has been difficult. "Since feelings were meant to predict behavior but could only be assessed from behavior, economists realized that, without direct measurement, feelings were useless intervening constructs" (Camerer, Loewenstein, and Prelec 2005, 10). Economists themselves are generally aware of the modeling character of their analyses, its underlying assumptions, and its deficits (Ulshöfer 2001, 75ff).

Nevertheless, there is a long tradition of criticizing *homo oeconomicus* as inadequate when making "real-life-decisions," leaving out important aspects like the sociality of human beings and emotions—as can be seen in sociology or when looking at the history of economics (Ulshöfer 2003, Rammel 2002). *Homo oeconomicus* has been characterized critically in many different ways—for example, as a "lust machine" as nineteenth century British economist Francis Ysidro Edgeworth called the model (Tietzel 1981, 117).

The focus of present-day critiques of the economic brain lies as well on the lack of emotions, the individualism, and the self-centeredness of this model. These critiques can be seen in "post-autistic economics" (PAE) and in most of feminist economics,[1] for example. At present, one of the most popular descriptions of *homo oeconomicus* is "autistic"[2]—taking up a description from the natural sciences to refer to a behavior, which is assumed similarly self-centered. Autists' lack of a "theory of mind," that is, "to make attributions about the mental states (desires, beliefs, intentions) of others" (Singer and Fehr 2005, 340), is brought into relation with the individualistic, nonrelationalist characteristic of a market participant in economic theory. Autism as a characteristic of and within the "science"[3] of economics has been exposed by the newly emerged *"post-autistic economics" movement*, and it is also used in neuroeconomics to describe those people who act in line with the individualism of the economic theory.

In 2000, economics students at the Sorbonne in France wrote a petition entitled *Autisme-Économie* (Dürmeier 2006, 14), calling for a more pluralistic economic theory. Their protest spread to universities in other countries, like the United Kingdom, Germany, and the United States, gaining support among renowned scholars like James Kenneth Galbraith (Galbraith 2001), and has reached an international audience with its online journal *Post-Autistic Economics Review*.[4] Besides the critique of methodological individualism in economics with its self-centeredness as well as the lack of social and cooperative characteristics in *homo oeconomicus* (Arbeitskreis Postautistische Ökonomik 2006, 29), their critique also referred to the uncontrolled use of mathematics, the lack of pluralism in the economic approach, the paucity of realism, and, at the pedagogical level, the need to teach more than the established skills (Fullbrook 2003, 13f). By labeling the well-known critique of economics "post-autistic," the French students managed to attach their demands to the ongoing dialogue on the role of emotions in capitalist societies. Hollywood films like *Rainman* (1986), for example, thematized the topic of individuals who are unable to get into a proper relation with other people by using an autist as the main character in the film, and so autism found its way into the public realm (see also Karafyllis, this volume, for details). This critique also stands in relation to standard critique of capitalism for nurturing egoism, exclusive self-interest, and self-centeredness (Boltanski and Chiapello 2006, 79ff).

Although feminist critique does not use the "label" autistic, there are similarities between PAE and feminist economics. In 1993, Marianne A. Ferber and Julie A. Nelson edited a "pathbreaking collection" (Jacobsen 2007, 21) of feminist critiques of economics called *Beyond Economic Man* (Ferber and Nelson 1993), in which the assumptions of neoclassical economics were also under attack. Paula England, for example, describes the characteristics of *homo oeoconomicus* as expressing a "separative self" (England 1993, 37), that is, a self which is not emotionally connected to others, lacks empathy, and is autonomous. However, feminist analysis goes further than PAE by detecting the underlying gender bias in economic models and revealing them as "androcentric," that is, that the existing system of gender relations has been chosen because it is biased in favor of men's interests (England 1993, 37), which are often considered to be different from women's interests. This imbalance is especially clear in Gary S. Becker's "new home economics" (Becker 1991), where he applies the neoclassical model to the household. Here, market and family behavior are differentiated: "In the family, individuals (particularly men) are presumed to be altruistic. Thus, empathic emotional connections between individuals are emphasized in the family whereas they are denied in analyzing markets" (England 1993, 37). Becker refers to the paternal altruism of the "family head," traditionally the man, who takes financially responsibility for the family, in order to be able to go on with a single utility function for the family, without mentioning that the "head of the family" also traditionally controls the resources. With this assumption a gender bias is implicit. Although both forms of criticism are similar, gender issues are not a priority for the PAE movement—a fact criticized by feminists (Nelson 2001).

In a way, neuroeconomics can be seen as a reaction to these forms of criticism of economics, although no direct references are made to them. In neuroeconomics the role of emotions for economic decision making is researched, which also relativizes the *homo oeconomicus* concept. In some of the neuroeconomic studies, economic rational behavior is labeled "autistic" as well. However, it is never declaring itself as being radically critical of economics. Neuroeconomics can be seen in the tradition of adding new and other methodologies to economics. In this sense, "behavioral economics" can be understood as its forerunner.

For the last two decades, "behavioral economics" has been doing psychological and cognitive science research on economic behavior and its relation to economic topics such as finance, game theory, macroeconomics, and so forth (Camerer, Loewenstein, and Prelec 2005, 9). This way of taking up psychological and particularly cognitive insights into economic theory and of also using laboratory experiments in economics was acknowledged by the broader scientific community in 2002, when the Nobel Prize committee awarded the prize for economics to two scholars who have challenged neoclassical economics: Daniel Kahneman and Vernon Smith.[5] Although these approaches are further developing economics (Ross 2005), in general, the neoclassical paradigm is still dominant in economics.

The transdisciplinary field of neuroeconomics also deals with the topic of emotions in economic decision making but challenges the "economic brain" in a different way: Instead of merely observing behavior, brain functions are measured in vivo while subjects are active with economic decision making. With brain- and neuroimaging technologies, emotions and feelings are thought to be empirically verifiable and can, therefore, also be taken consideration for economic decision making and economic theory, that is, for a "science" like economics (Gächter 2005, 2).

Since PAE as well as feminist economics do not put the brain at the center of its analysis or critique of economic theory, and since the focus of this chapter is on the "economic brain," it is neuroeconomics which will be analyzed here in depth in order to show the ways in which brain research stands in relation to economics and economy.

10.3   Flexible Capitalism, the Economic Brain, and Gender

In neuroeconomic research, biological, medical, economic, and business issues merge. This merging also has a problematic side: For research, functional magnetic resonance imaging (fMRI) scanners are needed, which are usually found in clinics. With the possibility of carrying out commercial studies, there is, on the one hand, the chance of financing these expensive instruments and apparatus. On the other hand, it is said that the effects of research done in this setting have to be evaluated very carefully (Steinmetzer and Müller 2007). The intermingling of business interests and scientific research is one of the critical points concerning this connection, as is, for example, referred to in the critical letter of Consumer Alert, that has been criticizing Emory University for allowing neuromarketing research on its campus.[6]

These networks between business corporations and universities can also be interpreted as part of flexible capitalism which Richard Sennett (1998, 2006) describes in his analysis. One characteristic of this kind of capitalism is "networks." The cooperation needed in neuromarketing can be understood as networking—with the effects that power is diffused. The two other characteristics of the underlying power system of flexible capitalism are an ongoing restructuring of organizations, institutions, and corporations. And this means also for production that it has to be more flexible and more specialized, so that there can be more innovations in shorter time periods (Sennett 1998). The organizational structures correspond with characteristics which are needed by human beings living in this era of flexible capitalism—as flexible employees who can easily adapt to changing situations (see also Baumeler, this volume) and who need to have a certain attitude in order to be able to survive. They should be short-term oriented, looking toward the future, neglecting past experiences, and having their potential abilities and their development in mind rather than real achievements (Sennett 2006, 83ff). The ideal of a market with its individualized market participants with economic brains seems to have become reality.

However, for employees as well as for the elites and leaders in this setting, their abilities have become more important, since flexibility and change are the most relevant features in this economic world. Sennett makes this clear by referring to testing culture and what it tests: the "innate abilities" of human beings (Sennett 2006, 117). The employees need the potential abilities and not so much the "craftsmanship," as Sennett calls the deeper knowledge about something. This situation also has an influence on human beings on a more personal level: "Potential ability focuses only on the self. The statement 'you lack potential' is much more devastating than 'you messed up.' It makes a more fundamental claim about who you are" (Sennett 2006, 123).

In this setting, emotions are considered to be important and play two different roles. On the one hand, they can be seen as needed in order to improve one's situation in this context. Since abilities have become relevant, emotional abilities might be considered important now as well—for this interpretation of the situation we can name Daniel Goleman's idea of Emotional Intelligence (EI).

On the other hand, emotions play an important role in coping with the challenges this situation provides—thereby, three challenges can be distinguished. First, how can the individual handle unstable life situations (how to deal with uncertainties and risks)? The second question is how is one to survive in the situation and make the most out of it, as an individual, but still relate to others—be it in a business or in a personal context? How is one to maintain relationships when moving from one town or even one country to another is required by the job in short time periods? And the third challenge is how is one to learn to adapt to the social environment, also emotionally, and still find one's own way with respect to how to do things?

In Arlie Russell Hochschild's book *The Managed Heart* (1983), she analyzes the situation of "emotional labor" in the workplace. Her concept of "emotional labor" refers to paid work which requires adapting one's emotions and feelings to the working situation where a certain emotion is required (Hochschild 1983, 7). In the occupations of care which are often held by women, part of the professional education is learning to manage emotions (Colley 2003). However, emotional labor in society is not restricted to women; men are also part of this both societal and social demand (Soares 2003, 37). If a person does not have the demanded emotion in his or her repertoire of emotions, she or he obviously has to train it, that is, make it emerge or suppress it. In this way, the economic brain is challenged, economic rationality is no longer sufficient, and emotions seem to be required. Emotional labor in times of flexible capitalism is not restricted to service jobs (Zapf et al. 2000; Zapf and Holz 2006). Leaders are also required to refer to emotions—or does leadership mean using an economic brain? And what role do organizations play, especially if we see them as social contexts where gender roles are inscribed (Acker 1990), so that gender, race, and class all play a role? Differences between the behavior which is accepted and how the pay for work and labor is determined run along the lines of sex, race, and class (e.g., Rhode 2003a, 2003b). There are parallel processes concerning gender and race groups, and exclusion mechanisms: In top positions, women and people of color, in European and U.S. contexts at least, are in a minority; they are assigned a lower social status and are subject to negative stereotypes in relation to important competencies for top positions (Parker and ogilvie 2003, 182). We can still see a gender and race gap concerning wages in the United States[7] as well as in Europe (European Commission 2007). Equal pay for equal work is not the rule. In the European Union, the gross wage per hour for women is between 63% and 90% of that of men, depending on the work area (Eurostat 2007). The wage gap is where gender discrimination is most obvious (see also the Introduction to this volume).[8] Affirmative action, which is positive discrimination for the benefit of those groups in society which have traditionally been discriminated against—for example, women, homosexuals/lesbians, persons of color, and so forth—was one strategy in the 1980s to improve their political, social, and economic situation. In the 1990s, "comparable worth" was a political strategy to ensure equal wages for men and women in their occupations in order to abolish sex-based differences. In her description of the development and implementation of "comparable worth," Joan Acker—a professor of sociology and member of its legislative task force—shows just how difficult it is to transform a system, because, among other reasons, the techniques used are also political (Acker 1989). This is something the Gender Equality approach of the European Union is emphasizing at present as well. Gender mainstreaming has become an important E.U. policy since the beginning of the 21st century, focusing on equal treatment and equal opportunities for women and men by legislative, mainstreaming, and political actions.[9] The details of the strengths and weaknesses of these concepts will not be discussed here, but the concepts show that important criteria for improvements of participation in leadership, for example, are the ways and principles for admission to these positions.

In the era of flexible capitalism, with the possibilities afforded by the neurosciences, the questions concerning how to get into top positions are put anew: Will there be brain scans in the future for detecting the perfect flexible employee, in addition to the traditional achievement and ability tests, and what about the influences and tests possibly to be developed by the neurosciences on the behaviors of consumers?

Before we come back to the relation of the economic brain, neuroeconomics, and leadership, a closer look is needed at how neuroeconomics deals with this situation in flexible capitalism. The brain has become a central subject in flexible capitalism because it stands for the stability and continuity of the individual and can also be seen as his or her "instrument" to adapt to uncertain situations. Neuroeconomics focuses on the brain and tries to reveal the emotional elements of economic decision making. In order to be able to understand the underlying ideas concerning neuroeconomics, I will focus now on the research methods in this discipline.

10.4 Neuroeconomic Research

10.4.1 Introduction

In general, neuroeconomics researches the connection of brain activities with certain forms of economic behavior. Individual decision making could be considered, as well as social exchange, or behavior in relation to institutions such as markets; taken together, "the working hypothesis is that the brain has evolved different, but interdependent, adaptive mechanisms for each of these tasks involving experience, memory and perception" (Smith 2002, 550). With this broad description of a potential research field, Vernon Smith opens it up, but at present mostly economic decision making in the broadest sense (including marketing issues) is researched in neuroeconomics. The brain, and especially those areas in the brain which are considered to be emotion related, and which can be seen as being active during economic activities as well, are at the center of this research, which takes place in a laboratory.

The focus on economic "decision making"—which means having the choice between different options, generally framed as an investment or noninvestment of money, or, to describe it differently, as a decision about how to use the money provided in the game—can be seen as a reduction of economics and economic issues: Abstract tests or games, like the ultimate game,[10] are typically designed for one or two players with a certain task which is theorized to detect an "emotion," that is, activities in brain regions ascribed to emotional processes. In some of the experiments, a questionnaire is used after the scans to detect what the person says verbally in relation to the researched hypothesis (e.g., Singer et al. 2006). Blood is sometimes drawn before and after the games to detect hormonal reactions; thus, at least part of the body is taken into consideration (Zak, Borja, Matzner, and Kurzban 2005, e.g.). However, the focus lies primarily on the brain.

10.4.2 The Four Main Topics in Neuroeconomic Testing

Neuroeconomic experiments in general deal with four topics, although one experiment might deal with different topics at the same time. These topics can be seen on a broader level as generated within the framework of flexible capitalism—since the three basic questions mentioned above with respect to how individuals can cope with this economic situation is also relevant in them.

First, there are experiments which deal with central categories of economic theory like utility, preferences, and incentives, and the question of which role "emotions" or other nonrational elements, like, for example, attitudes, play in the tests which are oriented toward these concepts (Sanfey, Loewenstein, McClure, and Cohen 2006,

109f). A comparison is made between *homo oeconomicus* and "living people," also trying to understand basic elements in modern economic theories—like game theory (Camerer 2003). This implies a comparison of science and society (see the Introduction to this volume). As an example for a new understanding of a basic economic issue, research on the utility of money and the reactions of the brain to financial gains can be mentioned here. The reactions to the gains are found to take place in the reward center of the brain and elicit the same activation as other attractive things. This result stands in contrast to economic theory because here money is considered a medium, not as something which represents a direct reward. The idea underlying the study on money might have been to give "physiological evidence" for a feature in capitalism that money is a direct reward and with it to make economic theory more realistic.[11]

The second topic refers to the basic situation of human beings in flexible capitalism. The question is how to deal with uncertainties and ambiguities. The "economic brain," being a present-oriented utility maximizer, does not take time aspects into account in general. Therefore, decisions under this premise cannot give a clue how to handle these situations in real life. Neuroeconomic researchers bring the temporal aspects of decision making into view (e.g., Huettel et al. 2006). However, there is a long tradition in economics about the exposure to risk and uncertainty and economic decisions made in relation to them. In economics, exposure to risk and uncertainty has often been dealt with as a problem of probability calculation. In neuroeconomics, the question of how people make decisions in situations where there is risk (defined as "uncertainty with known probabilities") and ambiguity (defined as "uncertainty with unknown probabilities"; both Huettel et al. 2006, 765) is considered by testing the reactions of the brain in relation to decisions affecting the future.[12]

And third, human beings in individualized, flexible capitalism have the problem of how to keep up their social life, which communities they want to join, and what brings the communities together. Therefore, in neuroeconomics, researchers also look at "social" issues in experiments which deal with topics described by neuroeconomists as trust, altruism, cooperation, strong reciprocity, empathy, and fairness (e.g., Fehr and Fischbacher 2004). These behaviors, which are oriented toward other people, are of special interest for neuroeconomic research, because some of the behaviors, like altruism, for example (Ahlert and Kenning 2006, 38), are considered "abnormal" behaviors by economists and in the sphere of economics, since a behavior such as altruism does not fit with the "economic brain" and its utility-maximizing self-centered rationality.

On the other hand, seen from a societal point of view, as some neuroeconomists do, a number of these behaviors—like trust—are understood as being basic for the functioning of an economy (Zak 2004). One of the outstanding scientists dealing with trust is Paul J. Zak from Claremont, California. He also brings the social dimension of his research into view and emphasizes that trust is one of "the strongest predictors of whether a country will successfully develop: poor countries are by-and-large low-trust countries. This occurs because low trust inhibits investment and thereby the creation of wealth" (Zak, Borja, Matzner, and Kurzban 2005, 360). Trustworthiness for him means "cooperating when someone places trust in us" (Zak 2007, 2). In this quote from Zak, we can see that in these experiments a transgression of the economic paradigm, that is, the *homo oeconomicus*, takes place and a broader view on society is taken into account.

Fourth, neuroeconomic experiments focus on learning and reward mechanisms, sometimes in relation to the regulation of social relationships and sometimes with regard to marketing issues (Erk et al. 2002, 2499).

These four research areas in neuroeconomics show the relation of this new discipline to flexible capitalism, and the urge to take up the topics of emotions and nonrational reactions in economic decision making. In this sense, neuroeconomics looks at the deficits of flexible capitalism. In order to see how neuroeconomics approaches these issues—and if they really refer to a change in the "economic brain" and lead to a change in economic theory, and perhaps even in economic policy, and thus, maybe, resolve deficits of economic theory as well as capitalism—we need to take a closer look at the experiments and their experimental designs.

10.4.3 Test Persons and the Laboratory

The test persons involved in neuroeconomic experiments are often students,[13] considered to be "healthy," and they are recruited for playing games or solving the tasks put to them by scientists. Both men's and women's behaviors and emotions are researched, but only some of the tests are gendered. In neuroeconomic experiment descriptions, sometimes there is the contra-intuitive usage of "normal" and "autistic" for the test person: The category "normal" is used for the test person as long as she or he does not behave according to economic theory; otherwise, he or she is labeled "autistic."

The autistic person seems to have the perfect "economic brain"—which is in this context pathologized. Camerer and colleagues give an example of a student test person who is astonished at the noneconomic behavior of counterplayers in an "ultimate game."[14] They comment, "Ironically, while the subject's reasoning matches exactly how conventional game theory approaches the game, it sounds *autistic*, because this subject is surprised and perplexed by how normal people behave" (Camerer, Loewenstein, and Prelec 2005, 47).[15] "Normality" is defined here in a very narrow sense—the "norm" is just the majority of the researched persons' behavior. The small number of participants— approximately 20 to 30 volunteers or fewer in the experiments (e.g., Huettel et al. 2006, 772; Moll et al. 2006, 15626)—is probably due to the costly experimental settings: The experiments are carried out with technologies like fMRI, positron emission tomography, and magnetoencephalography (Ahlert and Kenning 2006, 32).

The person who takes part in an experiment with fMRI is put inside the fMRI test tube and answers questions or reacts to a game while his or her brain is scanned, that is, the blood flow in a specific brain region is measured. The images of the brain which are made with this technique are representations of reconstructions, created by algorithms and special software for image data processing on the computer. Therefore, it is problematic to say that these images are images of the real brain, representing brain functions and how they are really structured (Schmitz 2003). Also, the placement of the test person inside the fMRI machine might influence his or her behavior and the possible outcome of the experiment.

In his article "Mind Games: What Neuroeconomics Tells Us about Money and the Brain," in the September 18, 2006, edition of *The New Yorker*, John Cassidy describes his experience in a scanner at New York University's Center for Brain Research, where a graduate student, Peter Sokol-Hessner, guided him to the laboratory and through the experiment: "After an hour inside the machine, I was more concerned about getting out than I was about making a few dollars. . . . 'That's the terrible thing about MRIs,' Sokol-Hessner conceded. 'You are in a long tube, and you might feel tired or claustrophobic. There's definitely other stuff going on in there besides the experiment. We have to be very careful about how we interpret the evidence.'" However, there are some experiments in situations which are close to real-life situations, and which use not fMRI, but, for example, psychophysiological characteristics like skin conductance, blood volume pulse, heart rate, electromyographical signals, respiration, and body temperature as described in Andrew Lo and Dmitry V. Repin's field study. Lo and Repin measured foreign exchange traders while they were trading and making contracts in a volatile market in their "natural environment without disrupting their workflow while simultaneously capturing real-time financial pricing data from which market events can be defined" (Lo and Repin 2002, 232). They found out that "rapid market movements provoked traders' sympathetic nervous system; this can be interpreted as emotional response" (Zak 2004, 1743). In the field experiment, in which society became a "natural environment" of the actor, the question was also raised about the relationship between rational economic decisions and emotions.

As for individuals in flexible capitalism, it is also in these experiments that their own histories and individual experiences (i.e., the unique person) are not what is important here. The focus in the experiments is on the reaction of the human being in his or her brain, which everybody has. In contrast to the therapeutic use of brain scans, where the individual image is of importance for the diagnosis, and for finding deviations from health norms, here neuroimaging is used to set up economic and societal norms.

How is the "test person" seen—is he or she an "object" or a "subject"? Participants in the experiments are called "subjects" or "volunteers" (e.g., McCabe 2003) rather than "objects." The labeling refers first to the fact that the experiment is not a mass scanning, which is forced on the population, but a voluntary decision to participate in the experiment. It also alludes to the point that participants in the experiments might only be part of a certain group in society, for example, students. Second, by using "subjects," the idea might still resonate that human beings are the participants, that is, persons with their own individual history and experience. On the other hand, the boundary between subject and object is vague here, because while subjective processes are experienced by the person, neuroscientists look for a causality-related effect in the brain which can be generalized and thus made objective. Therefore, the neuroimage resulting from a scan should allow scientists to make inferences about abstract generalities of human economic behavior. In this sense, "objectification"[16] (Nussbaum 1999b, 218) takes place here through fungibility: Although the persons tested are subjects, the experiments turn them into objects because their brains are seen as interchangeable. It is not their individuality which is observed and focused on, but the common reaction of all volunteers in the test. The search for the localization of emotions in the brain by scanning and by testing also implies, in a way, a "standardization" of reaction patterns a priori and a posteriori. By taking the majority of the neural activations' region, size, and intensity as the "norm," this kind of behavior comes to be seen as the standard for human beings in this situation. Due to the small number of test persons in the experiments as well as the special laboratory setting, these standardized conclusions about humans are difficult to evaluate.

10.4.4 Two Experiments: Detecting Emotions and Sexualizing Brains in Neuroeconomics and Neuromarketing

In this chapter I will focus on two experiments: one on empathy in neuroeconomics and the other on reward related to neuromarketing. In these experiments, the transgression of *homo oeconomicus* is most obvious because they deal with aspects which lie outside of the traditional economic rationality paradigm, and they also thematize differences between brains of men and women directly as well as indirectly.

The empathy experiment which will be described here was undertaken by the research group of Tania Singer and was published in *Nature* in 2006 (Singer et al. 2006). Empathy is understood in a neuroeconomic sense as enabling one "to share the emotion, pain and sensation of others" (Singer et al. 2006, 466). The study researched empathy reactions in the brains of men and women in relation to the fairness of others.

This kind of experiment is interesting for the field of economics for two reasons. First, it seems to reveal that the behavior in decision-making situations influences our perception of the person on an emotional, noncognitive level. This understanding contrasts with the assumptions of *homo oeconomicus*. Second, this experiment is an example of how a game—like the prisoner's dilemma game (PDG)—which is also used in economic theory becomes part of a test of empathy. The prisoner's dilemma game involves two players. The rules are that each one can choose to either defect or cooperate. When both defect, they will lose (lose money, lose the opportunity to go free, or lose the opportunity to be assigned some other fate, depending on how the game is structured); if both cooperate, they will both win; if one defects and the other cooperates, the defector wins more. Adding *homo oeconomicus* into this situation, the only rational answer to the PDG is the defection of both. On the other hand, people frequently cooperate in real-life situations. In the context of neuroscientific experiments, the PDG is often employed in order to thematize the willingness of the test persons to cooperate.

Here, the game has been used in the first part of the experiment with 16 men and 16 women as test persons and four actors, two men and two women. The aim at this stage of the experiment was to induce liking or disliking of players. The game was set up so that a sequentially iterated PDG was played. The "first player can trust a second player by sending 10 starting points (subsequently converted to money) to the other player knowing that each point sent will be tripled. The second player (confederate) then reciprocates by sending an amount between 0 and 10 points back, which is also tripled" (Singer et al. 2006, 468). The professional actors were the scientists' "confederates." Based upon previous findings, the researchers expected that the test persons would like fair players and dislike unfair ones.

The second step in the experiment was the scanning of participants in the fMRI in order to look for responses in the brains of the test persons to determine whether having seen the liked or disliked person in the game receiving a pain stimulus elicited different responses in the brains, that is, empathy for pain.

The third step was filling out questionnaires, that is, giving a rating on a standard empathy scale "to rate the intensity of the low and high stimulation, their liking for the two confederates, and their desire for revenge on the two confederates" (Singer et al. 2006, 468).

Focusing on the second step again, there were two important findings: Just seeing the pain produced in the other player elicited the pain-sensitive activation networks in the brain, but these brain regions reacted differently according to whether the recipient of the painful stimulation was a fair player or an unfair player. In the experiment, the results were differentiated along the lines of sex: Women's reactions to the pain inflicted on fair and unfair players were nearly the same. In men, the results were different: "the knowledge that an unfair player was in receipt of pain elicited no increase in empathic activity in FI [fronto-insular cortex]" (Singer et al. 2006, 467; see also figure 1.2, this volume), that is, part of the pain center. The second point is that seeing pain inflicted on unfair players is not the only difference between men's and women's brain activities. Men also have an increased activation in the left ventral striatum/nucleus accumbens (NA) (see figures 1.3a and 1.3b, this volume). The NA and the orbitofrontal cortex were correlated in the experiment with the desire for revenge (see figure 1.3d, this volume) since in the after-scan questionnaires, men showed a stronger desire for revenge than did women, so that this correlation was acknowledged, too. Although the questionnaire data showed that women said that they also felt a desire for revenge (lower than men; see figure 1.3c, this volume), their NA showed no further activity. Image results and questionnaire results for women thus were contradictory.

The focus of the study's interpretation lay on the men and their higher NA activity. The men's increased activity in the image suggested a correlation with the results of the questionnaire. Since there was no such correlation on the side of the researched women, their lower desire for revenge was not of further interest for the paper. The reactions of the men were generalized and brought into relation with theories of social preferences that "people value the gains of others positively if they are perceived to behave fairly, but value others' gains negatively if they behave unfairly. This pattern of preferences implies that people like cooperating with fair opponents but also like punishing unfair opponents" (Singer et al. 2006, 467f). The authors realize the generalization which lies in this interpretation by expressing a need for further research on the different emotional evaluation of men and women, but the sexually biased interpretation goes further and becomes even gendered: Singer et al.'s conclusions rely on a certain understanding of how women usually behave.

Here, the authors offer two possible interpretations: While admitting that their research design might be biased, they refer to stereotypes about female behavior, since the pain induced was physical pain. Their idea is that this might have influenced the desire for revenge in women. They wonder if, with a psychological or financial threat, women might have answered differently. Women are here associated with the "emotional" and the "nonviolent." Another interpretation explores the relation with the structure of society. This can be viewed as an example of how neuroscientific research is not free from ideas of society which can have an influence on the way we perceive not only *homo oeconomicus* or our individual behaviors but also society: "Alternatively, these findings could indicate a predominant role for males in the maintenance of justice and punishment of norm violation in human societies" (Singer et al. 2006, 468). What conclusions can be drawn from this statement? The friendliest one would be that this is not an emancipatory statement but a sexist one. One can assume that the norms of society are derived from biology. Political life and public life seem to be determined by biological differences.

Another research area in the field of economics and business is marketing, where emotions are already in the focus (Kenning et al. 2005, 57). In order to improve advertising and sales, neuroscientific methods are used to make the emotional effects of advertisement observable and measurable.

In a study carried out in a clinical setting at the University Clinic Ulm, Germany, in cooperation with the Daimler Chrysler Research Center Berlin, the focus was on the effects sports cars have on the brain reward regions. The assumption was that sports cars, as "cultural objects," signal "high social rank, social dominance and wealth, and can be regarded as the human equivalent to the peacock's tail" (Erk et al. 2002, 2500).

Twelve men were questioned about their car preferences. While they were being shown photographs of cars from different categories, their brain activity was measured. The results of the brain scans showed that the reward circuitry was more active when seeing sports cars than when seeing other types of cars. In order to explain this reaction, these results were compared to the higher activation of the reward center of heterosexual males when looking at attractive female faces—with the underlying idea that these faces "can be regarded as a potentially rewarding stimulus, that is, the initiation of a social interaction" (Erk et al. 2002, 2501).

After the test in the scanner, the test persons went through an interview, which was in part quantitative, about "preferences and indifferences concerning cars in general and their individual criteria for the evaluation of a car" (Erk et al. 2002, 2500).

In this experiment a typical connection is made between men, cars, and attractive female faces. The assumption is that men might need some signal of social status or wealth to become attractive to others. Although this is not directly addressed in the study, by referring to "the peacock's tail," the underlying idea is that the purpose of acquiring this attraction is to impress women. The researchers mentioned in another article that the "tail thus fulfils no meaningful function except for signaling that its owner is obviously strong enough to be able to invest energy in such a superfluent structure . . . peacocks that are able to produce the most fancy and ornamental tails are 'fitter' in the Darwinian sense. . . . In human societies, it is known that the demonstration of wealth and superfluity is also a strong signal for social dominance" (Walter, Abler, Ciaramidaro, and Erk 2005, 370). Following the line that underlying the image of the peacock's tail lies a description of the relation of men and women, I will interpret the relationship between men and women modeled here as being that the woman seems to be able to choose the attractive man, who needs some social status symbols in order to make himself attractive. But at the same time, the point is that the man still remains in the dominant position, having power and wealth, and seems to need the woman as another attribute of these categories.

The problems concerning neuromarketing do not at present stem only from the possibility that the techniques of brain research might be misused and people directly manipulated by a neuro-based marketing campaign (Ziegenfuss 2005). These fears might be justifiable, but more in the long term, since, at present, the research on the brain cannot provide clear explanations about how the brain really works. Of utmost importance currently is the question of which images of society and individuals are promoted by neuroeconomics and neuromarketing. The underlying evolutionary concept of the survival of the fittest seems to leave out those who are not able to compete in the market. No research on social interaction is carried out on those who are on the fringes of society. The aim seems to be to control and improve oneself—in order to join the group of the "fittest."

10.4.5 Gender and Emotions in Neuroeconomic Research

Taken together, what we have seen concerning the test settings as well as the experiments in neuroscience, and taking into consideration the two experiments described above, paradigmatically, there is only a rudimentary sensitivity to the sex of the test persons in neuroeconomics. Although the descriptions of the experiments refer to the sex of the test persons, and the findings are also sometimes described in relation to the sexes, there seems to be no or little reflection about the way in which the behavior of men and women as test persons might be influenced by their cultural or historical context as well as their gender roles. Sexual stereotypes, for example, that women are considered more empathetic, might have played a role in research setups. There also seems to be no reflection about the question of what constitutes a "female brain" and a "male brain." Neither transsexuals nor homosexuals/lesbians apparently play a role in the experiments. This reductionist view of society and its groups corresponds to the relatively small number of test persons in each experiment and the problematic that the conclusions are often generalized. The gender problematic of flexible capitalism is not explicitly referred to here. On the contrary, sexual stereotypes and traditional gender roles are written ahead in the structures of these experiments (see also Vidal and Benoit-Browaeys 2005).

Second, the experimenters want to show that "emotions" play a role in economics. This is done, for example, by referring to empathy as the way to "share the emotion, pain and sensation of others" (Singer et al. 2006, 466). It is not clear, however, how the relation of emotions and sensations as well as something like empathy is understood. On the level of basic research, the "status of emotions" in the brain and its relation to deliberation is not clear. In an article on neuroeconomics, Alan G. Sanfey and his coauthors argue the "greatest immediate ramifications for economic theories is between systems supporting emotion and those supporting deliberation, which closely parallels the distinction between automatic and controlled processes" (Sanfey, Loewenstein, McClure, and Cohen 2006, 112).

Some experiments show that empathetic response is automatic and that the brain regions activated are also observed when an unknown person shows pain reactions, but there are different individual empathetic abilities (Singer and Fehr 2005, 339ff). In the latest research, for example, Tania Singer and Frederique de Vignemont have questioned the assumption that "individuals automatically share the emotions of others when exposed to their emotions" (Vignemont and Singer 2006, 435), proposing instead that there are "several modulatory factors that might influence empathic brain responses" (Vignemont and Singer 2006, 435).

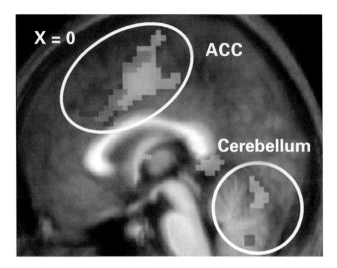

Plate 1
Pain-related activation associated with either experiencing pain in oneself or observing one's partner feeling pain: activation in anterior cingulate cortex and cerebellum. Areas in green represent
significant activation ($p < .001$) for the contrast (pain–no pain) in the "self" condition and areas
in red for the contrast (pain–no pain) in the "other" condition. The results are superimposed on
a mean T1-weighted structural scan of the 16 subjects. Activations are shown on sagittal slides.
(Source: Singer, Seymour, O'Doherty, Kaube, Dolan, and Frith. 2004. "Empathy for Pain Involves
the Affective but Not Sensory Components of Pain." *Science* 303, no. 5661: 1157–1162, 1158;
reprinted by permission from the American Association for the Advancement of Science: *Science*,
© 2004.)

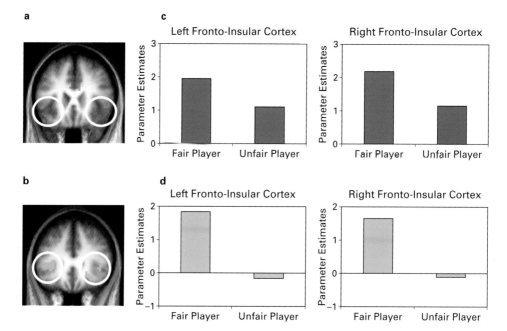

Plate 2

Pain-sensitive activation networks to the sight of fair and unfair players in pain. (a, b) Conjunction analysis between the contrasts pain–no pain in the context of self and the fair condition at $p < .001$ for women (pink; a) and men (blue; b). Increased pain-related activation (asterisk indicates whole-brain corrected) for women in ACC* [9, 18, 27], left fronto-insular cortex* [–42, 15, –3], right fronto-insular cortex* [30, 18, –18], left second somatosensory area (SII)* [–60, –30, 18], right SII* [63, –30, 24], and brainstem* [3, –18, –18]; for men in left fronto-insular cortex* [–33, 33, 3], right fronto-insular cortex [42, 33, 3], and brainstem [3, –33, –30]. (c, d) Average activation (parameter estimates) in peak voxels of left and right fronto-insular cortex for the painful–nonpainful trials in fair and unfair conditions for women (pink; c) and men (blue; d). (Source: Singer, Seymour, O'Doherty, Stephan, Dolan, and Frith. 2006. "Empathic Neural Responses Are Modulated by the Perceived Fairness of Others." *Nature* 439: 466–469, 468; reprinted by permission from Macmillan Publishers Ltd.: *Nature*, © 2006.)

Painful trials in unfair — painful trials in fair

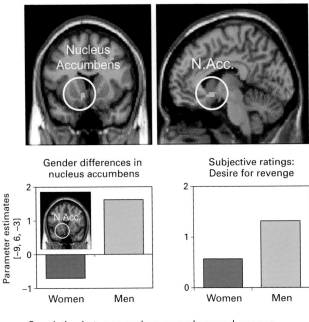

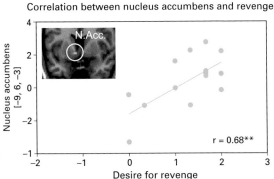

Plate 3
Gender differences in brain activity in nucleus accumbens (N. Acc.) specific to the perception of an unfair compared to fair player in pain. (a) Increased activity ($p < .005$) in nucleus accumbens [–9, 15, –9] for painful trials in the unfair/fair condition for men but not for women. (b) Average activation (parameter estimates) for women (pink) and men (blue) in left nucleus accumbens [–9, 15, –9] when testing for gender differences. (c) Men (blue) compared to women (pink) indicate stronger feelings of desire for revenge, $t(30) = 2.40$, $p < .05$, measured on a scale ranging from –2 ("not at all") to +2 ("very much"). (d) Correlation ($r = .68$, $p < .05$) of parameter estimates at peak of nucleus accumbens activation [–9, 6, –3] for the (pain in unfair–pain in fair) contrast in men with expressed desire for revenge in men. There was no correlation for women. (Source: Singer, Seymour, O'Doherty, Stephan, Dolan, and Frith. 2006. "Empathic Neural Responses Are Modulated by the Perceived Fairness of Others." *Nature* 439: 466–469, 469; reprinted by permission from Macmillan Publishers Ltd.: *Nature*, © 2006.)

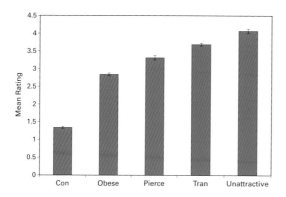

Plate 4

Mean disgust ratings: post hoc individual ratings, reverse scored such that 1 = "not at all disgusting," 5 = "very disgusting." Con, control; Tran, transsexual. (Source: Krendl, Macrae, Kelly, Fugelsang, and Heatherton. 2006. "The Good, the Bad, and the Ugly: An fMRI Investigation of the Functional Anatomic Correlates of Stigma." *Social Neuroscience* 1, no. 1: 5–15, 9; reprinted by permission from the publisher Taylor & Francis Ltd., http://informaworld.com: *Social Neuroscience*, © 2006.)

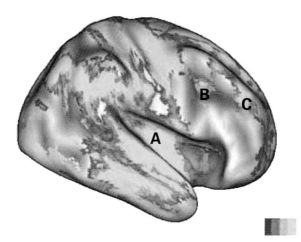

Plate 5

Parametric modulation of disgust ratings: analysis conducted with individual disgust ratings modeled linearly as a covariate of interest. An inflated voxel-by-voxel cortical rendering of the right hemisphere with a minimum threshold set at T = 3.53 and maximum set at T = 7 for $p < .001$ uncorrected (Van Essen, Drury, Dickson, Harwell, Hanlon, and Anderson 2001). Region of interest analyses extracted activity in the right inferior frontal gyrus (A; BA 45: 53, 24, 18), right medial frontal gyrus (B; BA 9: 50, 8, 36), and anterior cingulate gyrus (C; BA 32: –9, 22, 35) activity. (Source: Krendl, Macrae, Kelly, Fugelsang, and Heatherton. 2006. "The Good, the Bad, and the Ugly: An fMRI Investigation of the Functional Anatomic Correlates of Stigma." *Social Neuroscience* 1, no. 1: 5–15, 10; reprinted by permission from the publisher Taylor & Francis Ltd., http://informaworld.com: *Social Neuroscience*, © 2006.)

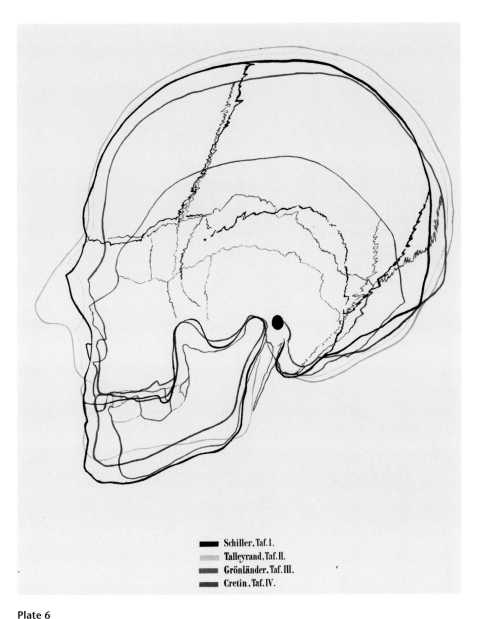

Schiller, Taf. I.
Talleyrand, Taf. II.
Grönländer, Taf. III.
Cretin, Taf. IV.

Plate 6

Carl Gustav Carus, facsimile drawing of four skulls. (Source: Carus. *Atlas der Cranioscopie oder Abbildungen der Schaedel- und Antlitzformen beruehmter oder sonst merkwürdiger Personen.* 1843–1845, table IX.)

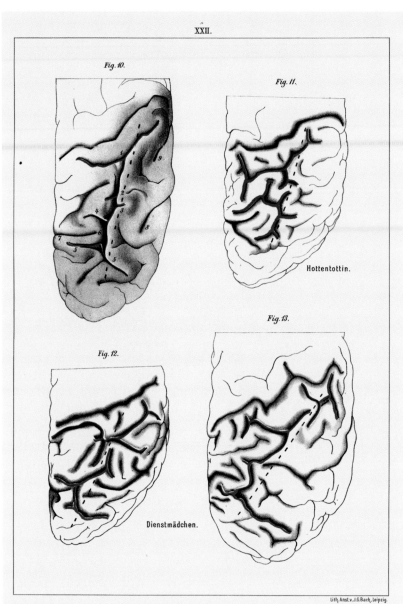

Plate 7

Nikolaus Rüdinger, brains of women. Hottentottin, Hottentot woman; Dienstmädchen, handmaiden (Source: Rüdinger. Ein Beitrag zur Anatomie der Affenspalte und der internen Interparietalfurche beim Menschen nach Race, Geschlecht und Individualität. In *Beiträge zur Anatomie und Embryologie als Festgabe Jacob Henle zum 4. April 1882 dargebracht von seinen Schülern*. 186–198. 1882, table XXII.)

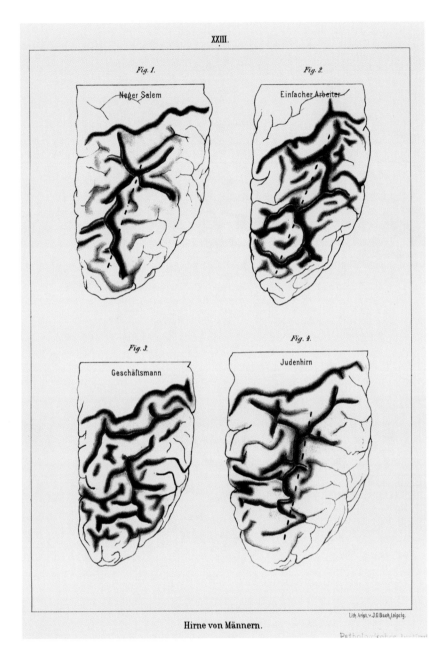

Plate 8

Nikolaus Rüdinger, brains of men. Neger Salem, Negro Salem; Einfacher Arbeiter, unskilled worker; Geschäftsmann, business man; Judenhirn, brain of Jew. (Source: Rüdinger. Ein Beitrag zur Anatomie der Affenspalte und der internen Interparietalfurche beim Menschen nach Race, Geschlecht und Individualität. In *Beiträge zur Anatomie und Embryologie als Festgabe Jacob Henle zum 4. April 1882 dargebracht von seinen Schülern*. 186–198. 1882, table XXIII.)

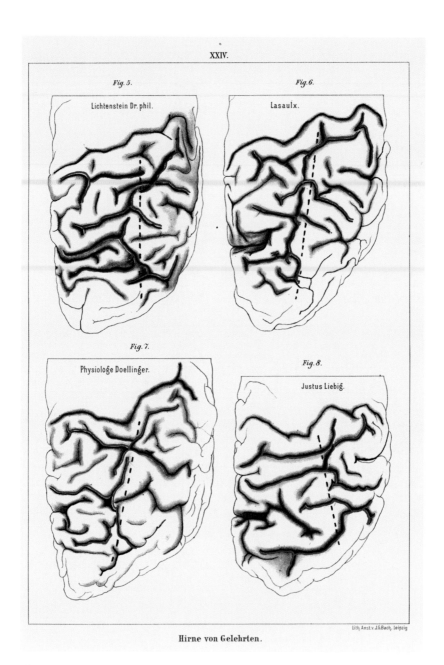

XXIV.

Fig. 5.

Lichtenstein Dr. phil.

Fig. 6.

Lasaulx.

Fig. 7.

Physiologe Doellinger.

Fig. 8.

Justus Liebig.

Lith. Anst. v. J.G.Bach, Leipzig

Hirne von Gelehrten.

Plate 9

Nikolaus Rüdinger, brains of scholars. (Source: Rüdinger. Ein Beitrag zur Anatomie der Affenspalte und der internen Interparietalfurche beim Menschen nach Race, Geschlecht und Individualität. In *Beiträge zur Anatomie und Embryologie als Festgabe Jacob Henle zum 4. April 1882 dargebracht von seinen Schülern.* 186–198. 1882, table XXIV.)

As can be seen from these different interpretations, neuroeconomics is still a new research area, and there are many different possibilities for interpreting research findings. However, sometimes research possibilities are declared which lead to a direct explanation, for example, in Camerer et al.'s statement that via neurosciences "direct measurement of thoughts and feelings [are made] possible for the first time" (Camerer, Loewenstein, and Prelec 2005, 53). This diffusion makes the status of emotions in neuroeconomic findings and their relevance for economic theory problematic. On the one hand, neuroeconomics has taken up issues like emotions and noncognitive activations in the brain—and with them it goes beyond the model of *homo oeconomicus*. On the other hand, no real differentiation is made concerning the role of emotions in economic issues.

This gap also has to do with a functionalist understanding of emotions. The functionalist idea is that having a certain mental state is an output and a reaction to a certain input (on the concept of function in social science, see Radcliff-Browne 1952). However, as we can see in the empathy example as well as the reward example, even if certain input (cut/pictures) stands in relation with pain or empathy and reward, the question is whether the quality and the experience of the emotions can really be shown in these settings (the *qualia* problem, e.g., Searle 1992; see also the Introduction to this volume). In these examples, in order to detect the "quality" of the emotions, questionnaires are needed. But then, as Tania Singer's research shows, for example, the feeling of desire for revenge, expressed by women, is not extensively referred to in the interpretation of the experiments. And by calculation, they become "statistical" qualities. This narrow view on the relation of economic problems and emotions can become problematic when applied to "real-life situations" like leadership.

10.5   Neuroeconomics, Leadership, and Elites

Neuroeconomics has not yet explicitly focused on leadership.[17] This lack of research might be due to a functionalist understanding of economic decision making, which is not sufficient in order to deal with leadership problems. Leadership, that is, being in charge of others in a group, institution, or company, can be described as dealing with the decisions concerning the group or the organization, referring to each member of the group (most often the subordinate employee) as well as convincing stakeholders of the organization. The problems in these settings might be too complex and refer to elements which cannot be easily measured with brain scans.

Although neuroeconomics itself does not refer to leadership, there are two approaches which are inspired by neuroscientific findings and which relate to leadership issues. One is Daniel Goleman's *Primal Leadership* approach, coauthored with Richard Boyatzis and Annie McKee (Goleman, Boyatzis, and McKee 2002), which refers to his EI concept and applies it in leadership contexts. The other approach is Simon Baron-Cohen's

(2004) systemizing leadership style (see Karafyllis, this volume). In both approaches, emotions play a role, one in their presence, the other one in their absence.

In Goleman et al.'s approach, the improvement of the individual leader in his or her emotional skills is central. The authors present a concept of leadership which they call "primal leadership," and they argue that "the fundamental task of leaders . . . is to prime good feeling in those they lead. That occurs when a leader creates *resonance*—a reservoir of positivity that frees the best in people. . . . Primal leadership demands we bring emotional intelligence to bear" (Goleman, Boyatzis, and McKee 2002, ix). The relation between leaders and their employees is defined by means of emotions. For the leader, key aspects concerning EI are self-awareness, self-management, social awareness, and relationship management. Although Goleman and his coauthors refer to the neurosciences in order to present "scientific" arguments for the importance of EI (Goleman, Boyatzis, and McKee 2002, 103), it is from the field of psychology that the concept of EI in Goleman's sense has been heavily criticized for not providing scientific empirical proof (see also MacCann et al., this volume) about how leadership effectiveness can be successfully measured by EI (Antonakis 2004). In this sense, EI including brain science is understood as pop science.

The other approach also refers to neuroscientific findings but has "autistic" brains, which are declared as the "perfect male brains," at its center. With respect to relating his "extreme male brain theory" to leadership, Baron-Cohen (2004, 126) shows that although he is referring to neuroscience as well, his ideal leader is completely different. For him, a leader is a good systemizer who knows how to control situations and does not empathize too much with subordinates. So, Goleman as well as Baron-Cohen refer to neuroscientific findings as proof for their ideas but arrive at different results. This difference has to do with the norms and images which are attributed to leaders and which are different in economic contexts and in those of the neurosciences.

To describe different kinds of leadership is a task of sociology or psychology, to evaluate them normatively, an ethical task. The sociologist Max Weber differentiates between three types of authority (*Herrschaft*). Alongside tradition and rational authority, he puts charisma (Weber 1956, chapter III, § 10). This differentiation resonates within some of the theories of leadership of the last decades. In the 1980s, leadership was constructed as a model in opposition to management. Managers were seen as lacking vision for the future. Bernhard Bass, building on the approach of James G. Burns, emphasizes a theory of leadership based on the charismatic and visionary leader (Antonakis, Cianciolo, and Sternberg 2004, 9): *transformational leadership* has at its center a strong identification with the leader and a vision which is shared; raising "one another to higher levels of motivation and morality" (Burns 1978, 20). *Transactional leadership* is differentiated from this approach: it "creates the leader–employee relationship on the basis of the contingent positive and negative reinforcement in a sense of the exchange theory" (Kroeger and Tartler 2002, 126).

Bass developed a test on which facets of transformational and transactional leadership, as well as nonleadership behavior and outcomes like satisfaction, effectiveness, and extra effort, were measured using a set of questions on 45 items concerning how subjects evaluate their own leadership style, their own reactions, and the reactions of others to their own behavior (Bass and Avolio 2000). This Multifactor Leadership Questionnaire (MLQ), based on Bernard Bass and Bruce Avolio's Full Range Leadership Model, is one of the most often used tools in the measurement of transformational leadership (Heintz 2006, i). Although within the context of flexible capitalism, the achievements are not so much tested on the MLQ, the test is at least not only based on an evaluation of the subordinate leader by a superior but takes different aspects of leadership into account as well. On the other hand, only a certain set of leadership styles are tested, and an MLQ evaluation identifies which of these leadership styles best describes the individual being tested. Therefore not the individuality of the leadership style is appreciated but a certain standardization of leadership styles is developed. The ideal seems to be an emotionally open-minded, democratically oriented person who is sympathetic and comfortable with his or her surroundings. Bass and Avolio suggest that female leaders tend toward the transformational leadership style (Bass and Avolio 1997). However, different studies on the evaluation of men and women in leading positions questioned with the MLQ have yielded differing results. Sometimes the leadership style of men and women (e.g., Australian bank managers) is rated equally by subordinates (Carless 1998). Other studies show differences in the evaluation of female and male leadership styles by subordinates.[18]

The idea in flexible capitalism is that self-improvement strategies like EI or the orientation provided by an MLQ-type measure suggests to leaders, as well as to employees, that it is possible, by their own energy, to improve their position in society's hierarchies (see also Bandura 2003). As can be seen from the MLQ evaluations, the leadership styles of women are perceived differently and probably are also different. However, the measurements of abilities are often problematic since they not only interfere with the employee's personality but seem also to refer to patterns and stereotypes of how men and women are perceived and often do not take into account the organizational structures of the workplace.

In a study on female design engineers, Joyce K. Fletcher shows that although organizations may propose an emotional and relational behavioral style for their leaders, the reality is different: This kind of behavior is not recognized when decisions are made concerning rewards and promotions because it contrasts with powerful behavior (Fletcher 1999). Often the definition of a power position is already "contaminated" with gendered connotations (Powell, Butterfield, and Parent 2002), which excludes women (Bourdieu 2005b (1998), 110ff), as well as other persons who do not fit into these concepts.

Since women are generally associated with caring roles and more "communal strategies" (for an historical overview see Allen 2005), in contrast to men who are associated with more aggressive behaviors and more "agentic strategies," it might be that women are not seen as being capable of ensuring success in leadership positions—as role congruity theory explains (Eagly and Karau 2002). These expectations concerning women and men have become injunctive norms, so that women or men who break out of these roles might get into trouble.

The above-mentioned tests, as well as neuroeconomic research on empathy, for example, fit into this setting: The individual's abilities to react and empathize with others are tested—and generalized from a gender perspective as well, while ignoring that sexual stereotypes are social constructs (Konnertz, Haker, and Mieth 2006). The individual who has to optimize himself or herself, in order to fit into an unstable society, can be seen as the underlying societal construct in neuroeconomics as well as in EI and modern leadership theories.

What are the effects of brain scans in relation to the development of the understanding of leadership? One could imagine that a brain scan of, for example, empathy, could also be used for testing and thereby the simplistic biologistic image of empathy would be brought into the realm of leadership qualification. And would the use of brain scanning then change leadership styles or change the composition of leadership groups? Leaders can be seen as elites. However, not all members of elite classes are transformational leaders who are responsible for a certain group of people and have vision. In elite groups, as well as nonelite groups, leaders seem to have the task of giving advice and meaning to the actions of others. They seem to have this power because they can give meaning to what is important for the society, the organization, or the group that they are leading. These definitions exclude others not only from leadership but also from joining the elites, which is something that could also change if brain scans were made available to a broader public, since the myth that neuroimaging provides more "objective" data than are obtained using other measures would also be brought into play.

However, up to now, in general, the U.S. power elite, for example, has not become as diversified, with respect to ethnicity, gender, race, and sexual orientation, as expected, although there are members of "minority" groups who have made themselves acceptable to the establishment as Richard L. Zweigenhaft and William Domhoff (2006) show in their analysis of American power elites, which follows in the tradition of C. Wright Mills (Mills 1956). The same effect is seen in the European Union (see, e.g., Imbusch and Rucht 2007).

Will this closure of elites change due to brain research? In the past, elite brains have been detected a posteriori (see Hagner, this volume), but could the idea come up that "brain elites" can also be detected a priori via brain scans? And would this be a desirable perspective? Answers to these questions depend on the metalevel and which anthropological premises are taken up (Gräb-Schmidt 2002) and which answer is given to the question of what constitutes a human being. On a more practical level, answers also depend on which role is attributed to the "fetish" brain and on how findings in neuroscience make their way into public realm and are converted into "general knowledge."

10.6   The Pop-Scientific Side of Neuroeconomics

As the foregoing sections have shown, neuroeconomics takes place in a certain form of capitalism, being influenced by its economic and political system. But what about the other way around? How does neuroeconomics influence society? This broad research question cannot be taken up here in its entirety, but I will focus on an article which can be seen as idealtypic. Often neuroeconomic findings make their way to a broader public, in a pop-scientific way, through articles in newspapers and magazines. "Pop-scientific" means that scientific findings are simplified and also interpreted for a broader audience. The images produced through neuroimaging also have their own quality and fascination, which might lie in the way that an image from inside the body is presented with a certain coloring—which helps popularize the neuroscientific findings (Groß and Müller 2006).

Let us look at an article which can be seen as an example of presenting neuroscientific findings to a broader public. In "Taxes a Pleasure? Check the Brain Scan," John Tierney, in *The New York Times* from June 19, 2007, reports the neuroscientific finding that human pleasure centers in the brain respond to doing good not only for ourselves but also for others and interprets this finding. Tierney himself takes on a bemused distance—and is also skeptical about the validity of the generalizations of the research—which is based on a neuroeconomic study done at the University of Oregon in which researchers measured 19 female students' brain reactions to decisions which were modeled as simulations of donations of money and paying taxes, voluntarily or involuntarily.

At one level, the article can be interpreted as showing that neuroeconomics also tries to deal with open questions in capitalism. Here the topic—already announced by the heading of the article—is taxes. The underlying question is: Why should individuals pay taxes? Paying taxes implies that private money has to be given to the state and therein to the "public," and this also means giving up control over it. The idea of taxes is that "public goods" like streets or military activities can be financed and a kind of redistribution of wealth takes place as well. For a hard-core *homo oeconomicus*, this last point in particular is not acceptable. Seen from the neuroeconomic perspective of this research which the articles describes, paying taxes is not a question of responsibility for the common good or a question of an ethical norm or even an economic question but rather a question of physiology: What is going on in the brain when paying taxes—or when a simulation of paying taxes is conducted? And I can formulate it also in this way: In this article the reason given to explain why paying taxes is a positive act is that it elicits activation of the reward center. On another level, an implicit political statement in favor of a libertarian society might be found in the statement of one of the researchers who conducted the study: Although the researcher admits that the proof might be vague, he sees a slight tendency toward more activity in the brain areas when making donations than when paying taxes. The way the experiment was structured, as well as the kind of interpretations given by the researchers, provides hints that neuroeconomics also influences society by dealing with issues of economic policy, and therefore I will have a closer look at which concepts of economics and economy and even biology can be found at the base of neuroeconomic studies.

10.7   Underlying Concepts of Economy, Economics, and Biology in Neuroeconomics

The research focus of some neuroeconomic studies on altruism and trust hints at one of the basic questions concerning an economic system: How is it possible to get an individualized market society to inspire united action? The old question of the relation between individual and community or society is addressed here, that is, sociality (Deuser 2004, Bedford-Strohm 1999, Parsons 1977).

   An element which is seen as important in different economic theories is trust (e.g., for a libertarian approach, see Fukuyama 1995). Neuroeconomist Paul J. Zak focuses on trust in his research and often takes up trust games, where trust is understood in a monetary sense, and the individual is the DM (decision maker): "The consensus in the literature is that the transfer from DM 1 to DM 2 is a (costly) signal of trust" (Zak 2007, 23). In these games the point is to show that human beings trust one another in economic situations as well. In one of his descriptions of an experiment, Zak concludes with his vision for society: "At the national level, trust can be raised by emphasizing the importance of education, reducing inequalities, and promoting freedom and democracy. National institutions that allow and encourage individuals to achieve their goals directly promote trust and therefore the creation of wealth. . . . Friendships, confidence, empathy, mercy, love and faith all follow from trust and are likely mediated by oxytocin. As social scientists apply these findings to institutional design, not only will productivity be raised, but so will happiness" (Zak 2007, 32). First, this statement, with its allusion to an increase in happiness and its image of individuals building a society based on trust, resonates with Adam Smith's description of the "invisible hand," which leads to the happiness of everybody, in his *Theory of Moral Sentiments* (Smith 1759, part IV, chapter I). Zak refers to the need for education and reduction of inequality and combines it with the importance of freedom and democracy in relation to national institutions. Here, a market economic model informs neuroeconomics—it still refers to the need for institutions and the reduction of inequality. Second, in contrast to Smith, the ordering of society is not mediated by an "invisible hand" but by a hormone: oxytocin (OT). This hormone simultaneously acts as a neurotransmitter in the brain and is related to the body of women. In one of his studies, Zak refers to sex differences and concludes that women who were ovulating "were less trustworthy than other subjects" due to their higher progesterone level which inhibits OT uptake (Zak 2004, 1745). In the above-mentioned quote on society, OT leads people to engage in interpersonal relationships, that is, sociality is based in this view on a body-interior biological medium. Interpreting his findings, Zak writes that it is "nature" which has "designed" human beings to cooperate. A close theoretical and practical linkage between biology and economics can be seen in this approach. In Zak's view—quoting Thorstein Veblen—"'economics, properly understood, is simply a branch of biology'" (Zak 2004, 1746).

Let us have a closer look at the connection between biology, economics, and economy which can be found in neuroeconomics. There seems to be an ongoing struggle about which of the sciences is more influential in interpreting the results of neuroscientific research and which paradigms are challenged in the related sciences.

Without question, the main focus lies on economics and neuroscience, which is considered part of biology. Although neuroeconomics sees itself as a transdisciplinary approach of neurobiology, economics, and psychology, the last of these seems to be pushed to the margin because media, like tests and questionnaires, are taken from this discipline, but only to cross-check the scanned results or to make behavioral assumptions. Psychologists' research questions are hardly taken into consideration.

Economics is challenged by the neurosciences, since the "rationality" concept of *homo oeconomicus* is questioned, though for scientists like Colin Camerer, doing research in neuroeconomics, the reverse is also true. He proclaims that neuroscience "is shot through with familiar economic language," and suggests that an "economic model of the brain" could help to develop an overall theory of the brain and explain how it allocates resources.

Paul Glimcher draws the conclusion that economic theory can overcome the Cartesian model of mind and body, rephrased in modern terms as brain and behavior, with a cognitive model which is economics based (Glimcher 2003). Findings in scientific contexts are interpreted in an economic sense, and in this way the impression is created that economics and biology merge. For Glimcher, for example, decision-making processes are "holistic" and are present in other mammals as well. He and colleagues carried out experiments with monkeys, in which, for example, thirsty monkeys were trained via a visual stimulus to expect different amounts of juice in relation to eye-movement targets. The monkeys adapted their behavior to the setting so that they could maximize their payoffs. The firing rate of the neurons was close to the rewards the monkeys got. Glimcher interpreted their findings and those of other studies to suggest that the primates' brains acted as if monkeys were rational agents, maximizing their utility: "The final stages of decision making seem to reflect something very much like a utility calculation" (Glimcher, Dorris, and Bayer 2005, 31).

Is economic rational behavior then something biological? For Glimcher, economics is not a "pure" social science. Like the sociobiologist Edward O. Wilson (Wilson 1978), he thinks that economics and biology both address a single subject and will merge soon. This close relation between economics and biology has a long tradition in economics, and they have exerted influence on each other.[19] In neuroeconomics as well, reference is often made to evolution to explain the relevance of findings (e.g., Moll et al. 2006, 15626). From evolution theory, with its characteristics of variations, selection, and survival of the fittest, it is the idea of selection, re-envisioned as choice, which is considered important in economics (Haferkamp and Smelser 1992). "Ultimately, economics is a biological science. It is the study of how humans choose. That choice is inescapably a biological process. Truly understanding how and why humans make the choices that they do will undoubtedly require a neuroeconomic science" (Glimcher, Dorris, and Bayer 2005, 31).

Perhaps due to the underlying evolutionary framework, with its focus on selection and choice, neuroeconomics also makes choice and decision making its primary interest. It is the reformulated selection process of evolution. However, in order to be able to make the two sciences of biology and economics merge, the rational foundation of *homo oeconomicus* is questioned and emotions or something, which is "inscribed into the brain," is researched. So when neuroeconomics takes up questions of insecurity and freedom, it refers to self-optimization in order to improve selection processes within a society that is interpreted as nature. This also includes having underlying specific sexual stereotypes of men and women, with women being the ones who nurture and guarantee reproduction, and men the ones responsible for defense and law.

10.8 Final Thoughts

The foregoing analysis argues that neuroeconomics challenges the "economic brain" by taking into consideration the impact of emotions on economic decision making. However, neuroeconomics still has little influence on economic theory, perhaps because the findings are too recent—or are there other reasons?

Let us speculate, how might "the economic brain" develop from a neuroeconomic point of view? Will economic theory be completely transformed? In contrast to "post-autistic" and feminist economics, neuroeconomics is still bound to its underlying concepts of economy and biology, both of which are at present referring to the concept of evolution. At least for the moment, this common underlying reference frame makes neuroeconomics compatible with economics as well as with flexible capitalism. It is through neuroeconomics that economics and the economy respond to the criticism that in these areas emotions are not taken seriously. Neuroeconomics tries to make emotions "visible" and measurable, and the next step would be to integrate emotions into an economic paradigm. In this sense, neuroeconomics fits to economics.

In my opinion, the mélange of economics and biology in neuroeconomics is becoming problematic, especially when referring to evolutionary explanations for economic and social relations and societal issues, for then the border of Social Darwinistic concepts is easily transgressed. From a gender perspective this is especially problematic due to the different tasks of the sexes traditionally assumed by evolutionary theories (Miller 1993). In the discussion concerning access to leadership positions, for example, the question of how to handle personnel evaluations is also a political question. Should it be by merit or ability (Young 1990), the criteria which determine the access to leadership positions should be evaluated critically in relation to their underlying gender biases and discussed not only under a paradigm of competition but also of quality and of democratic structures (Huber 1996, 299f).

Even if one does not share this normative position, it is at least—when considering neuroeconomics—important to be aware of the anthropological premises, to realize the underlying reference frame, and to see that the results of neuroeconomics are often quite open to interpretation. The interpretation of these results is at first a task of the scientists. In order to maintain standards of good science (Fausto-Sterling 1994), greater sensitivity to sex and gender implications of the research results is needed. However, there are also other aspects concerning the interpretation of research results to be considered, especially when realizing how close economics, neuroscience, and business work together in neuroeconomics. The influence on research, which runs over the finances, is to be taken into consideration in order to thematize its underlying power relations.

This leads to the point that we also have to become aware of how neuroeconomic results are used in the scientific community as well as in the realm of the general public. What kind of knowledge is communicated here—and what kind of explanatory value is it thought to have? Neuroeconomic research gives, at present, interesting hints as to which brain regions are active during decision making in abstract decision-making models. However, the functionalist explanations of neuroeconomics are not adequate to understanding economics in general and to solving economic problems within society and between societies, particularly not from a gender perspective.

Acknowledgments

I would like to thank Nicole Karafyllis for valuable comments on drafts of this chapter as well as Carmen Baumeler and Thomas Ulshöfer for helpful advice.

Notes

1. Feminist economics is not monolithic. Research has also been done on economics and gender which remains within the economic paradigm (Jacobsen 2007). In this chapter "feminist economics" refers to the more foundational critique of economic theory.

2. For a critical analysis of the difference between autism and economics, see Devine (2002). The use of "autism" in the economic context is not considered to be discriminating against autists.

3. Uskali Mäki recommends differentiating between "the ontological convictions of an economist and the ontological presuppositions of an economic theory" (Mäki 2002, 6).

4. http://www.paecon.net (accessed January 7, 2007).

5. In his basic studies together with the late Amos Tversky, Kahneman developed *prospect theory*, demonstrating that human behavior in decision making under uncertainty does not always correspond to economic theory but is influenced, for example, by the frame given to a choice. They also showed that human beings focus more closely on relative gains and losses than on changes in their overall welfare (Rick and Loewenstein 2007).

6. www.commercialalert.org/issues/culture/neuromarketing/commercial-alert-asks-feds-to-investigate-neuromarketing-research-at-emory-university (accessed June 8, 2007).

7. See, for example, http://www.census.gov/prod/2005pubs/p60-229-pdf (accessed July 25, 2007).

8. This discrimination can even be seen in the description of the wage gap: It is analyzed from the perspective of men—and it is often not analyzed in relation to the complexity of the underlying social injustices (Kreimer 2006, 163).

9. http://ec.europa.eu/employment_social/gender_equality/index_en.html (accessed July 25, 2007).

10. In this game a fixed sum of money has to be divided between two persons. The proposer makes an offer about the division of the sum to the other person, who can accept or reject it. If rejected, none of the players gets any money; if accepted, the offer is taken.

11. The twentieth century libertarian economist Ludwig von Mises, for example, supposed that money is not seen as having utility in and of itself, but only indirectly (Mises 1981, HP 15). With neuroscientific findings, some "evidence" is assumed for a connection between money and "hemodynamic acitivations overlapping those seen previously in response to tactile stimuli, and euphoria-inducing drugs" (Breiter et al. 2001, 627).

12. In the study by Huettel et al. (Huettel et al. 2006), the researchers show that "different attitudes toward perceived risk and ambiguity in decision-making situations may reflect a basic distinction in brain function," as *Science Daily* reported in March 2006 (http://sciencedaily.com/releases/2006/03/060303113346.htm, accessed July 20, 2007).

13. Colin Camerer describes the participants in experiments for behavioral game theory, for example, as "college students playing a couple of hours for modest financial stakes" (Camerer 2003, 4).

14. For a description of the "ultimate game," see endnote 10. In general, the actions of most proposers are economically nonrational, because they offer nearly half (40% to 50%) of the money, somehow anticipating the observed fact that offers of less than 20% are rejected by nearly half of the responders.

15. Autists are stereotyped here, because there are studies which show that adult autists also cooperate in strategic games—although there are behavioral differences in real-life situations between autists and nonautists (Hill and Sally 2003, 50ff).

16. For Martha Nussbaum "objectification" has seven notions: instrumentality, denial of autonomy, inertness, fungibility, violability, ownership, denial of subjectivity, but not all have to appear together. Fungability is defined as "The objectifier treats the object as interchangeable (a) with other objects of the same type and/ or (b) with objects of other types (Nussbaum 1999b, 218). Note that Axel Honneth (2005) emphasizes that the tradition of "objectification" goes back to Georg Lukács and Karl Marx, but in this tradition, "Verdinglichung" is called "reification."

17. Although there are conferences on "neuroleadership" where neuroscientific findings are applied to leadership questions, this is done more on a "practical level" than on a scientific or scholarly basis; see, for example, http://neuroleadershipsummit2007.blogspot.com/ (accessed July 7, 2007). On neuromanagement see Senn (2004).

18. At a police academy, police students at the beginning of their training evaluated female and male leaders differently, but at the end of the education leaders of both sexes were evaluated about the same. http://www.aic.gov.au/conferences/policewomen2/Panopoulos.pdf (accessed July 27, 2007).

19. British economist Adam Smith, as a central figure in the development of modern economics, influenced Charles Darwin in his "theory" on the origin of species, which is now known as evolution theory (Gould 1982, 66). And in his work *Principles of Economics* (1890) British economist Alfred Marshall referred to biology as "the mecca" of the economist, emphasizing the importance of biology and evolution theory for economics (Hodgson 1993; see also Ghiselin 1974). The economist and social philosopher Friedrich August von Hayek also intensively worked on theoretical psychology (Hayek 1976) and developed a cultural evolution theory. There are a variety of different ways in which economics has incorporated evolutionary theory (e.g., Dopfer 2005, Faber and Proops 1997, Maynard-Smith 1982).

IV Self-Representations: The Human Person and Her Emotional Media

11 Emotional Intelligence at the Interface of Brain Function, Communication, and Culture: The Role of Media Aesthetics in Shaping Empathy

Kathrin Fahlenbrach and Anne Bartsch

11.1 Introduction

Emotional Intelligence (EI) is often thought of as the "wisdom of the body." We believe this view is generally justified, as a growing number of research findings suggest EI skills are rooted in evolved brain functions which comprise a part of our biological makeup (see, e.g., Gazzaniga 1995). As we argue, however, evolved brain functions tell only half the story. Brain functions and the resulting cognitions and behaviors are intelligent only in relation to the opportunities and demands of a given environmental situation. We therefore propose to consider brain function in the broader context of social communication and culture, including both individual communication and media communication.

Studying EI at the interface of brain function, communication, and culture requires an interdisciplinary approach that combines the perspectives of neuroscience with those of social psychology, media studies, and cultural studies. In the first part of this chapter, we outline possible key elements of such an interdisciplinary approach; in the second part, we focus on the specific insights a media studies perspective has to offer when it comes to the role of communication and culture in shaping EI skills, particularly empathy.

Mass media are a prominent sphere, within which the common cultural understanding of emotion, interaction rules, and other norms and values are communicated and negotiated. Audiovisual media use both innate and culturally established patterns of emotional communication in order to guide the emotional effects on their viewers. They provide viewers with a wide range of information about different emotional behavior patterns and their specific bodily appearances; they are therefore strongly involved in the cultural conditioning of skills related to EI. The aesthetic representation and performance of emotions in audiovisual media, especially in "scenes of empathy" (Plantinga 1999), appeal to all levels of emotional experience in the viewer. Media shape viewers' ability to understand and evaluate the emotions of others, to relate them to their own emotional experience, and to coordinate emotional behavior in adaptive and socially appropriate ways (Plantinga and Smith 1999).

11.2   EI at the Interface of Brain Function and Social Context

EI is usually defined as a set of emotion-related skills and abilities that include the monitoring, appraisal, and expression of emotion, emotion regulation, and utilization of emotion to motivate adaptive behavior (Salovey and Mayer 1990). If one looks for brain correlates of EI, it soon becomes evident that there is no single underlying brain mechanism for the entire spectrum of EI skills. EI seems in fact to be subserved by a large number of neural networks distributed all over the human brain and body. We still do not fully understand all facets of EI at the brain level, but existing research clearly points to the modularity of underlying brain functions. We are going to briefly review some of the existing findings, and we will then turn to the question of how modular skills and brain mechanisms might be integrated to function as a holistic intelligence. From a media and communication studies perspective, EI can be characterized as a normative concept that goes beyond modular skills and brain functions and involves the idea of a unitary person or self who is able to integrate modular skills in a socially and culturally meaningful way.

11.2.1   Brain Correlates of EI

Emotional self-awareness   The ability to monitor and discriminate between emotions in the self has been related to the representation of bodily reactions in the somatosensory association cortex of the right hemisphere. According to Damasio (1994), this brain region is critically involved in people's "gut feelings." Extended scripts or schemata of prototypical emotions that integrate gut feelings with representations of eliciting situations, action tendencies, verbal labels, and so on are assumed to rely on large associative networks that are coordinated by convergence zones in the frontal cortex.

Emotional expression   Several brain regions are involved in people's ability to communicate emotions. Spontaneous expression of emotion is based on limbic and subcortical brain structures like the amygdala and cingulate gyrus, whereas intentional expression (including suppression and masking of spontaneous expression) is based on different regions of the motor cortex depending on the muscle groups involved in the expression (Rinn 1991, Brothers 1997, Damasio 1994).

Emotion regulation   It is widely assumed that the prefrontal cortex plays an important role in emotion regulation (LeDoux 1996, Rolls 1995). Emotion regulation is not restricted to cortical structures, however. Subcortical structures seem to be involved as well—for example, the hippocampus is involved in the regulation of amygdala responses to emotionally arousing stimuli (LeDoux 1996).

Motivation   The motivating force of emotion is thought to arise from the connection of subcortical emotion systems (e.g., the amygdala) with two motivational brain systems—the behavioral activation system and the behavioral inhibition system (LeDoux 2002, Rolls 1995, Gray 1995). The behavioral activation system motivates and reinforces behavior that has led to positive emotions, whereas the behavioral inhibition system inhibits behavior that has led to negative emotions in the past.

Decision making   According to Damasio (1994), gut feelings play an important role in decision making. He proposes that a neural network including the amygdala, prefrontal cortex, and right somatosensory cortex is critically involved in guiding the process of intuitive decision making based on prior emotional experiences.

Empathy   Several brain regions have been related to people's skill at recognizing and empathizing with the emotions of others (see the editors' Introduction to this volume). Simple stimulus features of emotional expression can be processed at a subcortical level, for example, by the amygdala—this is the case with cries (LeDoux 1995) or the staring eyes of the fearful facial expression (Morris, deBonis, and Dolan 2002). Recognition of more complex patterns of facial expression is based on a specialized region of the temporal sulcus (Rolls 1995, Brothers 1997). Forms of empathy that go beyond discriminating between facial and vocal expressions and include recognition of another's intentions further involve the mirror neuron system of the frontal cortex (Gallese 2005). At this cognitively elaborate level, the brain correlates of empathy seem to overlap with those of self-awareness, as mirror neurons respond to intentional acts regardless of whether the act is executed by oneself or others, or is merely imagined (Seitz, Nickel, and Azari 2006).

11.2.2 Putting Brain Function in Context

This overview on brain correlates of EI is far from exhaustive. Nevertheless, it seems fair to conclude that EI is based not on a single underlying brain mechanism but on a wealth of modular brain structures and neural networks, each of which makes a specific contribution to the toolbox of EI skills. It is worth noting that most of the modular skills are not adaptive in and of themselves. Expressing emotions openly and spontaneously can be helpful in some situations but counterproductive in others; relying on one's "gut feelings" and intuitions can lead to good or bad decisions, and so on. We therefore propose that EI is not only the sum of modular skills and brain functions; rather, it is a characteristic of a unitary person or self who is able to integrate modular skills in a meaningful way and to choose from his or her toolbox the skills required to meet the demands of the current situation (see Karafyllis, this volume).

But how can a unitary person or self arise from modular skills and brain functions? We propose solving this problem by drawing on the skill theory of Fischer, Shaver, and Carnochan (1990; Fischer et al. 1993). According to Fischer et al. (1993), higher order skills related to personhood like self-reflection, strategic planning, and self-control arise from the stepwise integration of innate skills and brain functions. Simple reflex skills are integrated to form sensorimotor schemata, sensorimotor skills are integrated to form symbolic representations, and representational skills are integrated to form abstract concepts and ideas. This hierarchy of skills on different levels of cognitive complexity emerges in a fixed sequence during child development. It is assumed that the superordinate skills do not replace the skills on the more basic levels but serve instead to regulate and reorganize these skills.

A comparable approach to emotional communication has been proposed by Bartsch and Hübner (2005, 2006). This model of emotional communication comprises three interrelated levels of complexity: (1) reciprocal activation of emotional stimulus–response patterns, (2) reciprocal attribution of emotions based on sensorimotor emotion scripts, and (3) social negotiation of emotions based on symbolic representations. It is assumed that the three levels of emotional communication have an interlinked construction and coordinate via bottom-up and top-down-processes.

Both Fischer et al. (1993) and Bartsch and Hübner (2005, 2006) point to the fact that EI is not a property of isolated individuals but a property of a person in a specific social context. The quality and efficiency of EI skills is critically dependent on the quality of the context and feedback information provided by the person's social environment. Fischer et al. (1993) distinguish between an optimal and a functional level of skill development. The functional level consists of skills that a person can use both spontaneously and with minimal social feedback. The optimal level consists of skills that a person can use on his or her own when provided with rich social input and feedback information. According to Fischer et al. (1993), children's optimal level of development is often years ahead of their functional level. The considerable gap between the functional and optimal levels of EI raises doubts about the usefulness of studying EI solely as a matter of brain function since the performance and functionality of the same brain or brain circuits can vary substantially depending on the social context. Rather, we suggest considering brain function in the broader context of personal development, social communication, and culture. We contend that nature and nurture should not be regarded as competing explanatory frameworks but as complementary processes that interact in shaping EI. Several authors have argued that the brain circuits involved in innate skills need to be trained and fine-tuned by adequate environmental stimulation in order to attain full functionality (LeDoux 2002, Schore 1994). Due to the brain's plasticity and the constant growth and decay of neural connectivity, innate skills and brain circuits either are used and are thus subject to environmental influence or are not used and consequently decay.[1] It thus seems fair to speculate that social deprivation and abuse can have devastating effects on innate brain functions, whereas a rich and supportive social environment can help individuals to function at a much higher level of EI than they could achieve on their own. In the following sections we turn to research on the role of family communication and media communication in shaping EI.

11.2.3 Meta-Emotion: How Social Environments Support and Motivate the Acquisition of EI Skills

The many studies which have dealt with the role of the family in the development of emotional skills are too numerous to be discussed in detail here. We focus instead on a concept we find particularly useful for modeling general patterns of emotional communication which shape EI above and beyond the development of modular skills. Drawing on the seminal work of Mayer and Gaschke (1988) on the meta-experience of mood, Gottman, Katz, and Hooven (1997) used the concept of meta-emotion to describe the overall emotional climate in a family and its influence on the development of EI in a child.[2]

Gottman, Katz, and Hooven (1997) studied meta-emotion using qualitative interviews. They asked parents about their thoughts and emotions concerning their own anger and sadness and that of their children. Parents with a generally positive attitude toward their own emotions reported that it was important for them to teach their children how to make sense of and deal with emotions. They engaged in a set of supportive behaviors that the authors called "emotion coaching." According to Gottman, Katz, and Hooven (1997, 280), emotion-coaching parents are characterized by the following:

1. The parent is aware of the child's emotion.
2. The parent sees the child's emotion as an opportunity for intimacy and teaching.
3. The parent helps the child to verbally label the emotions the child is having.
4. The parent empathizes with or validates the child's emotion.
5. The parent helps the child to problem solve.

In contrast, parents who felt uncomfortable with emotions reported that they ignored or downplayed the child's emotions, distracted the child's attention from the eliciting situation, and criticized the child's emotions and emotional behavior.

It can thus be assumed that children who grow up in emotion-accepting and emotion-coaching families get ample opportunity to practice and refine their EI skills. Parents with negative meta-emotions, by contrast, engage in a variety of behaviors that actively interfere with the development of EI skills: They teach their children *not* to attend to emotions and emotion-eliciting events, *not* to react to such events, and *not* to express or talk about their emotions. Consistent with predictions, Gottman, Katz, and Hooven (1997) found that parents' meta-emotions were related to a number of developmental outcomes in the child. Children who grew up in emotion-accepting and emotion-coaching families were able to recover from physiological arousal more quickly, were less vulnerable to negative daily moods, engaged in cooperative peer interaction more often, and achieved better academic results than children who grew up in emotion-avoiding or emotion-dismissing families. Parental meta-emotion even had an influence on the child's physiology—for example, on basal vagal tone, an index of the functionality of the parasympathetic branch of the autonomic nervous system that regulates sympathetic arousal. Gottman, Katz, and Hooven (1997, 287–291) took this to indicate that parental emotion coaching is—more or less directly—involved in training the brain circuits that EI skills are based on.

Perhaps most important of all, children seem to internalize parents' meta-emotions due to the communicative feedback they get when experiencing an emotion. Children of parents with positive meta-emotions learn to greet emotions in themselves and others with warmth, interest, and self-confidence, whereas children of parents with negative meta-emotions learn to react to emotions with concern, avoidance, denial, and (self-)criticism. We suggest that internalizing parents' positive meta-emotions promotes the development of EI in the child over and above the coaching of modular skills and brain functions. This is because positive meta-emotions act as a general motivation to approach emotion-eliciting situations, to be aware of and communicate about emotions, and to find solutions and actively cope with emotion-eliciting situations (Maio and Esses 2001). This can be seen in contrast to the internalization of negative meta-emotions, which interfere with the development of EI, as they motivate avoidance, denial, and suppression of emotions and prevent the child from confronting and actively coping with emotion-eliciting situations.

The family is only one of the social institutions that shape people's meta-emotions and EI skills. As children grow up, the family's role in the "education of the heart" is gradually replaced with that of peer groups and the unwritten "feeling rules" of professional life (Hochschild 1983; Bartsch and Hübner 2006, 190f; Baumeler, this volume). In the next section we extend our focus beyond the role of interpersonal communication to that of culture and media communication in the socialization of meta-emotion and EI skills.

11.2.4 Meta-Emotion and Gender-Specific Media Use

Like the family, media do not merely communicate emotions; they also communicate specific attitudes and feelings *about* emotions (Bartsch and Viehoff 2003) which can either encourage or discourage the employment and further development of EI skills. When it comes to meta-emotions during media use, two points are particularly noticeable:

1. Meta-emotions involve emotion-specific preferences and aversions—for example, a person may enjoy the experience of sad, melancholic emotions (as evoked by melodramas) but avoid the experience of suspense, fear, and disgust (as evoked by horror films);

2. Meta-emotions generally conform to gender-specific norms and expectations.

Oliver's (1993) research on sad film preference provides a prime example of these points. Oliver constructed a Sad Film Scale that measures people's preference for melodramas. As expected, this pattern of media use was much more frequent in women than in men. In people who scored high on this scale, the reported degree of sadness while watching sad film scenes was positively related to enjoyment of the film scenes. Low scorers, in contrast, showed a reverse pattern of correlation. Oliver therefore concluded that feeling sad while watching "chick flicks" and "tearjerkers" is a rewarding experience for a specific (predominantly female) audience group while for others it is rather aversive. She explains this in terms of social norms concerning other-directed forms of sadness such as empathy, sympathy, and pity. Empathy is morally valued in our culture—especially in the female gender stereotype, whereas it is associated with ambivalent meta-emotions in the male stereotype. Thus, especially for women, empathy should be gratifying because it has been constantly rewarded during their socialization and is associated with self-enhancing thoughts and emotions.

In a similar vein, the predominantly male preference for film genres that deal with fear and aggression such as action, thriller, or horror might be explained by gender-specific norms and values that lead to a particular fascination with these emotions in men. Unfortunately, meta-emotions related to fear and aggression have not yet been sufficiently studied in the context of media use.

Thus, in the remainder of this chapter, we focus on the role of media in the socialization of empathy. While empathy is not the only domain of EI skills shaped by a society's media culture, the following considerations provide a case study of how a specific domain of EI skills might be applied to and shaped by media portrayals of emotion. A particular focus will be on the integrating function of media use with regard to EI skills. As we will argue, entertainment media typically communicate positive meta-emotions and engage the recipient's empathy skills on different levels of complexity, thereby coaching the integrated functioning of these skills.

11.3 Aesthetics and Performance of Emotional Interaction in Audiovisual Media: The "Scene of Empathy" in Audiovisual Media

The aesthetics involved in the audiovisual representation of emotion and emotional interaction are an important key to understanding the function of media use in the acquisition of EI skills in a specific culture. It is by creating aesthetic and narrative *conventions* of emotion representation that the media confirm and create emotion-related norms and values and guide recipients' meta-emotions. Media strategies for creating empathy are therefore closely related to the cultural conditioning of meta-emotions and EI skills.

Drawing on the three-level-approach to emotional communication mentioned earlier, we argue that audiovisual media engage recipients' empathy skills on different levels of complexity and thereby invite and coach the integrated functioning of these skills. Three levels of empathy skills and corresponding aesthetic and narrative devices of audiovisual media are considered: (1) perceptual empathy based on innate stimulus features in relation to aesthetic devices of emotion representation, (2) intentional empathy based on sensorimotor emotion scripts in relation to audiovisual narration, and (3) normative aspects of empathy in relation to character[3] evaluation. Engaging these different aspects in varying intensity, media may invite different kinds of empathy, depending on the degree to which the different facets of empathy are activated and related to each other in meaningful ways.[4]

11.3.1 The Sensorial Design of Empathy in Audiovisual Media

Audiovisual media offer their public dense compositions of visual, acoustic, and linguistic emotion cues that activate networks of sensorial and affective associations and experiences. Sensory emotion cues basically rely on innate perceptual mechanisms. Following G. M. Smith (1999, 2003), we argue that these sensory cues produce initially diffuse moods and feeling tones that prepare the viewer for the more intense emotional episodes to follow. At the same time, sensory emotion cues within an empathetic scene may intensify the effect of prototypical elements of emotion scripts, activating higher cognitive processes of emotional understanding and experience.

As previously stated, facial expressions of fear, sadness, happiness, and so forth can be experienced on a subcortical level and may trigger innate reflexes and reactions that are linked with these emotions. Since facial emotion expressions are strong emotion cues, audiovisual media widely use them in their emotional design in order to trigger empathic reactions in viewers.

The representation of emotional expression in audiovisual media not only relies on the innate gestalt characteristics of these expressions (as represented by the actors) but also refers to well-established aesthetic codes that selectively perform and intensify these gestalts (see also Tan 2005, and see Reddy, this volume). As direct and bodily interaction with the on-screen characters is impossible, the aesthetic simulation of media interaction has to be all the more intense.

The acting has to follow specific aesthetic codes in order to guide the empathic effect in the recipient. The aesthetic conventions of acting tend to "underacting," especially in cinema. The closeness and size of emotion expressions on the screen maximize the stimulus features of a prototypical emotion expression in a generally unnatural way. Every mimic movement is intensified on the large screen of the cinema. Overly explicit emotion expressions therefore tend to be experienced by viewers as exaggerated and artificial. By toning down their performance, actors forestall the eventuality of viewers distancing themselves from the screen characters' emotions.

With acting reduced to a few single prototypical mimic elements, the camera and audiovisual setting are free to compensate for this constraint. First, the duration of a shot is relevant for the empathic effect. On the one hand, it has to be long enough so the viewer can develop empathic emotions toward the film character (Plantinga 1999, 249–250). On the other hand, it must not be too long: According to the continuity-editing code, the duration and sequence of single shots have to simulate a natural viewing process. The permanent and close focusing on one person is experienced as unnatural, so the viewer becomes aware of the camera's presence and backs out of the "audiovisual contract" of illusion (see also Tan 2005).

Thus timing of both camera and editing is a key element in the audiovisual performance of emotional interaction in the media, as well as between the media and the public. In particular, the cinema has only to carefully set in scene the emotion cues that are prototypically and innately rooted in our brains, and their very presence will automatically trigger emotions. For this reason, the cinema has established complex aesthetic codes and conventions which focus on the whole audiovisual setting and context of the represented emotion cues—that is, on associated emotions and bodily experiences which are connected to these primary emotions and can be triggered by the audiovisual design itself. While the mimicry of the actors and the camera only show us a few single and prototypical facial elements of an emotion expression, they provide us the opportunity to *project* our own emotional experiences and emotions on the characters' situation. This projection is encouraged by other, implicit and associative elements of the audiovisual setting that are mostly perceived unconsciously by the viewers.

On the sensory level, audiovisual media convey the physical and affective intensity and dynamic of emotions via synesthetic compositions of vision and sound in the audiovisual setting (see also Plantinga 2007). The synchrony of the diverse visual and acoustic elements such as sound, music, tempo of editing, visual effects, colors, light, and so forth mostly relate to basic sensory and physical patterns of emotional experience that are closely related to the mimic and gestural expressions of film characters.

The forging of vision and sound in audiovisual media basically relies on an innate mechanism of human perception, namely, the cross-modal processing of sensory stimuli. Referring to qualities such as tempo, intensity, duration, location, and so forth, visual and acoustic elements in audiovisual compositions can refer to intermodal or suprasensory qualities which can be processed by all senses (see Anderson 1996; Flückiger 2002; Fahlenbrach 2005, 2006, 2007). The coordination of vision and sound along these categories not only ensures a unitary perception of reality but also provides a fundamental guide for emotional communication. In an emotional interaction, for example, the loudness of speech and the tempo and intensity of a gesture are as a rule coherently coordinated in relation to a specific emotion. This offers observers a coherent emotional gestalt that they recognize and that simultaneously allows them to coordinate their own emotional experience and behavior in an interaction affectively and bodily (see also Stern 1985).

Returning to the performance of empathetic interactions in audiovisual media (especially in narrative film), the coordination of vision and sound in reference to patterns of cross-modal processing is of crucial importance. The spaces of an empathic scene and their audiovisual atmospheres are loaded with affective qualities which ultimately relate to the primary emotions indicated in the facial expressions and the bodily behavior of the characters. While viewers recognize the prototypical emotion in the mimic and gestural behavior, their empathic projection is intensified by the related affective qualities that further visual and acoustic elements communicate cross-modally.

In scenes of empathy, *music* plays a prominent role in mediating the intensity and the dynamics of the inner emotions of a character on the screen. Music strengthens viewers' projection of their own emotional experiences onto those of the characters (see also J. Smith 1999). This effect relies on the double nature of music. On one level, music is abstract because it lacks a discrete reference (setting aside musical stereotypes). Therefore, it is adaptable to varying situations. On another level, it may mimic innate patterns of emotional experience which are very concrete in their reference to specific physical dynamics of prototypical emotions (emotions such as overwhelming, powerful, upgrading intensity, fading of energy, etc.). Film music effectively uses amodal qualities such as rhythm, duration, intensity, and direction—as well as significant gestalt patterns (e.g., regular–irregular, harmonic–disharmonic, etc.) in order to communicate the specific emotional state of a protagonist. Melodic contour, modality, tempo, and dynamic (see J. Smith 1999) are key facets in music used to express emotions. By directly depicting supramodal qualities of emotional expression, these facets provide the opportunity to forge the diverse audiovisual elements within an empathic scene into a unitary, coherent affective gestalt.

As Cohen (2001) has argued, music guides the cross-modal coordination of picture and sound. In densely composing those supramodal qualities, music may be the leading medium guiding the emotional tone and mood in an atmosphere, thereby reinforcing the facial and bodily expression of the protagonists. In this dominant function, music may trigger complex physical and affective associations and connotations that go far beyond the audiovisual representation on the screen. These associations are rooted in the emotional experience of the viewer herself. Thereby music intensifies the empathic emotions toward the affected characters.

Apart from the music, the acoustic atmosphere primarily maintains the emotional tone and mood in a scene of empathy and serves as an intensifier of the emotion cues communicated in the characters' emotional expressions. In cinema, sound has a significant effect on the filmic space (see Chion 1994): It affects both the visual space within the film and the interior space of the cinema, namely, the space of the reception. Whereas the visual space is restricted to the screen in front of audiences, the acoustic space surrounds them. Sound, thus, integrates the viewer into the filmic space and has a strong influence on his or her affective immersion.

Guided by sound and music, the moving pictures are affectively loaded with acoustic qualities that may intensify in the recipient the physical and affective anticipation of the emotional dynamics of the characters on the screen. The intensifying effect of pictures and sound also refers to another aspect of synesthetic perception: Visual and acoustic stimuli may activate multisensory associations on the base of mirror neurons (see Gallese 2005), including all kinds of sensory associations. Affective movements in vision and sound therefore trigger complex sensorial associations which may initiate in the viewer holistic physical and mental experiences of the emotions performed on the screen (see Fahlenbrach 2007).

11.3.2 The Performance of the Emotional Interaction on the Level of Sensorimotor Emotion Scripts

Emotion scripts are associative and dynamic schemata which include prototypical characteristics of eliciting situations, emotional action–reaction tendencies, and self-regulation strategies. Due to their associative structure, only one or a few significant elements represented in a film scene may trigger the whole script (see Fahlenbrach 2005, 2006).

In scenes of empathy, the facial expressions of the affected characters stand at the core of the whole setting, representing the main emotion cue. The perception of the facial expression automatically triggers the whole emotion script of the specific primary emotion. Therefore, it is crucial that the attention of the viewer is guided toward the facial expression and viewing perspective of the affected character (see Plantinga 1999, Tan 2005).

A general aesthetic code for scenes of empathy is the continuity-editing code. By constructing a coherent point-of-view perspective, the camera indicates to us the inner emotions of a character by showing a facial expression in a close shot, and, in addition, we are usually shown the object and person the affected character is looking at (see Plantinga 1999). In so doing, camera and editing provide us with intimate information about the emotional state of a character and its object or cause. Thus the viewer may already anticipate mentally (and affectively) the intentions and reactions prototypically related to this emotion.

This mental anticipation of the emotional intentions performed by the actors on the screen is a basic precondition for the viewer's empathy. Even if it does not suffice to arouse intense emotions in viewers, it can activate basic emotion scripts that let them anticipate specific action tendencies of an emotion.

The anticipation of intentions and causes of emotions is, again, intensified and directed by the whole audiovisual design. This also affects the anticipation of intentions in the emotional expression shown on the screen. While the facial expression of the protagonists already communicates prototypical intentions, their body movements, intensified by the audiovisual setting, indicate further intentional information. Significant movements activate sensorimotor action simulations (based on mirror neurons) in viewers which make them experience the intentions linked with these movements.

The creation of coherent and affectively significant audiovisual scripts further relies on *kinesthetic image schemata* that structure our bodily, emotional, and cognitive experience of the world. These image schemata refer to patterns, such as in–out (container), strong–weak (force), from here–to there (path), up–down, near–far, balance, and others (Johnson 1987, 79). These embodied schemata essentially guide our spatial orientation and kinesthetic coordination. At the same time, we refer to them in order to articulate complex experiences and concepts. Following Lakoff (1987) and Johnson (1987), we thereby produce conceptual metaphors in our thinking, perceiving, and feeling. By referring to metaphorical image schemata—for example, progress toward a goal is like progress made traveling on a road—audiovisual media translate inner emotional processes into outwardly visible action, thereby making them more tangible and easier to understand (Fahlenbrach 2005, 2006). If these image schemata are integrated with prototypical emotion scripts, they may activate higher cognitive processes that include a deeper understanding of the characters' emotional situation.

11.3.3 Symbolic Meanings in the Scene of Empathy

Empathy is further related to aspects of identification and sympathy which are based on social values, rules, and so on. Empathic emotions are therefore grounded in social and cognitive evaluations of the characters and symbolic rules of emotion expression (see Reddy, this volume). Consequently, the characters' emotion expression, and behavior must conform to emotion rules that are part of the viewers' social and cultural makeup in order to elicit empathy (or even admiration; Plantinga 1999, Gaut 1999). Sympathy and antipathy are based on processes of social comparison; the recipient compares the behavior and the reactions of a character with her or his own experiences, social values, and norms. Accordingly, sympathy and antipathy are cognitively driven evaluations that may also affect the empathetic emotions felt toward a film character (Zillman 1991). Yet, sympathy differs from empathy in a fundamental way. While empathy is *feeling with someone*, sympathy is typically experienced as *feeling for someone* (Plantinga 1999). While we experience a shared emotion with a film character empathically, we may feel sympathetically toward a film character who is experiencing a different emotion. In the case of antipathy, we feel resentment or contempt for a film character and often experience "counterempathic" emotions in which the valence of character emotions is reversed, for example, with gloating or malignant pleasure.

Yet as we react automatically during scenes of empathy to innate physical and mental emotion cues that we can barely control cognitively, we may even experience a weak form of empathy with characters we dislike or who may even disgust us (e.g., Plantinga 1999, Gaut 1999). Accordingly, we may experience different degrees of empathy toward a character, depending on the levels of emotional and cognitive experience involved in the empathetic anticipation (see also Zillmann 1991).

The cognitive and moral evaluation of a character's behavior and emotion expression is not restricted to individual scenes of empathy but is based on the development of a character's profile within a narrative. It is in the narrative development of a film or a TV show that we may be informed about the social and cognitive background of the characters' actions and behavior, about their inner emotions and desires, and about the contexts of their actions. Of course, the density of narrative information differs in every genre and with regard to different characters. Thus media can influence the cognitive and emotional anticipation experienced toward a character by information strategies (e.g., Alfred Hitchcock's famous suspense techniques).

Two final aspects remain to be mentioned which influence the symbolic and cultural dimensions of emotion expression in the scene of empathy: the viewer's knowledge concerning both the context of emotion expression and genre-specific emotions.

As Plantinga argues, our cognitive knowledge of emotion expression is fundamentally structured by the difference between the public and private sphere. In our (Western) culture, we presume that people tend to control their emotion expression in a public situation and may even hide or feign their inner emotions. Emotions expressed in public therefore seem generally to be less authentic than privately expressed emotions. Empathy, therefore, tends to be more intense if a character is shown in a private situation.

Furthermore, knowledge of genre-specific characteristics guides the viewer's allegiance and empathy toward media figures, even when the empathy may be experienced in a weak, automatically generated form toward characters we dislike. Recipients actively search for genre-specific gratifications among the very different kinds of media gratification available. The viewers' choice may also include experiencing affective and cognitive empathy with characters whose behavior and values differ widely from their own. Audiences of action films or horror films, for example, often enjoy the vicarious experience of emotions that are culturally and socially proscribed. In these cases, they actively share the perspective of a character they would probably condemn in their everyday life (see also Carroll 1990, M. Smith 1999).

11.4   Outlook

Obviously, empathy is performed on both sides of the screen by both media producers and media recipients. Empathy includes every dimension of emotional experience: the reflex-like sensory anticipation and physical experience of emotions, perspective taking and understanding of emotionally motivated actions and intentions on the level of sensorimotor emotion scripts, and the cognitive allegiance and moral evaluation on the level of social and cultural norms and values.

Through a dense and artful composition of emotion cues on different levels of emotional communication, media coach a number of different EI skills in an integrative manner. First, the stylistic and narrative conventions of emotion representation in audiovisual media help the viewer to coordinate self- and other-directed skills on an equal level of complexity. On a stimulus level, expressive cues that are indicative of emotion from a third-person perspective are combined with cross-modal mood cues that evoke experiential qualities of emotions from a first-person perspective. On the level of associative schemata, narrative information about the unfolding of emotional scripts and character intentions is combined with concrete metaphorical images that appeal to viewers' image schemata of physical interaction with the world, thereby helping them to grasp the inner forces and dynamics of emotion. On a symbolic level viewers are invited to evaluate characters from an empathic perspective by disclosing the characters' intimate thoughts, perceptions, and emotions, even if these are flawed or morally objectionable. All of these aesthetic and narrative devices strongly encourage the integration of first- and third-person perspectives on emotional experience. Second, by simultaneously appealing to skills on different levels of complexity, audiovisual media coach the integrated functioning of EI skills. Thus, in the long run, the aesthetics of audiovisual media appear to shape human empathy—by integrating and reorganizing innate brain functions in culturally meaningful ways.

The aesthetic and narrative devices for creating empathy analyzed above are not unique to "women's films" such as melodrama and romance, but they are used by these genres to a significant extent and with considerable sophistication. We are cautious to interpret this as an explanation for the proverbial superiority of women's empathy skills. Suffice it to say that women's empathy tends to be socialized to a higher degree than men's (Rosenthal and DePaulo 1979; Buck 1984 264–281) and that gender-specific meta-emotions and media preferences are critically involved in this socialization process. Considering the potential impact of media on the conditioning of EI skills, especially in the performance of empathetic scenes, they may implicitly regulate the emotional rules of communication and interaction within a culture.

However, as media offerings typically appeal to multiple aspects of emotional experience simultaneously, their emotional effects can be complex and even paradoxical. Spectator emotions are not simply a mirror image of emotions performed on the screen; they also evaluate, make sense of, and reflect upon these emotions (Bartsch, Eder, and Fahlenbrach 2007). As mentioned above, cognitively elaborate reactions like sympathy and antipathy involve emotions that differ from the emotions on the screen and may include counterempathic reactions. Aesthetic emotions and meta-emotions provide further examples of emotional phenomena that go beyond the coperformance of portrayed emotions.

Furthermore, it is important to note that media users take an active part in the process by which the media unfold their emotional effects. Audiences seek out and select certain media offerings, they decide whether they should welcome or reject a media offering's invitation to experience emotions, and they manage their level of emotional involvement by using a number of regulatory strategies—like selective exposure to emotionally arousing media stimuli, selective adoption of an empathetic or distanced mode of reception, and selective interpretation of symbolic meaning (Bartsch et al. 2006). Recipients' active involvement with the media, their selective emotions, cognitions, and behaviors, need to be taken into account as codeterminants of emotional socialization effects. People would not expose themselves voluntarily to emotional media effects if they did not expect the media to satisfy certain emotional needs and desires—be it hedonistic pleasure and well-being, playful application and refinement of emotion-related skills and abilities, or validation of personal norms, values, and self-ideals concerning emotion.

The efficient use of media-related competencies to satisfy emotional needs may be considered a form of EI in its own right. At this point, however, the normative significance of the EI concept comes into play. The phrase "emotional intelligence"—as it is used in academic and public discourse—implies that emotion-related skills and brain functions are used for the "good" of individuals and society as a whole. But what is "good" and, consequently, "intelligent"? Is it "intelligent" to seek pleasure and well-being during media use? Is it "intelligent" to learn the emotional lessons that the media have to offer? Is it "intelligent" to adopt the emotional norms and values that have come down to us as part of our media culture? Psychological research—including research on the neuropsychology of emotions—might help us to better understand emotional communication and to use the media more effectively to meet certain ends, but it cannot tell us whether it is really "good" or "intelligent" to do so. Defining desirable and "emotionally intelligent" forms of communication and media use is a task of society and media culture as a whole.

Notes

1. A classic study by Sackett (1966) on emotional communication skills in monkeys provides an example of this point. Sackett (1966) was able to show that monkeys have an innate ability to discriminate facial expressions of conspecifics even if they were reared in social

isolation prior to the experiment. If isolation ended early, the monkeys recovered quickly and developed normal communication skills. If isolation was prolonged after the fourth month, however, the innate skills began to decay, leaving the animals socially handicapped for the rest of their lives.

2. In the early work of Mayer and Gaschke (1988) and Salovey et al. (1995), the concept of meta-mood is closely related to that of emotional intelligence. Mayer and Gaschke (1988) define meta-mood as "the possible outcome of a regulatory process that monitors, evaluates, and changes mood" (Mayer and Gaschke 1988, 109). Contemporary approaches to emotional intelligence focus primarily on the skills and abilities that are involved in this regulatory process, whereas research on meta-emotion has specialized in the experiential, evaluative, and motivational aspects of higher order mental processes that accompany and regulate emotion. We think that the study of emotional intelligence could profit from drawing these divergent lines of research together again.

3. The term "character" is used in this chapter in the sense of media or film character, not in the sense of personality characteristics.

4. There are several approaches in film theory that differentiate in a comparable way the different levels and degrees of empathy in films (e.g., Tan 1996, Plantinga 1999, Gaut 1999, Wulff 2002, just to mention a few). Due to space limitations, we cannot discuss the different approaches here.

12   Oneself as Another? Autism and Emotional Intelligence as Pop Science, and the Establishment of "Essential" Differences

Nicole C. Karafyllis

The female brain is predominantly hard-wired for empathy. The male brain is predominantly hard-wired for understanding and building systems.
—Simon Baron-Cohen, British psychopathologist (2004, 1)

12.1   Autism: "Othering" Emotional Intelligence

12.1.1   Autists as Human Aliens: A Control Group for Science and Society

What do Dustin Hoffman in *Rain Man* (United States, 1988), Jodie Foster in *Nell* (United States, 1994), and Sigourney Weaver in *Snow Cake* (United Kingdom, 2006) have in common? They all belong to the elite of Hollywood actors, and they all play the role of different types of autists.[1] It is a challenge for the best of actors to bring a negative social performance to the screen *by* an act of performance, stressing both of the meanings of "performance" in ordinary language today. One might add Jack Nicholson as Melvin Udall in *As Good as It Gets* (United States, 1997), but he appears to portray more a sociophobe than an autist; nevertheless, he has the "typical" autist's difficulties with communicating his feelings and responding adequately to his social environment while simultaneously being obsessed with ensuring that everything around him is in perfect order. The ambiguities of the real world are much too complicated for his personality structure. With the help of a woman he feels attracted to (a role played by Helen Hunt), he learns to open up and finally wins her love. However, maybe he trained his emotional intelligence (EI) to become accepted by the ones he wished to be accepted by—who knows what his emotional potential might have been? This positive change within a "monster" is a leitmotif already familiar from *King Kong* (1933) and the *Alien* movies.

However, in the films mentioned above, the focus is not on gorillas (Griem 2008), monsters, or cyborgs but on human beings. Nevertheless, the films do not fall into the category of psycho-movies (Fellner 2006). The protagonists' mental lives are concealed, as they rarely show emotions by gestures or mimics, or, as in the case of the film *Nell* (Nell Kellty, a female Kaspar Hauser), they have developed a private language because of an upbringing in solitude. The film borrows ideas from François Truffaut's *L'Enfant Savage* (1969). Even if Nell Kellty is not an autist in every medical sense, as her brain has *been* "normal" at birth and developed abnormally because of social isolation, she at least *behaves* like an autist to some extent, exhibiting ritualistic behaviors, for example, as Nicholson's Melvin Udall does. The cinema audience has to make inferences from social representations, that is, the behavior observed in various situations, and popular diagnostic categories, in order to make sense of the agentic abilities of the protagonists on-screen. Biological representations of abnormalities in the brain like neuroimages or gene scans (which would allow for conclusive findings about whether Nell is "neurotypic" or "genotypic" and has a "regressive phenotype") are not available to the viewer. However, they are also not available to scientists, as will emerge in due course. In the cinema, the audience seems to be aware of the *reasons* for deviant behavior (if the plot allows this), or—already saturated with diagnostic categories from psychology due to an overall therapeutic culture (Illouz, this volume)—it does not even think of reasons but rather focuses on the protagonist's therapy, whereas science has to determine the biological *causes* in its laboratories.

In *Nell*, the female protagonist gradually adjusts to the daily presence of the caring scientist Dr. Jerome Lovell (played by Liam Neeson), making the world of science part of the young woman's life after her sick mother's death. Initially, she had fought him. Dr. Lovell tries to ensure that she is not reduced to a mere scientific object. In *Backstreet Dreams* (1990) the gender relation is the other way around, and this is the typical gender relationship—but not only in the movies. Brooke Shields (*Backstreet Dreams*) plays a psychiatrist caring for an autistic boy. Kirstie Alley plays *David's Mother* (1994), Dede Tate (played by Jodie Foster) mothers whiz boy Freddy in *Little Man Tate* (1991), and so forth. Through the lens of gender, many autism movies are mother movies. In only a handful of the many films on autism is the diagnosis "autism" made explicit. Maybe this reflects more on how difficult a correct diagnosis is and how diffuse are the *Diagnostic and Statistical Manual of Mental Disorders* (*DSM*) criteria developed in the last 50 years than on social stigmatization. How should filmmakers know when even scientists do not know? The lack of concreteness both in science and in the media is one of the reasons why Web sites promoting the autism rights movements also often refer to Tom Hanks in the sympathetic role of *Forrest Gump* (United States, 1994) as one of their icons, though his behavior—and assumed IQ—differs substantially from that of the phone-book-memorizing genius Raymond Babbitt in *Rain Man*.

Back to the "real" world. This chapter will deal with scientific approaches to reduce "the" autist to "an" extreme male brain, and with the pop-scientific and pop-cultural discourses that accompany and legitimize this modeling. What autists really suffer from—if they *suffer* at all—is determined by medical doctors, psychologists, and psychiatrists, who can only describe these isolated interior worlds symptomatologically, or by biologists, who can make neuroscientific images to represent what is happening inside the brain at a particular moment—but none of them can enter these worlds.

The guiding questions of this chapter thus include the following: How is an abnormal "social" brain condition scientifically modeled and tested, and how are normal and abnormal brains viewed through the lens of sex and gender? Which *Menschenbild* is employed? Why should we worry when particular forms of autism are described by scientists as "hypermale" and "high functional" (Baron-Cohen 2004, 184), while "the normal autist" (quasi-diagnostically categorized as "low functional") is left behind in the public perception? With reference to pop science: Do you have to accept your brain as it is, or can you work to enhance its capacities? Which particular role does the female brain play, and what role do women play, in the pop science of the brain?

Apart from offering a brief account of the status of autism research, and of the related fields of developmental and social cognitive science, in light of the declared need for EI (Goleman 1995, 2006), I will also outline possible outcomes of these research areas. I will then conclude by summarizing the findings and exploring ways of "othering" related kinds of selves in the market of pop science.

Some caveats are in order at the outset, however. First, although I use the terms "autism," "cognitive science," "neuroscience," "psychology," and so forth, and also "man" and "woman" and "male" and "female," I am aware that this use of generalities involves problems. Each of the concepts and disciplines (and more) mentioned above can be divided into numerous subgroups and related to multiple and heterogeneous discourses. Second, categories like "brain" or "body" or "Western society" are generalities themselves and can easily be affiliated with holisms, which is a weakness inherent to discourses on normality and on the self and the other. In this chapter, I cannot avoid painting a picture of the encounter between scientific and public views of EI and autism in broad strokes, though I will eventually go into detail, particularly where scientific models and philosophical concepts are concerned.

I arrived at the research topic of autism by a detour. During the last years, I intensively questioned whether the two main anthropological models of the twentieth century, the animal (for the body model) and the robot (for the brain/mind model), would be sufficient for future explanatory contexts in science, particularly when psychology was supposed to be embraced (Karafyllis 2008a). Questioning whether the machine is not simply corresponding with the human any more, rather than embodying it, is, of course, not new; neither is it new to connect the machine to a mental disorder put on a societal level (in relation to schizophrenia, see Deleuze and Guattari 1983, e.g., 36). Still, prominent critiques have often dealt with symbolisms rather than material entities and had the animal as its material "other," needed for guaranteeing "the flow" inside the human and society, while the machine was said to be responsible for the controllable disturbances of the flow, for instance, the rhythm and the pulsing. After several centuries in which human nature and society was more and more understood by means of models and metaphors borrowed from technology (Keller 2002; Köchy 2003; Lewens 2004; Karafyllis 2006a, 2007a, 2008e; Zittel, Engel, Nanni, and Karafyllis 2008), revealing that what is referred to in science as human nature is actually better described as "human biopsycho(techno)logy," the use of autists' brains as epistemic models has introduced a new issue into the debate—because autists are not simply epistemic models, they are real human persons. Both their brains and behaviors are under scientific scrutiny within the field of developmental and social cognitive neuroscience. So, what is really new?

Simply put, first, what is new (in an epistemological sense) is that autists are already there. Autists are real, or better: People with autistic behaviors are real as insofar as there is a consensus on what autistic behaviors are (on the problem of how "real" can be defined in relation to psychology, see Hacking 1998, 8–20). Scientists and engineers do not have to physically create them—they can find them; however, they can create them scientifically, that is, model them as more or less deviant, according to intentions of powerful elites who might be keen on "social engineering." Not only has the autist's brain obtained the status of some *essence* in the material world but so also has his (modeled) a-sociality. Both seem to be real because of the real human person that "embodies" it (this term, in the brain context, derives from the cognitive sciences). Autists are a living control group for science as are likewise, on the opposite side of the so-called extreme male brain of the autist (Baron-Cohen 2004), women and their female brains (Brizendine 2006). In a society which is seen as a laboratory space of *real* experiments (Krohn 2007), and as an epistemic object itself, the category of abnormality is constantly being redefined around an inert core of power: male-encoded intellectuality, corresponding to the brain of a "normal" man as an epistemic object. In social neuroscience, society is an epistemic object of inquiry and of modeling, as is deviant behavior—be it high functional or low functional, in reference to society's proclaimed needs. The approach of using society as an extended laboratory space, as an enhanced environment for transforming neurosciences into social neurosciences, rests upon the *malleability* of natural objects (Knorr-Cetina 1999, 26f), which must, at the same time, be describable as social agents (Cole 2005). The autist is such a malleable, "natural" object. He has no illness, neither a physical nor a mental one. Thus, there is no problem of scientific creditworthiness of his statements within the laboratory context. His purported asocial behavior while still being situated in society makes him a purified "social" agent with a natural core which remains biologically and scientifically "normal."

Second, the rhetoric is new as, in the case of Baron-Cohen's science and pop-science writings, the category "gender" is embraced—though "sex" is meant. The adoption of the analytical category "gender" from the social sciences hides the fact that gay and lesbian "brains" do not exist in a biological approach because lesbian and gay bodies also do not exist. Earlier studies *comparing* women's and men's brains, and, for example, their different language-processing capacities and verbal fluency, were primarily based on the brain's different laterality and interhemispheric exchange of information (Kimura 1999). Turning to scientific ontology, in Kimura's studies, it remains clear that the heterosexualized category body is superior to the category of the brain, that is, she analyzed brains *of* women and *of* men. In a variation of this approach, after discussing the findings reported by Kimura, Baron-Cohen adds the argument that "Homosexual men are also reported to have a larger anterior commissure than heterosexual men, and as large as heterosexual women" (Baron-Cohen 2004, 112), which, following the previous line of argumentation, provides an explanation for why gay men are empathic and both good listeners and talkers. He does not explicitly draw this conclusion but places this single scientific finding on the brains of homosexual men in a row with the findings on women's brains. This suggests to the reader that gender issues are involved, though all of the argumentation with respect to essential brain differences is based on the biology of dysmorphic heterosexuality. Baron-Cohen then adds a new category of sex ("brain type"), to which he adds a new criterion which also functions in terms of a causal explanation, "sex-typical behavior": "this follows from your brain type" (Baron-Cohen 2004, 98f). In the end, then, he made his biological determinism of sexualized brain and social behavior explicit.

Above all, what is relatively new is the possibility of genetic engineering to *materially* let the human be a reproductive animal and a high-functional machine at the same time, that is, a triangulation of human soul, animal body, and machine. This triangulation incorporates both flow and disturbances while still allowing the individual to have a separate development and a unique history, in which had been technically interfered before he/she existed (i.e., the making of "biofacts," rather than artifacts; Karafyllis 2003, 2004, 2007a, 2008d). Animal and machine comprise also gender-coded female and male capacities, and we will come across these codes again in this chapter.

The autist as a long-wished-for union of animal and machine did not come as a surprise. Once Baron-Cohen, in the late 1980s, asked whether social deficits of autists are cognitive or affective (Baron-Cohen 1988) and attributed to autists' brains a defective theory-of-mind module, borrowed from artificial intelligence (AI) research (see Turing [1950] and Jefferson [1949] for the classic controversy), humanoid robotics, and cognitive psychology, the way was paved for all that was still to come in his research and the research of some others on autism—which deals with far more than autism and is thus adopted in various scientific and popular contexts, ranging from the concept of autists' mindblindness in philosophy of language (Kristin 2002) to the extreme male brain as boundary object for new "manliness" (Mansfield 2006) and artists, poets, and politicians of the past who are now thought to have been autistic (Fitzgerald 2005). In a philosopher's view, at least within a limited analytical perspective (which I do not share), the autist is the best evidence that the mind–body problem can be solved, if the mind and body are hypothetically reduced from substantial corelations, particularly those to themselves, to other persons, and to nature (Karafyllis 2001).

However, there is something missing even in the publications critical of either animals or robots as models for humans (e.g., Orland 2005): the plants. Looking across cultures, in ontologies of nature the activity of soul, and thus life, starts with plants, that is, what Aristotle regarded as (Latin) *anima vegetativa* (or Greek: *psyché threptiké*). As the plant metaphor has always guaranteed the processual vegetative capacities of growth, development, and emotionality, both in the body and in what was later called the "psyche" by psychology (note: Sigmund Freud's "drive" reads "*Trieb*" in the German original, which means "shoot" as opposed to the invisible root, and this metaphor played with the ancient idea of the root of *physis* in Homer's *Odyssey*), it survived in many psycho-relevant contexts, not least in the term "vegetative nervous system." It is responsible for the "essentials" of human life, digestion, pulse, and so forth and also emotional stability (maybe some remember the old medical term "vegetative dystonia" for depression, and the Latin *tonus* leads back to music metaphors for emotional states—thus depression was formerly seen as a disharmony autonomously caused, rather than as a disorder). The vegetative nervous system was named the "autonomous nervous system" by John Newport Langley (1852–1925), thus reminding medical doctors and psychologists even in the twenty-first century of its uncontrollable and self-empowering processes (see also the experiments on plants and emotions of Haviland-Jones, Rosario, Wilson, and McGuire 2005). The genuine plant capacities, their mediality, is also essential to the instruments used in genetics (as they import one core concept of the Greek plant soul, i.e., the *genesis*), in a very material sense, because without this mediality no gene, or organ, could be "transplanted" or "cloned." There has to be something that *makes* bodies, body parts, cells, genes, and so forth integrate into and assimilate to something, accompanying the technical interventions of scientists—something which has no fixed body itself. In scientific representations of bodies and particles, the vegetative mediality shows in what is *not* visualized and represented. The invisibility of the medium's own materiality and potentiality is the reason why organs appear to function context free in science, for example, the gray matrix in which organs or faces seem to be embedded in photographs, the black background of neuroimages, the purified DNA which comes out of the blue, or even the imagined "brain in the tank/vat" in the philosophical traditions of dealing with skepticism (based on a thought experiment from René Descartes).[2]

Therefore, though I refer to robots and computers in this chapter, I do not argue in favor of the known machine/animal tradition. And I do not use autists to exemplify a philosophical case. At present, it is more relevant to analyze how autism is used, and how autists are used, to manifest this blindness to autonomous abilities (a crucial point that Ian Hacking also stressed in relation to psychosciences; Hacking 1998). With the animal/machine approaches tacitly euphemizing plants as a modern utopia for romanticists, a critique on modern biopsychoscience ideologies of systems and their inputs and outputs will never reach the status that critique matters in regard to a biopsychologization of autonomous potentials. Plants are not only nature's body (Schiebinger 1993) in the sense of material, they are—metaphorically—what *enables* the soul to be a time–space continuum and to finally reach the state of personal autonomy (or not). They are not definite and concrete, but potentials. In Western cultures, we have no other terms with which to imagine these *potentials* of life's flow, growth, and emotionality than water, music or plant metaphors, and plant metaphors always accompany the movement metaphors which are used for describing behaviors and functions of fixed entities (bodies, brains, machines, etc.): emotions, motivations, and drives.

To give an outlook on autism research and its relation to the invisibility of growth: Simon Baron-Cohen's "extreme male brain" of an imagined idealtype of an autist is not autistic from the start of "its" life, rather it *becomes* essentially male because, while *growing* in the mother's uterus, it receives an overdose of testosterone from the mother's blood via the placenta. This hypothesis about the relation of intrauterine development and disorder was introduced back in 1985 (Geschwind and Galaburda 1985), and at that time too much testosterone in the womb was also thought to influence the development of left-handedness and dyslexia. Here we see that neither the theory-of-mind module (in which autists are supposed to have deficits) nor the brain is a constructed system built in an empty space but rather has to grow somewhere, fostered by other potentials, in order to acquire the status of a human. The psychobioscientific power structure of autism research is the control of growth and development, including its media of potentiality like blood and amniotic fluid, as early as possible and the epistemological design of essences. Male brains are not identical with autistic men, as Baron-Cohen purports. When you read Baron-Cohen's writings on the male brain and subtract the dominant murmuring of brains, pregnancy, gonadal hormones, and so forth, the core concept of this assumed identity is genetic: the XY-chromosomal genotype (i.e., the "normal" man, not the chromosomal abnormalities XYY, or XXY, the latter known as Klinefelter's syndrome). Biologically, there can be no sex difference *in* the brain (Baron-Cohen, Knickemeyer, and Belmonte 2005) which was not already there before, rather there is the potentiality of its essence (the genetic determination of sex) more or less developed. In Baron-Cohen's approach, you have to *be* essentially a man, before you are able to *become* an autist with an essentially male brain, which is, in Baron-Cohen's sense, a disability that fosters exceptional intelligent abilities. Genetics, when fused with hormone research (an area known as psychobiology since the 1970s), is a scientific couple sharing the power to define essences (genetics) and potentials (hormone research). In the neuroendocrinological approaches (Hines 2004,

Brizendine 2006), these potentials are modeled—by means of "invisible" blood containing invisible hormones—as crossing the border of body and brain and creating new essences in the brain: emotions. And they also cross the border of the body and the skin and create new essences in the social world: behaviors. Thus, following Baron-Cohen's line of argumentation, if you are the XX type, you will neither grow to the full bloom of a male brain nor to a male behavior, though his use of the word "gender" rather than "sex" veils that (see also Nye, this volume).

For this reason, I stress the relation of autism research, gender, and future genetics. Media and its representations (or the lack thereof) are at the hidden core whenever we talk about physical or psychical capacities, abilities, or disabilities or even something like healing. Robots do not have genes or hormones, but they have still been modeled as idealtypic males (regarding body anatomy, morphology, and labeling with male forenames; see also Weber 2003). For a thorough critique, we should not overestimate popular analogies which are all too visible.

If there ever was a film which really envisioned how the material union of robot and animal model could take place by the medium of plants' vegetative soul capacities, for the sake of controlling humans and societies, it is *The Invasion of the Body Snatchers* (United States, 1956, 1978). The original film offered a critical comment on an alleged communist invasion of the United States during the McCarthy era, the second on the imagined invasion from outer space. It shows how plants' potentials are used as technical means to control the sphere of the body and the psyche, and how this control results in a lack of emotions, high-functional autistic behaviors, and antisocial attitudes. It is about symbolizing the functionalization, rationalization, and homogenization of personal drives, emotions, and motivations by means of the "non-moving" plants, without throwing the audience off the scent by explicitly staging the movement imaginary implied in the modern psychological terms (e.g., "emotion"), for instance, by showing "cyborgs" or animal-like creatures. In a philosophy of science reading, this plot is the brilliant ancestor of what actually is taking place in the science of autism and with autism—though the film was not related to the disorder of autism at all. Examining the film from a gender point of view, it is disappointing that it had to be a woman who "instinctively" feels that something is wrong with her friends, who, at first glance, appear to be normal. Not surprisingly, she is declared insane by a (man) psychologist.

12.1.2 Constructing Autistic Selves

The autist's self remains hidden as, strictly speaking, does the self of any person. Moreover, scientists do not know how people like the ones portrayed on the cinema screen created these exclusionary states of intimate privacy: by chance (genetic and neurophysiological causes, e.g., related to the development of abnormal spindle neurons and serotonin levels), after a vaccination (containing thiomersal,[3] e.g., in vaccinations against mumps and measles), because of diet (e.g., mercury in the food chain; see Mutter et al. 2005), due to factors resulting from abnormal intrauterine child development (imbalanced maternal hormones; see Baron-Cohen 2004; or mercury from the mother's amalgam fillings or a rubella infection; see Chess, Korn, and Fernandez 1971), because of a lack of attention, education, or social stimuli and response?

While the causes are unclear, a "theory" has already been conceptualized about the outcome. The *extreme-male-brain theory*, put forward by Simon Baron-Cohen (1999, 2004; Baron-Cohen and Hammer 1997), claims that the increased ability to analyze systems and patterns of humans who have little or no empathy and understanding of other's feelings can be ascribed to an idealtype, the extreme male brain.

In the following, I will not focus on causes of autism but rather on a *cultural mentality* that produces both pieces of popular art, pop science, and science concerning the interface between intelligence and emotions within a limited understanding of "self"—and, with Ian Hacking (1998), within a merely empirical and thus undercomplex understanding of "soul" even in the psychosciences. In the discussion about what is autism, both limited understandings meet. As the idea of self always depends on the idea of another, a limited understanding of self implies a reduced recognition of the other. This reduced recognition of the other becomes obvious in the present research on autists and its communication to the public, particularly with regard to gender issues. It does not matter if we look in the laboratories, in the pop-science books, at TV, or at the cinema screen: The majority of autists presented are men. On-screen, autistic men are definite heterosexuals who can be aroused by the opposite sex—in fact, that is an element of most plots included in order to reveal their hidden emotionality, to weaken their control, and to show that they are "real" human beings who can be cured of their loneliness. However, is it really *their* loneliness or ours?

On a phenomenal level, there is an illness which represents something of an opposite to autism, the Williams–Beuren syndrome. Apart from medical students, hardly anybody knows about it. Children with this syndrome read earlier than others, are very intelligent, have an exceptional sense of hearing, and love social interaction. However, the syndrome has long-known genetic causes, has a definite phenotype, and is a rare illness involving physical (e.g., cardiovascular) problems. It is not a disorder or an epidemic. Therefore, it does not inspire the fear that everybody might potentially have it. Neither does it encourage thinking about a dark, unsocial part of us. Above all, it implies no sex ratio.

The title of my essay is borrowed from French philosopher Paul Ricœur's masterpiece *Oneself as Another* (1992). The idea of the "self" is generally based on a *reflexive* structure. With this concept, one can outline strategies of "othering" in neuroscientific and related discourses because "to say self is not to say myself" (Ricœur 1992, 180). This is why a self-organizing network of neurons does not imply that this network knows that it *is*. Within a phenomenological approach, this difference is referred to as essence (Latin: *essentia*), that is, knowing *what* an entity is, and existence (Latin: *existentia*), that is, knowing *that* it is (e.g., Heidegger 2005, 128ff). In modeling "essential differences" (Baron-Cohen 2004) within the idea of a human being, this difference is touched upon though not explored. What do these insights imply for autism research? According to Baron-Cohen (1999), the impairment in the capacity to "mindread" can be regarded as "mindblindness" and "is defined as the ability to attribute mental states to oneself and others, and make sense of and predict behaviour on the basis of mental states." The primary thing obvious in comparing this statement with a phenomenologist's statement is that Baron-Cohen's "oneself" does not imply "myself." Baron-Cohen's perspective of the individual does not provide any causes or reasons as to why there should be an "I," a first-person perspective; rather, it stresses the singularity and objectivity ("oneself") of the individual body and brain.

The awareness of existence remains within the sphere of the subject and its personal relations to the life world (Schütz and Luckmann 2003). This also relates to the important difference between what is real and what is actual (e.g., Hubig 2006), and what is implied by the term "empirical" knowledge. As philosopher W. v. O. Quine (1951) has analyzed, one of the false claims of empiricism is that the meaning of a single proposition is its verification conditions. Science can model autism in terms of real knowledge, but only the autist himself or herself, and the ones who belong to his or her life, can actually experience that there *is* an "autist"—by experiencing resistances to what others consider to be normal. Only for the autist and his or her family, friends, and caretakers, autism actually matters. Autists can say "I" and "myself." They are real human persons, and neither brains nor robots, herewith an objection to Baron-Cohen's hypothesis of autists' *mindblindness* (Baron-Cohen 1999). If we think in a cultural dimension, autism, derived from the Greek word *autos* for "self," can be seen as a cultural metaphor for a general *self-occupancy*. This implies that even if we do not know what it is like to be an autist, we at least seem to be able to imagine it. Autism as a phenomenon has something to say about self-occupancy and loneliness to "normal" people, and, when looking at the pop-science texts on autism, it is a challenge to keep in mind the needs of the autists and those who care for them.

Is there a cure in sight? No. Let's take a brief look at the science of autism, a topic which will be discussed in detail in section 12.3 of this chapter. After several huge genome scan initiatives, such as the Autism Genome Project (AGP; AGP Consortium 2007), geneticists can now describe a watered-down version of "self," that is, the autist's genome, which is particularly interesting because it is, in fact, the autists' genome (on the population level). Still, geneticists have no idea about what really causes autism. There is no definite genotype, and there is no definite phenotype for autism (not even an agreement on phenotypic traits; see, e.g., Dawson et al. 2002), while, at the same time, hundreds of people are diagnosed as autists every day. Health politicians have described autism as an epidemiological threat (in an economical sense, because, fortuitously, autism is not contagious). And the Baron-Cohen group primarily analyzes the development of the extreme male brain in the womb, which means that the many autists already walking around will hardly profit directly from this research.

Establishing fetal autists and their brains as scientific objects not only provides a real opportunity for backlash gender politics (to which the rhetoric of an extreme male brain belongs) but also presents a challenge primarily for the transformation of bio–cogno–neuro– and psychosciences to fuse into "big science," that is, an even bigger science than before. This big science will have a fundament of "hard science" with genetics, statistics, and computer science rather than neuroscience. "Neuro" is always high-end. What really matters in empowering bioscience lies in the *beginning* of human development, and thus it makes strategic sense that the extreme-male-brain theory was created in the area of developmental psychopathology (dealing with fetuses and children), and not, for instance, in gerontology (note: there are hardly any costly functional magnetic resonance imaging [fMRI] studies on how the old brain "feels"). The medical subdiscipline of developmental psychopathology (in which Baron-Cohen's autism research is situated) was recently renamed *developmental cognitive science*, a category already suggested by Andrew Meltzoff (1990), or perhaps even earlier. As it is partly supposed to focus on analyzing socially relevant disorders in the cognition and expression of emotions, another new label for the ongoing research in which autism research is embedded is *social cognitive (neuro)science*. The latter works under the premise that it is important to be socially effective (see, e.g., Singer et al. 2004a).

However, the public self-fashioning of many sciences involved in autism research (and its other: emotions research) orbits around the brain, both a fetish object and a normative icon (Wassmann 2007) of Western culture. The brain is part of the rhetoric surrounding the emerging science of systems biology, which, on the explanatory levels of science, ranges from genes to social behaviors, based on heterosexuality (whereas on the methodological level in genetics, it is necessarily based on asexual forms of reproduction, e.g., cloning). The initial rhetoric of "neuro," and the representation of the brain in the neuroimage, demarcating systems biology's high end, relates to the organizing process of high-functional life science, which encompasses all "life" structures, starting from the gene and the cell, passing tissues and organs, and ending up with the brain, body, and even society.

Initial rhetorics and imagery of science formations are nothing new. Ian Hacking (1998, 5) argues that photography in the late nineteenth century was part of the initial rhetoric of multiplicity, shaping the scientific discourses and the research field for what was nearly a century later known as multiple personality disorder (MPD). Moreover, the related idea of a "second self" in the interior of the soul was easily adopted in popular culture because of its purported connection with early child abuse, criminality, spiritism, and reincarnation. The second, dissociated self was in fact a second subject. Conversely, the idea that there is a "pure" mind system feeling alone with itself ("autism") can be connected easily with an all-encompassing systems approach to scientifically model mental life in an exclusive third-person perspective. Cognitive sciences model a second object as situated in the brain, that is, the mind which potentially covers the full range of analyzing systems in the "world."

In this modeling process, the "second self," who has been inscribed into the psyche with painstaking effort by psychology during the last century, is likely to be subtracted. In the 1970s, it was modeled as a dissociated *Inner Self Helper* (Hacking 1998, e.g., 47f), a medium of cure which could, when applied correctly, help the individual to reintegrate both with herself or himself (the first, unhappy self) and society. After all, the imagined second self was gender neutral, that is, a man might possibly have a female second self (an idea that led to the rhetoric of "coming out"). Bio–psycho–cogno–info–neuroscience currently promotes a process of purifying the mind, of abandoning "the second" in the self by describing a *static*, second "self," seen as an entity occurring in the outside world, as a natural category which the brain can intellectually "grasp" and integrate into its system (Lakoff and Johnson 1999). Moreover, the second self's representation is (owing to earlier biosemiotical approaches in cognitive science) considered to be identical with the materiality of the brain (or some of its "modules"), thereby blurring important distinctions such as those between signals and symbols (Cassirer 1944/1972) and the environment and world. Simulating an entity from outside the person as something inside a person is carried out in the field of neuroscience by the relatively new concept of mirror neurons (see the Introduction to this volume, Gallese 2005, and below).

As there is no brain area defined for "feeling lonely" or "being alone," functional neuroimages for visualizing what is publicly described as the core of the autism disorder, "loneliness," do not really make sense yet. The aforementioned self-occupancy does not necessarily imply a preference for loneliness, not even in autists (see Jobe and White 2007). Moreover, there is a difference between feeling lonely (though people are there and care; as, e.g., in some cases of ADHD) and being socially excluded, which, in fact, many people with autism are due to a lack of social skills. From this lack of social skills, one could infer a broader phenotype of autism (as Jobe and White 2007 vote for), encompassing autistic behaviors which "normal" people also exhibit. In contrast, in a cognitive approach, loneliness would imply that there is nobody else in the mental world (solipsism). But, in fact, other people *are* "there."

Behind the public fashioning of autism with "the brain," most autism researchers know that the results on how autists' brains differ from "normal" ones are limited. The differences found in autists' brains are still mainly based on neuroarchitecture (see Waiter et al. 2004; Baron-Cohen, Knickemeyer, and Belmonte 2005), imaging (by

MRI, not fMRI), for example, an increase in gray matter volume in brains of autists with IQs above 80 (high-functional autists; HFAs). These differences relate to high-functional adults (mainly men, e.g., Waiter et al. 2004). On the other hand, a neuroscan of the developing hypermale autist in the uterus is not, at present, possible. However, a German–Swiss team of psychiatrists recently carried out experiments with (only) the HFAs (individuals with Asperger's syndrome) on curing an extreme male brain. Neuroimages were not necessary. By sniffing a nasal spray which contained the hormone oxytocin (OT), subjects' capacity for mind reading in psychological tests increased significantly (Domes et al. 2007).

Why might these facts be important to know? Scientific modeling depends on what is technically possible to model, that is, it depends on the apparatus and instruments. Hacking (1983) describes this as the relation of representing and intervening. Laboratory work follows distinct orders of visibility (Geimer 2002), established by a technical apparatus like the microscope. Over the last four centuries, advances in microscope technology have increased the resolution of images, but the perspective, and thus the order of visibility, has not changed. What happens if the visualization technique is not applicable or does not exist? The lack of a technical opportunity to scrutinize the object of interest *in statu nascendi*, for example, the fetal brain *developing* abnormal (e.g., "autistic") brain structures and functions by means of a hypothesized high exposure to testosterone in the womb, often results in the remodeling of the phenomenon suggested to be abnormal (e.g., autist's behavior in the social world).

Therefore, within science, you presently find many competing definitions of what kind of abnormality autism actually *is*, ranging from an "extreme form of the neurodevelopmental pattern" (of men) (Baron-Cohen and Hammer 1997) and a "neurodevelopmental disorder," to an "abnormally functioning social cognitive neural network" (Waiter et al. 2004) and a "global social disability" (Hamilton and Krendl 2007, who are actually critical of that term). What is involved in these definitions are different sample sizes, genders, tested IQs, and ages of autists examined, and different degrees of severity of autism at the phenomenal level. Therefore, "autist" represents a very heterogeneous category both in the scientific and the social world.

The above juxtaposition of "neurodevelopmental" and "social" implicitly contains the continuum of biological systems which have to be passed to arrive at the very beginning of an individual's life at the social level. The main medium for passing through these "systems" is hormones (neurotransmitters), including sex hormones, which are thought to be responsible for organizing both brain structures and behaviors (e.g., Geschwind and Galaburda 1985; see also Hines 2004, Geher and Miller 2007). In order to use the method of fMRI in autism research, the autist's disorder has to be modeled such that it corresponds with the brain areas for which functions have already been defined: the areas for "intellectual" capacities in a broad sense. Current brain areas of interest in autism research are as follows:

1. Anterior cingulate and superior temporate sulcus (responsible for mental state attribution, e.g., "theory of mind").
2. Right fusiform gyrus (face recognition).
3. Superior temporal gyrus (eye gaze; Waiter et al. 2004).

Seen in a quantitative sense, autists' own emotions are not a research topic in the neurosciences, which suggests that the neuroscientific community has already accepted that autists do not feel at all, particularly the male ones (there are hardly any neuroscientific studies on female ones). Neuroscientific studies of autism and emotion generally analyze how autists recognize *the others'* emotions (mainly fear, happiness, sadness, disgust), as expressed in faces in photographs (e.g., Deeley et al. 2007). Probably, this disproportion is also due to methodological constraints, because autists are predefined as being unable to understand the questions "How do you feel?" or "How did you feel when seeing *X*?" (related to the dominant concept of a "deficit in theory of mind," not necessarily to other concepts such as "executive dysfunction" and "weak central coherence"; see Hill and Frith 2003 for an overview; see also Happe 1994). These kinds of questions are crucial for the experimental design of fMRI studies of emotions; they are normally asked after the image run. Normally, answers are scaled to correspond to the intensity levels of feelings. However, none of this allows for the conclusion that autists do not feel. Rather, they do not express emotions, which is an important difference.

Similar to intelligence (IQ testing), emotion is considered a graduated property in neuroscientific and psychobiological approaches. In contrast to their emotions, the intelligence of autists can be measured and scaled. And as in endocrinology, "sex" is also seen as a graduated property, graduated by sex hormones; methodologically, it is simple to relate sex and intelligence. The HFA's extreme male brain (which has an IQ above 80 and received extra testosterone in the womb) is the outcome (see also Schopler and Mesibov 1992).

However, what about the relation of autism research to emotions research in social neuroscience? It becomes clear through the lens of gender. The results of autism research, regarding the hypermale brain, also reflect how the "normal" man and the "normal" woman are envisioned by scientists (see below). The predominance of autism studies focusing on the "male brain" (e.g., Waiter et al. 2004, Baron-Cohen 1999) and the lack of scrutiny of autists' own emotions contrasts with the present dominance of emotion studies (e.g., Singer et al. 2004a) and sexual arousal studies in which women are under scientific scrutiny (e.g., Brizendine 2006, including detailed literature). Science actors engaged in both research areas, neuroscience of human emotions and of autism (of "nonemotions"), are often found to be associated with the emerging field of neuroeconomics (e.g., Hill and Sally 2003, Singer and Fehr 2005, Singer et al. 2006), in which the ideal market participant, the *homo oeconomicus*, is modeled (see Ulshöfer, this volume). Autists' "lack" of emotions guarantees optimal behavior for economists' modeling of the human idealtype, a (mostly male) human who makes purely rational decisions and has control over the disturbing power of emotions. What seems to ordinary people as a caricature of a human being is a godsend to researchers who have to make humans fit to their theories.

To put it bluntly: Within the neuroscience of emotions and of autism, the abnormal man is conceptualized as emotionally incapable of understanding others, whereas the abnormal female is modeled as sexually (not emotionally) dysfunctional. When we think of it from the perspective of overfulfillment, the hypermale is a brilliant calculator and analyst ("systemizer") and the hyperfemale is a highly reproductive mother with emotional capacity for everyone. Empathy, according to Baron-Cohen, is a combination of mothering skills, self-control (which he defines as being able to forget oneself for the sake of another; one could label that self-abnegation), and verbal abilities (including gossip; Baron-Cohen 2004, 129), which lead to a higher understanding of situations in which emotions are involved. A challenge for attempts at social engineering is thus the unsolved task of how both this man and this woman should meet and be able to reproduce.

We might be under no illusion: The "systems" rhetoric of Simon Baron-Cohen (2004), that the idealtypic male brain of the autist is an exceptional "systemizer," goes along with the new science rhetoric of an all-encompassing "systems biology." It is driven by the engine of genetics, proteomics, and bioinformatics. Whoever thinks that this idea of social engineering is far-fetched is invited to read the article by Satoshi Kanazawa from the London School of Economics (United Kingdom) and Griet Vandermassen from the Center for Gender Studies at Ghent University (Belgium), with the provocative headline "Engineers Have More Sons, Nurses Have More Daughters," in which the authors fruitfully expand Baron-Cohen's findings with regard to the paternal ability to regulate the sex ratios of offspring (Kanazawa and Vandermassen 2005).

Simon Baron-Cohen explicitly regards the spectrum of autistic disorders as a category of *abnormality* (e.g., Baron-Cohen 2000, 3) and renames it mindblindness, or the lack of a theory of mind. In his pop-science book, he omits "abnormality" and instead refers to autism as an *empathy disorder* (Baron-Cohen 2004, 137). Simultaneously, he regards the idealtypic female brain as related to "systemblindness" (Baron-Cohen 2004, 184). This proposition relies on an understanding both of "system" and of "female," neither of which is explicitly defined in Baron-Cohen's writings. Taking a closer look, female and male represent the two poles of woman and man, and same-sex sexuality (understood as behavior) is considered to fall within these two poles as well. Though Baron-Cohen states that theoretically a woman can have a "male brain," this is a false claim. She can only have a man's brain, as will emerge in due course.

In Baron-Cohen's approach, which is paradigmatic for the research field, the category being referred to is biological sex (determined by the sex chromosomes, gonads, and genitals) and gender (encompassing emotional styles, behaviors, and sexual identities of various kinds "in between") which results from abnormally balanced hormones. As a consequence, a woman with a male brain is set identical with being lesbian, as it is, biologically, the same hormone (testosterone) that enables her to think like a man and to "behave" like a man. This theoretical consequence of biological modeling is not stated explicitly. Since Baron-Cohen usually refers to "male"-encoded testosterone (rather than to estrogen, OT, or progesterone), the reverse argument with its implications for gays is even less recognizable.

According to Baron-Cohen, a system is described by the relation between input–operation–output (Baron-Cohen 2004, 112), employed in general systems theory (see, e.g., Ropohl 1999). In his writings, this operation can be applied to nearly all phenomena which can be modeled as systems: brains (neural systems, mirror neuron systems, emotional system, etc.), computers (information systems), robots (embodied information systems with agent capacities), organisms/bodies (organic systems, living systems), cells (physiological and genetic systems), populations (behavioral, genetic, ecological systems), societies (social and ecological systems), corporations (economic and social systems). In general, "system" is one of the most forgotten metaphors in scientific contexts (implying a metalevel perspective and artificial synthesis of elements and processes), which allows imagining a boundary where there may be none. In addition, a system depends on the possibility of external control, where in most cases none exists. The use of the word "system" always implies theoretical distance. And it neglects the processual perspective, which would include all modes of continuity in which modal concepts of agency and multiple realizations are embedded, such as: capacities, abilities, and drives.

In the sciences, system is often seen as analogous with self, for example, in the terms "self-organization" and "self-control." In contrast, psychological terms containing "self," particularly when related to personality research, often imply a reflexive structure which is partially due to its roots in phenomenology, for example, "self-awareness" and "self-esteem." They imply that you reflect on yourself as if your mind had an interior mirror which also reflects the broader perspective of the social world outside and how society's members might see you. These categories resist classical behavioral approaches, as well as those of the cognitive sciences (for counterarguments, see Lakoff and Johnson 1999).

Baron-Cohen himself, in his recent projects, turned to genetics (which does not contradict hormone- and neuroresearch) to find out if an autistic woman and an autistic man will have an autistic child. At present, there are insufficient data on autism's distribution across generations. There are many reasons for this: the mating rates of autistic persons is low, the chance of two autists of the opposite sex even meeting is low, the diagnostic category is not that old, and, finally, older autists often spend their reproductive years in mental institutions. Heredity studies are necessary for genetics, and, from a pathological point of view, that could be a science policy argument for, first, finally diagnosing more women as autistic (probably with the support of some autism rights movements; see below) and, second, scientifically invading self-help groups, as this is the place where autistic couples in general first come into contact. The implications of genetic research on autism are manifold, particularly with regard to behavioral genetics and social neuroscience (see section 12.3). These implications are disguised by a medical discourse on autists which provides an aura of healing and therapy. Many scientists and medical doctors are primarily concerned with helping both autists and those who take care of them, though.

Baron-Cohen himself uses the word "idealtype" for the extreme male brain. As philosophers of biology know, the hypothesis of an *idealtype* mediates between modeling of the phenotype and the genotype. And as researchers of gender in science (Schiebinger 1993, Ebeling and Schmitz 2006) know, the idealtype has an elder brother: the stereotype.

12.1.3 Autism Viewed through the Lens of Science and Gender Politics

The male autist emerged from a smaller variety of scientific sources than one might think. It is interesting to look at the figures. According to the scientific community, four out of five autists are men (Rutter 1978, Wing 1981, Ritvo et al. 1989). In the science on autism, for more than 20 years these astonishingly inert figures from the late 1970s and 1980s have been cited (see also, e.g., Baron-Cohen 2004, Reddy 2005). Most of these figures referred to patients in mental hospitals and not to a public screening. Maybe they are still accurate, or they have not yet been thoroughly questioned because autism research, historically, developed out of research on schizophrenia (Minkowski 1927, 1933), which has predominantly been regarded as a disorder of men. However, the unquestioned sex ratio of autism is part of modeling the "social phenotype" as male. Are there no new figures on the gender ratios (including same-sex orientation) of "normal" autists? In the (quite new) high-functional category of Asperger's syndrome, the ratio is even 1 woman to 9 men (Baron-Cohen 2004). Most likely the HFA is a man.

Surprisingly, neither feminist scientific researchers nor those with comparable political ambitions thoroughly question the gender imbalance of autism; it has not yet hit the radar of gender politics, which was engaged in gender "mainstreaming" in the last decade. Obviously, autists behave differently, and this can already be seen at a very early age. Of course, if the autist is categorized as disabled, nobody will want to belong to this category—but what if he is categorized as a male genius with a high-functional brain for future information technology (IT) economies, as, for example, by Simon Baron-Cohen (2004)?

There is considerable critique of the "male" aura of autism. However, it is most often addressed in the Internet forums of numerous organizations related to autism rights movements rather than in the academic world (and mothers of "low-functional" autists [LFAs] are engaged in particular). Unlike Asperger's disorder, HFA has not received approval as part of the diagnostic criteria catalogues. The former mainly differs from "normal" autism in that individuals experience no delay in verbal and cognitive development and exhibit a curiosity toward their environment. HFA, in contrast, is a quasi-diagnostic label, useful for proving that some persons, with PDDs, have an IQ above 80 and are not mentally retarded. HFAs not only speak clearly and are able to dress and wash themselves but are also hard workers, able to concentrate on one problem for many hours (diagnosed as obsessive behavior). The new label HFA and the new diagnostic category of Asperger's disorder in the *DSM–IV* (American Psychiatric Association 1994) caused quite a split within the movement, and thus some organizations now vote for "pro-cure" (generally those encompassing "normal" autists), and others—commonly those with a high percentage of individuals with Asperger's syndrome—for "anti-cure." The latter reasonably vote for *neurodiversity*, at least when not belonging to fundamentalist organizations which encourage their Asperger's syndrome members to be more proud of their intellectual superiority and to pity the mass of neurotypics for their normality. Looking at the Internet platforms of the autism movements, it can be seen that rather than being concerned with a gender critique of science, the mothers and fathers critically reflect on why their autistic daughters are less commonly diagnosed as high-functional "savants" by pediatricians or psychiatrists compared to their sons. Terms frequently used by "normal" autists in the Web logs are "HFA/Asperger's syndrome elitism," "neuroelitism," and "functional autist," othering the high-functional one. The heteronormativity of the sexes is mirrored in the heteronormativity of the autists' identities.

Theoretically, if the sex ratio before the new *DSM* category Asperger's syndrome was 1:4, and after 1994 more Asperger's syndrome autists (with the ratio 1:9) were transferred into the new category of HFAs, this should lead to an increase of women in the sex ratio of the old category. I found no figures on this possible mathematical effect, nor were there related questions from within the autism movements. The autists' discussions on the Internet show more concern for the attitude about diagnosis than about the attitude toward gender. Part of the reason is that one icon of Asperger's syndrome autism, Temple Grandin, is a very successful and popular woman who seems to prove that female high functionals exist, and that female geniuses are not disadvantaged. However, can you think of a second woman autist media star or even a gay autist media star? However, we will return to Temple Grandin later (in section 12.2) when discussing media influence on shaping the idea of what "female autism" is.

As far as I can see, few academic groups object to the *extreme-male-brain theory* put forward by the Baron-Cohen group. And there are a respectable number of critical journalists who do so (e.g., Cohen 2004). One academic group that has objected is the academic group of women mathematicians (e.g., Rodd 2006) who detected this old story of high IQ scores, superior skills in mathematics, and male-brain genius more quickly than feminist researchers working on the relation of gender and psychology. The latter still focus on disorders which are predominantly diagnosed in women (e.g., borderline syndrome, anxiety disorder, and anorexia). Ian Hacking (1998, 69–80) complains that feminists have already overlooked the imbalanced sex ratio in MPD, as the "wings of feminism" found in the "recall of past evil"—in the form of a woman's multiplied mental self which emerged from incest and sexual abuse—a critical source of empowerment, and the gay and lesbian movements were happy to be backed by the scientific idea that a second, more original self was able to "come out" (Hacking 1998, 213). Now, if there is a new disorder for males—what then? Bad for them?—or, possibly, good for them? This ignorance of how the psycho–bio–cogno and neurosciences, in tacit agreement with public media, are shaping a new male *disorder* is not only dangerous, as these sciences might also be driven by power structures which try to determine what is female *order* and, even more, what is social order. Ignoring unfavorable modeling of the opposite sex does not fit into the idea of justice, and ignoring the highly favorable modeling does not show a sense of realism.

For instance, in the Internet encyclopedia *Wikipedia*, the entry "People_speculated_to_have_been_autistic,"[4] lists 23 historical persons ranging from Isaac Newton and Charles Darwin to Albert Einstein and Alan Turing. Many musicians are also included. Needless to say, no woman is listed. This entry draws heavily on an interview that Simon Baron-Cohen and mathematician Ioan James gave to *New Scientist* in April 2003 (Muir 2003), suggesting Einstein and Newton as candidate autists because they were reportedly loners who were obsessed with their work (the knowledge of their genius seemed ubiquitous), and a book from Michael Fitzgerald entitled *The Genesis of Art: Asperger's Syndrome and the Arts* (2005). In his book, which cites Baron-Cohen, Fitzgerald also labeled existentialist philosopher Simone Weil autistic, and she is the only one of the geniuses chosen by Fitzgerald who does not appear on the *Wikipedia* Web page mentioned above. This absence might give an impression of how cultural selection functions. The male genius, an endangered species in the last decades, makes his way back into public life at the same time as research on essential human sex differences does (hidden behind the category of gender differences; see Nye, this volume). The selection of Einstein and Newton hints, first, at the scientific modeling of HFAs as mathematical "systemizers," and, second, at the hidden methodology of IQ testing as an influential element in the diagnostic criteria. Similar to the mathematician's brain, the musician's brain has long been a preferred object of brain-scientific inquiry (e.g., Hagner 2004, 174–175) and still is (Münte, Altenmüller, and Jäncke 2002). The mathematician's and musician's soul, as two complementary approaches for imagining the soul's matter and form, were already objects of discussion in Greek antiquity (Langton 2000; see also Wardhaugh 2008, with a reference to the musical instrument as a model for natural philosophy). Baron-Cohen holds the systemizing male brain responsible for making a man not only a good scientist, mathematician, engineer, banker, or lawyer, but also a "most wonderful . . . musician" (Baron-Cohen 2004, 185). Music and harmony obviously do not have to be felt by the musician; rather, the notes have to be systemized and learned by rote.

Another group which is inclined to object to the extreme male brain consists of researchers who work on gender of science and biological determinism and who see biology and psychology as interrelated (e.g., Greene 2004). They recognize that the common and distinguishing idea within the humanities, that psychology has rewritten the soul and biomedicine has rewritten the body, has many invisible "thirds," for example, behavior and memory.

A third group critical of the extreme male brain are neuroscientists themselves, as some of them do not want autists to become objects of research on social cognition, that is, they comment critically on colleagues who abuse autists in experiments on their special brains' capacities for categorizing gender and race stereotypes (measuring, e.g., their facial processing; see Deruelle et al. 2007). To this group of critics belong, for example, neuroscientists Antonia F. de C. Hamilton and Anne C. Krendl (2007), who reject Lawrence Hirschfeld et al.'s findings that autists learn more effectively by stereotyping than neurotypics (Hirschfeld, Bartmess, White, and Frith 2007). Given that autists are not interested in people, Hirschfeld et al. wanted to analyze how autistic minds "map" society, that is, how they analyze society as a system of social groups. The controversy was published in the journal *Current Biology*.

A fourth, yet very soft, voice of critique stems from women working in health care. Autism in fact *is* an emerging public health problem, and while the majority of diagnosed autists are boys, the majority of those who take care of them are women. This situation touches on the important question of qualification and payment for emotional labor in society (Hochschild 1983). The main qualification is empathy, which Baron-Cohen regards as a core identity of the female brain. It corresponds perfectly to the gender division of labor, but perhaps a bit too perfectly. As Anthony McMahon has brilliantly analyzed, the rhetoric employed by the ones who have privileges (men) is of some importance for the maintenance of these privileges, that is, *how* the public issue of autism is debated in public conversations: in terms of brains, minds, intelligence, and science. Thus, we have to look at the "way thought masks and thus protects the interests of the powerful" (McMahon 1999, 203) and how autism is depoliticized. As a philosopher, I might be allowed to add that the vast increase in "neurophilosophical" publications in the last two decades, often centering on the mock battle with the neurosciences about whether there still is a free will, contributes to this depolitization of what *is* actually researched and financed in the sciences and thus follows the rules of elites in economy and politics (Karafyllis 2007b).

Pierre Bourdieu (2005a) has argued that language symbolizes political ontologies and refers to power. It should thus be viewed not only as a means of communication but also as a medium of power through which individuals pursue their interests. Daniel Goleman's (1995) book title, *Emotional Intelligence: Why It Can Matter More than IQ*, is a perfect example of Bourdieu's thesis that new terms follow a "linguistic market" and deploy resources which are already there. Linguistic expressions bear traces of the social fields in which they are produced, understood, and reproduced. In highly rationalized Western cultures, there is a clear demand placed on the linguistic market to bring the disparate categories "intelligence" and "emotions" together, both relating to the fragile topos of "the human." Rhetorics of autism also supply this market as they constantly refer to both the emotional deficits and the intelligence surplus of (some) autists. Of course, there are other, overlapping markets, for example, knowledge and nonknowledge (Wehling 2006), and autonomy and freedom (remember the "free will" discussion; see Searle 2004), which are also depicted in the autism movies in the repeatedly recurring issue of whether the autist should be put into an institution or not. However, we should not be thrown off the scent: In most popular movies (I am not talking about less well-known short or independent films), the autist was taken in because there was no woman who could take care of him or save him—be it from himself or from society (e.g., in *David's Mother* and also in *Rain Man*).

In a review of two new books on living with autism (Schreibman 2005, Nazeer 2003), Ian Hacking (2006) reported recently: "Over the past fifteen years everyone has got to know about autism. Autism will figure this year in dozens, maybe hundreds of cheap novels, thrillers and maybe a good book or two, just as multiple personality did fifteen years ago. (Thank goodness that's gone!)."

EI and autism are now the objects of a general interest which was once devoted to MPD, and there is no end in sight now that the "emotional market" has been created. How can the structure of this EI market be described? The reference to emotions conveys a sense of *immediacy* and *originality* in the human sphere, which is desperately needed by people in high-tech Western societies who still believe in pluralism. Pluralism is the cultural antagonist of functionalism. The possibility that emotions are *not* controllable is both desired and rejected by people in Western societies, as can be learned from analyzing Hollywood films (see section 12.2). Obviously, in cinema people can momentarily identify with characters unable to express themselves in a socially acceptable way. This imprisoned self, living in a, so to speak, isolated world of its own, resembles the experience of many people in Western culture(s) based on individualism and self-control. These films depict the ambivalent situation unique to modern humans: to behave in socially acceptable ways and, at the same time, to believe in one's own personality. In the cinema, the viewer has the rare opportunity to be the psychologist rather than the patient. Diagnostic and therapeutic cultures, based on egocentric amendment and enhancement techniques, for the sake of society as an imaginary whole, lead to a schizophrenic situation. You know best who you are, according to your own values and potentials, but others nevertheless can judge who you are, according to social norms and the way you behave. In social psychology, this difference is referred to as the *individual* systems reference and the *collective* systems reference. Both systems create norms within a reflexive structure of the self and the other. Therefore, social actors themselves must be reflexive social actors (Giddens 1991). It was none other than Sigmund Freud, deeply influenced by the phenomeno-logical thinking of his time, who considered sociology to be "applied psychology" (Freud 1999, volume 15, 194).[5] Most social psychology approaches involve class and describe how they collectively adopt, or refuse to adopt, certain social norms. How social norms are generated, however, remains a blind spot. That public media, among others, play a crucial role in the process of generating social norms is widely accepted. Social norms appear to be historically fluid while still containing core concepts that shape both ethical theory and moral practice ("justice," "freedom," "autonomy," "personhood"). It is worth noting that social norms vary even within a single culture—for instance, between rural and urban areas, between males and females, and between young and old.

Thus, the pathology of a self can be interpreted according to a pathologization both of an individual and of society (Fromm 1955), its classes in particular. Of course, elites in general successfully resist being described as pathological or at least as behaving pathologically. It is against this background that Baron-Cohen's concept of an extreme male brain, idealtypically embodied by the autist man, is agreed to have the system-izing skills relevant for a scientist, mechanic, engineer, programmer, or lawyer—all jobs which are still dominated by men and rewarded with high incomes. However, the autist requires female assistance in adapting to present social conditions in order to be normalized. As society "needs both of the main brain types," according to Baron-Cohen, people with "the female brain make the most wonderful counsellors, primary-school teachers, nurses, carers . . ." (Baron-Cohen 2004, 185), that is, the classic jobs of emotional labor, dominated by women. It was almost with amusement, while keeping in mind who was speaking, that I read the conclusion that "people with the balanced brain make the most wonderful medical doctors, as comfortable with the details of the biological system as with the feelings of the patient. Or they can be skilled as communicators of science . . ." (Baron-Cohen 2004, 185).

However, what if you cannot or do not want to show your potentials related to social norms, because your personal values conflict with these norms? For instance, what if you do not want to pretend? Loneliness then seems to be the price to pay for being innocent and honest, and not everybody is willing to pay that price. "Tolerating solitude" is one of the features that theoretically go along with high-systemizing capacities in Baron-Cohen's approach (2004, 123). Because the autistic people moving across the cinema screen seem to have mental disabilities (scientifically diagnosed and healed or not), a sphere of abnormality is constructed which reassures audience members of their own normality. A gut feeling of doubt remains, however, and some viewers may question themselves further about this abnormal behavior and perhaps find themselves also lacking a "normal" connection between perception and expression. In this sense, it is comforting to know that the abnormal protagonists all have "a beautiful mind," to allude to another famous film (on schizophrenia) in this *sympathetic-antisocial-behavior category* (*A Beautiful Mind*, United States, 2001).

During the 1990s, the number of "autism" diagnoses skyrocketed (for the increase in the 1980s, see Gillberg 1992), and the turning point has probably not been reached yet. The early pioneers of autism research, Eugen Bleuler (1911), Leo Kanner (1943), and Hans Asperger (1944), considered autistic phenomena to be rare. Yet, even then they had linked these phenomena to boys while diagnosing different kinds of schizophrenias. Since the film *Rain Man* (1988), the autist has become part of public knowledge. Today, familiarity with the autist *man* has become normal. In the last few years, this image has been transformed into public knowledge about "the male brain," and autism research and its related pop-science books, predominantly Baron-Cohen's *The Essential Difference* (2004, hardcover 2003), have played a crucial part in this new version of the old story of superior male intelligence, supported by the cognitive "neurosciences" (including parts of psychology, behavioral biology, and AI research). Recently, they labeled themselves *social neurosciences*. Later in this chapter, I will refer to aspects of Baron-Cohen's science as "Hollywood science," and this also touches on the new research field of social neuroscience. There, social determinisms meet biological determinisms within a causal architecture. In this merging of sex and gender categories, related to biological and sociopolitical ontologies, a fast and nearly imperceptible change of what is structure and what is function takes place. In addition, one's self-identity, related to a subjectivation of the soul, is transformed into a mental model of the high-functional world which just has to be embodied (related to a continuing objectivation of the soul). This process leads to what Axel Honneth (2005), borrowing from Georg Lukács, has called the objectification of the human being. Men and women, however, face different kinds of objectification.

If one were to attempt to describe Baron-Cohen's theory in one sentence, the sentence would probably read: *The extreme male brain is extremely male because a boy's fetus has been testosterone-soaked during intrauterine development.* And this is due to his mother's imbalanced hormonal status, a prenatal form of bad mothering. What Baron-Cohen does not explicitly say is that an increased level of testosterone in women is often related to stress exposure. What does this imply in a political dimension? Would it be better for working women to stay at home, in order to give birth to "normal" males? But who takes care of the autists then (or would they all then disappear)?

I will suggest an answer after analyzing the scientific and pop-scientific discourses. There is another important research area which recently has been revived under the "neuro" label: sexual arousal studies. It deals in particular with the female brain. Taking a closer look, it deals, as usual, with the female body, and this research is often endorsed by "feminalists"[6] (e.g., Angier 2000). Like Baron-Cohen's main epistemology, it is not guided by the brain as epistemic object but by hormones and genes. While employing the aura of a reconnection with the feminine and of healing sexual dysfunction and aging, it implicitly offers advice to working women and calls for female passivity, as exemplified in the following passage from Louann Brizendine's *The Female Brain* (2006): "Multitasking women end up having more distractions, which occupy their brain circuits and get in the way of sexual desire. . . . Women do not necessarily need to experience orgasm in order to conceive, though it helps. Despite some scientists' belief that there is no purpose in female orgasm, it actually works to keep a woman lying down after sex, passively retaining sperm and increasing her probability of conception. Not to mention that orgasm is intense pleasure, and anything that feels good makes you want to do it again and again—just what Mother Nature had in mind" (Brizendine 2006, 82f).

I will avoid the temptation to comment on this passage with regard to the term "Mother Nature" which conveys a—moreover misinterpreted—masked Darwinism. Anyone who has seen copulating mammals knows that after copulation there is no need for the female participant to passively lie down for conception to take place— which goes to prove that even in a biological context this argument is complete nonsense.

The passage in Brizendine's book from which I was quoting is placed in the context of an—seen from the perspective of leading male elites—unsolved problem of Darwinism: female choice. According to Brizendine, women select partners who provide them with the most pleasure even before conception has taken place; because the sensation of pleasure before or during sexual intercourse is seen as identical with a feeling, and this feeling is again set as a unit of evolution, the arousal of good feelings within a woman guarantees the survival of the genes of both partners. *The feelings are considered units of evolution* as they seem to compete with each other. Like good genes, only the good feelings "survive." The same kind of argumentation is put forward in Tania Singer's pain experiments, mentioned in the Introduction to this volume, because pain (which, like pleasure, is just a sensation) seems to be avoided whenever possible according to an evolutionary understanding of feelings and emotions. This pure functionalism, which is often accompanied by a loss of materiality when entities other than organisms or populations are scientifically constructed as entities of evolution, results in "material features . . . [being] tacitly smuggled into the inferences made" (Griesemer 2005, 61).

To summarize, Brizendine models a man by means of gonadal hormones and brain: a man who is everything, a fantastic lover, a potent breeder, and a (part-time, i.e., before his polygamous drives again win out over his hunter instinct to feed his family) devoted father and husband. After menopause, a woman is advised to use anti-aging strategies to keep both her and his sexual arousal capacities potentially functional. By the same tokens (hormones and brain), Baron-Cohen models a man who lacks empathy, lacks morals, is a genius in systemizing, and has a desire for control. If one had to choose between the two model idealtypes of "brains," Baron-Cohen's human model might even seem preferable, because, ignoring the economic benefits of being high-functional, at least the autist man does not use sexuality to control women. He simply leaves her alone. However, as the autist man has not yet been discussed in terms of criminalization, once rape is also biologicalized as happening due to a "natural" hormonal pressure, a less advantageous relabeling of the high-functional and innocent male genius might be possible in the future.

Brizendine's book employs a rhetoric that appeals to the idea of women's sexual liberation while arguing in the extreme opposite direction with regard to women's role in society (and there was considerable critique of this book from many sides, including feminists). It is symptomatic of the new *feminalism* that it enthusiastically worships scientific findings regarding the female body and brain and simultaneously forgets that the socioeconomic and bio-ontological architectures from which this new biofemininity emerged, and in which it is implicated, is still the old one. The quotation of Brizendine's ideas displays a combination of gender stereotype, the passive female waiting to be inseminated after having seduced the active male, and sex stereotype, the man who only wants to distribute generous amounts of sperm among as many women as possible. This argument is also put forward by Baron-Cohen (2004), who uses the age-old story of male polygamy as a globally dominant social structure, forgetting for a moment that his idea of HFAs as leaders depends on urban social structures in the industrialized Western hemisphere. Such an argument reflects a lack of respect for both sexes, since human persons are the subject here.

Let's turn to the social dimension, the social division of labor. Brizendine describes one of her clients who had been experiencing problems in arousability: "The worries and tension of her new job were interfering with her ability to relax, feel safe, and allow her amygdala to deactivate" (Brizendine 2006, 82). Multitasking women had better stay at home or take a job that "suits" them, that typifies the still predominant, gender-biased social division of labor within most societies. In order to sell this old wine in new skins, the brain is made use of as a marketing label for well-known findings from the past of hormone research.

Brizendine also refers to autism, describing as "objective scientific" knowledge the assertion that an excess of testosterone during development is responsible for socially handicapping the brain—transforming it into the "extreme male brain." It is the "woman's social contract" that, according to her, should be renewed in line with powerful "biological truths" (Brizendine 2006, 161). What this actually means in detail remains unwritten. Should some women raise children while others earn money? Obviously she is voting for something like a female elite, as a counterpart to the male elite, since both seem to exist as a result of biological determinants.

In the end, both books about the essential male/female brain lead back to ideas of leadership and social rank, either by using emotions strategically (Brizendine) or by lacking emotions in general (Baron-Cohen). And this reconnects these two books to the linguistic markets of EI and "soft" leadership, which are supplied by Goleman's publications. In my reading, autism serves as a sort of *antithesis* to Goleman's concept of EI (Goleman 1995, 2006), nevertheless sharing the boundary object (Star and Griesemer 1989) of "the brain" and some related basic scientific assumptions, such as the importance of mirror neurons for responding to the outside world. Moreover, both concepts share the view that the private, inside world is the primordial one, stressing the individual systems reference and neglecting the collective one. Simon Baron-Cohen's explicit division of empathizing and systemizing skills in the mind— separating the essentially female from the essentially male brain, or making it explicit, modeling *the autist as a natural hypermale*—stands in direct opposition to the unifying strategy of EI. The latter strategy advances the notion that emotions can be managed in an intelligent way by all humans, as emotions naturally occur in all humans, serve biological, social, and economic functions, and can be made accessible and trained to improve—by the self.

There is no definitive answer about which particular element of rhetoric persuades people to adopt these pop-scientific propositions. However, part of the rhetoric is in all cases (1) a hint at "another," more complete way of knowing the self, (2) a visual-ization technology for hidden self-knowledge, (3) a vision of how this visible knowl-edge will enable one to function more effectively under present socioeconomic conditions, and (4) a prognosis with regard to the decline which will take place if this "new" knowledge is not taken into account. A random selection from the books of Baron-Cohen, Brizendine, and Goleman reveals the following "dangers": ignorance of these more complete ways of knowing oneself (and others) can lead to war, discrimi-nation, increasing divorce rates, social isolation, the ending of friendships, loss of sexual desire, and economic decline.

Goleman's concept of EI (1995, 2006) leads back to personality research (see MacCann et al., this volume) and the idea of multiple intelligences; and personality research, like autism research, is rooted historically in scientific scrutiny of schizophre-nia. The idea of an alternative and more fruitful intelligence still reminds readers of a second self and the idea, already mentioned, of an *Inner Self Helper* for the first, unhappy self, which developed from therapeutic approaches to curing MPD in the late 1970s (Hacking 1998, 47). In other words, the therapeutic approaches to healing MPD attempt to motivate the dissociated second self to fruitfully reunite with the first one. In Goleman's EI concept, there is no dissociated self but rather a hidden, emotional, and original one, which is able to cure the rational second one of its antisocial blindness.

Though promoting opposing views, Baron-Cohen and Goleman share common ground, particularly with regard to gender issues, the ontic status of the brain, the mind, the self, and the world, the idea from evolutionary psychology that emotions and behaviors adapt to the social environment, and the idea that *mind reading* is a normal human ability. Methodologically, both are inspired by IQ testing, and, historically, both approaches can be traced back to personality and classical hormone research far more than to brain research, though both Goleman and Baron-Cohen support their concepts with recent neuroscientific findings and the fascination with brain "imaging." That one does not easily detect this common ground is due to three strategies (borrowed from Hubig 1978, 5): *translation*, that is, using different terms and models for the same concept or phenomenon; *reduction*, that is, abstracting from phenomena and generalizing from models; and *trivialization*, that is, omitting important aspects of phenomena and background assumptions of models.

For instance, an example of the strategy of *translation* (and reduction) would be Baron-Cohen's understanding of sympathy in terms of empathy (see below), mind in terms of brain, and world in terms of system; *reduction* crops up in typifying the male brain as identical with the individual man and even with the group of all men at a population level; finally, *trivialization* becomes obvious when environmental hypotheses—for instance, the influence of mercury in the food chain or in vaccines for causing autism—are not even mentioned in his approach.

12.1.4 Diagrammatic Representations of Male and Female Intelligences and Brains
The following objection to pop-scientific infusions on the causal relation between autism and sex refers to the use of a graphic representation. The *bell curve* is a graph for generalizing a binomial normal distribution in statistics. Both Baron-Cohen and Goleman refer to bell curves, that is, a generalized shape of normal distribution (a Gaussian distribution) within a coordinate system which is a typical representation for studies in which populations are measured (e.g., referring to demography). Though a scientific method of diagrammatically interpreting different kinds of data, as a pop-scientific representation its use has become particularly widespread in the U.S. public media with reference to IQ test results of nations', states', and groups' (e.g., students') mean average intelligence and its standard deviations, and other entities in which

population is involved (e.g., related to age: cohorts). It is also popular as an economic figure for the distribution of income across a nation's population and a way of asserting what is normal and what is extreme.

The protagonists of this essay, Goleman and Baron-Cohen, use the bell curve for different purposes and in different ways. Goleman (1995) refers to the then recently published book *The Bell Curve: Intelligence and Class Structure in American Life* (1994) by Harvard professors Richard Herrnstein and Charles Murray, which aroused a spirited debate in science, politics, and the press about the methodology of IQ testing, the status of the national education system, and the economy. They claim, for example, that African-Americans score lower in IQ tests than Caucasian-Americans (see also Lynn 2006 for similar IQ test results related to racism) and that a low maternal intelligence is genetically heritable (this leads back to the outsold hypothesis that the X chromosome in fragile-X syndrome is the cause of low-functioning autists' mental retardation; see section 12.3.1). Moreover, they try to convince the reader that there is a need to relate "class" to IQ to obtain highly effective leadership (reminiscent of Cattell 1937; see also Mehler 1997, Cattell 1971). The study was criticized by a number of peers, some even from within the Harvard community (e.g., by Howard Gardner), and led to a number of follow-up books offering various objections to their results and interpretations (e.g., Jacoby and Glauberman 1995, Gould 1996). Even if the data of this study were later found to be scientifically invalid, the diagram of the bell curve is still used to make claims about the "normal" segment of the population with an average mean. The dominance of visual representation works as effectively as in the neuroimages, tempting readers to think that they are being addressed personally. The bell curve works as a transgressive image with the middle terms "population" and "society," both of which seem to include us all, and the neuroimages work with the middle terms "brain" and "emotions," which we think are essential parts of each of us. Since the mid-1990s, the bell curve has become a public image of society's condition. The imagery appeals to an individual's moral sense of social responsibility to help the nation keep up in global competition, and, at the same time, the bell curve represents an aggressive posture on the part of the leading elites in politics, science, and the economy.

Goleman also comments on Herrnstein and Murray's (1994, 66) consoling passages where they argue that the link between test scores and achievements is dwarfed by the "totality of other characteristics," and that even if not everybody—merely because they have average IQ scores—can become a "mathematician," "he" (!) "should not put aside his dreams." Goleman objects: "My concern is with a key set of these 'other characteristics,' *emotional intelligence*: abilities such as being able to motivate oneself and persist in the face of frustration; to control impulses and delay gratification; to regulate one's moods and keep distress from swamping the ability to think; to empathize and to hope. Unlike IQ, . . . *emotional intelligence* is a new concept" (Goleman

1995, 34). These statements, referring to the equity of emotions among all human beings, must have read like a long-wished-for delivery from pain for those who were average or below within the normal distribution of IQ scores. It is worth noting that in the U.S. edition of Goleman's book the graph of a bell curve is not printed because the editors expected even readers of pop science to be familiar with it, which is quite different for readers of other languages, for example, in the early German translation (1996).

Let's turn to the other protagonist in this essay. Baron-Cohen (2004, 3f), without offering further references or empirical data, shows two graphs with normal distributions which appear at first glance to be identical. The first depicts the empathizing skills and the second the systemizing skills occurring (measured in "percentage of population"). These two graphs, which are only published in his pop-scientific writings on essential sex differences, introduce his idea of the two cognitive styles (empathizing/systemizing) and brain types (E-type, S-type). In the graphs, neither axis is scaled; rather, the y-axis is labeled with "percentage of population" while the x-axis is not labeled at all but is marked "low" at the very left and "high" at the very right. The bell curve stands context free, like the brain in the neuroimages. With this visual trick, the bell curve becomes a representation of "high and low" which *can—by visual abstraction—unite both the high and low levels of prenatal testosterone exposure in the womb, and high and low test scores of the empathy quotient (EQ) and systemizing quotient (SQ) tests.*

Referring to the normal distribution of empathy skills (Baron-Cohen's use of emotional "skills" is already to be found in Goleman's EI key set), Baron-Cohen argues: "Most people fall in the centre of the range. But the tails of this bell curve show that some people may have significantly less empathy than others (those at the left-hand tail of the distribution), while those at the right-hand tail may be blessed in this regard. We will discover whether females really are blessed with the brain type E (for empathizing) as we go deeper along the trail" (2004, 2f). The graph suggesting normal distributions of systemizing skills is accompanied by the following explanation: "Most of us fall in the centre of the graph . . . , but a few lucky individuals fall in the extreme right-hand end." And now comes a surprising statement: "Others find systems (like car engines, computers, science, maths or engineering) really puzzling, and they are at the other end—the left-hand tail—of the distribution" (Baron-Cohen 2004, 4). Why did he write "left-hand tail"? Left-hand tail in a normal distribution implies lower capacities/abilities in reference to any attribute which can be claimed to occur in a low percentage (here: of an imagined global population). Is he describing lower abilities as a systemizer as a disability, or even systemizing itself as a disability? The reason for this purposive confusion becomes evident more than 80 pages later, after discussions of the testosterone, the brain structures, the genes, and so forth of women and men. Then, he inserts the two graphs into one coordinate system with the same labeling (*y*-axis: percentage of population; *x*-axis: high/low) and shows their intersections and deviations. The caption for the figure is: "Male and female scores in systemizing," referring to the SQ test (measuring the systemizing quotient), which is outlined in section 12.2 of this chapter. In the SQ test, men were found to score higher, in general. The bell curves are then relabeled as "female" and "male." A new, fused graph reveals that the two formerly separate ones were not identical on the opening pages of the book, as the "male" graph now unveils a lower gradient angle at the beginning, that is, the gradient on the left-hand side of the bell curve, "low," is not as steep as in the "female" graph, but the mean (average) is equally high. This turns out to be the opposite on the right-hand side, where, on average, more men than women are said to score high in systemizing. What at first sounded like a disability in men turns out to be a male ability, according to the graph placed in the middle section of the book. The autist male genius rears his head.

At this point I would like to summarize Baron-Cohen's line of argumentation. The first premise is that there are two main cognitive styles inside a brain.

(A) *A brain possesses capacities for empathizing and systemizing.*

Both women and men are thought to have normal brains, when these capacities are in equilibrium ("balanced brain"). This balance implies a construction of *normality* in brains of both sexes, with mixed cognitive styles as an idealtype of the normal brain. The normal brain is obviously considered androgynous, while the bodies in which the brains are situated remain either woman or man. However, normal women reach the point of balance at lower levels of systemizing capacity. A reverse figure comparing "female" and "male" bell curves representing *empathizing* capacities in percentages of population is not provided. Moreover, it remains unclear which population is meant. The loss of the empathy argument within his line of argumentation represents a strategy of trivialization. The category of the HFA man then enters the arena of brain talking, and this implies again a trivialization by excluding all less functional people with autism:

(B) *HFAs' brains possess capacities for systemizing, not empathizing.*

The category HFA reveals a strategy of reduction, similar to that in the modeling which focused only on empathy (instead of sympathy, see below). The HFA man now, once empathy has been subtracted from his brain's capacities, seems to have no feelings at all. This second construction of *abnormality* is based on a single cognitive style and is correlated with sex. Note that the category of generality has changed from "a brain" in (A) to the plural form "HFAs' brains" in (B). This is in response to the empirical finding that 90% of those individuals with Asperger's syndrome, which is considered to be a high-functional group, are men. Baron-Cohen then arrives at the following conclusion:

(C) *The HFA's brain is the idealtype of the male brain.*

The group of HFAs, with their individual's brains, are reduced to a brain which functions in a certain way that is an attribute of the new group (autists/geniuses). Because the autist's brain is put in singular again, moreover using the essential category of "to be," proposition (C) refers to premise (A) again. *HFA men* are thus transformed to *male* idealtypes, revealing a strategy of translation. This structure shows how models, as categories of abstraction and singularity, can shape normality.

12.2 Hollywood Science—Overcoming the Nature–Nurture Debate

12.2.1 Autists, Computers, and Sexual Objectifications
The discursive strategy of trivialization belongs to what I will now characterize as the "Hollywood science" of autism. This phrase should stress the impact of pop-cultural stereotyping in science and, in particular, the use of scientific findings in popular culture media productions which deal with autism. Popular culture, with all its present stereotypes, interacts with scientific inquiry and eases the strategies of reduction and translation. Science and the popular film industry are by no means the same. Yet, their differences should not conceal what their peers take for granted. In the realm of pop science, both sell facts and fiction. There are exceptions and breaks with traditional stereotypes on both sides, in science and the media industry, but in most cases the match of facts and fiction is perfect. An examination of media representations of sex and gender in the context of autism is important because sex and gender roles are learned particularly by watching TV and cinema productions (e.g., McGhee and Frueh 1980).

As we have already seen, according to Baron-Cohen, there are two main cognitive styles which are in balance in normal brains: *empathizing* and *systemizing*. These two cognitive styles comprise the framework for making the autist's brain a model of the male idealtype. Empathizing involves a "drive to identify emotions and thoughts in others and to respond to these appropriately," whereas systemizing consists of a "drive to analyze and build systems, with the aim of understanding and predicting non-agentive events" (Lawson, Baron-Cohen, and Wheelwright 2004, 302). The last part of the definition is not only a relict demarcating autism from schizophrenia (and its manifestation via hallucinating agentive events) but also a supernatural upgrade of autists, as "predicting" skills are not included in the *DSM–IV* criteria for autism. Scientific actors, like media actors, work with categories of the imagination.

Autists are said to be "naturally drawn to the most predictable things in our world—such as computers" (Baron-Cohen 2004, 139). The analogy of brain/computer in a male autist had already been adopted by Hollywood and related autism to control of society and national security (long before 9/11). In the film *Mercury Rising* (United States, 1998), the protagonist Simon, a small autist boy, is the only U.S. citizen able to crack an encrypted code at the National Security Agency (NSA). He therefore becomes a risk. He spends most of his time with computers and avoids social contact. Nevertheless, although Simon naturally trusts women (after his own mother and father had been killed), he learns to trust Art Jeffries (a character played by Bruce Willis), who protects little Simon from the NSA. This observed social phenomenon of autist children sticking to computers, in correspondence with other findings such as more than only above average mean IQ scores and particularly high scores in mathematics, leads a number of scientists in autism research to hypothesize that autists' brains (made analogous with the autist self) seem to understand computers better than normal people. Is it possible, we might ask from a discourse perspective, that the network systems of computers and of autists are identical? But if so, why are they only identical in "male" networks?

Technologies are gender encoded, for example, cars and computers are still male encoded, while washing and sewing machines are not (e.g., Wajcman 2004, Cockburn and Ormrod 1993), though both genders can and do use them. Probably, autist boys would also get obsessed with the repetitive movements and patterns produced by a sewing machine. However, the sewing machine did not inspire cognitive science to create a theory-of-mind module as the computer did in AI research.

The computer metaphor trivializes the fact that in life science contexts of "the human," two other models are far more powerful: the savage and the animal. Autists fall into the epistemic category of apes and "savages" (see, e.g., Baron-Cohen 2004, 124–126, for the reference to the Yanomamo) at the phylogenetic level of explanation (social cognitive science) for understanding the "nature of their brain type" (Baron-Cohen 2004, 139): It is extremely male. The background theory is an evolution of culture from the Stone Age to the Computer Age, in which the survival of an extreme male brain made sense, thereby tacitly downgrading the survival of the female "brain" to an empathy-upgraded body of reproduction (see, e.g., Brizendine 2006). At the ontogenetic level of explanation (developmental cognitive science), autists fall into the category of the child, because, first of all, they still cannot manage to behave according to social norms when they are adults, which means that they quite often unintentionally offend people. Second, "normal" men are already considered to generally be less empathic than women, an inclination already observed in male newborns with reference to eye contact with subjects and objects (for details and further references, see, again, Baron-Cohen 2004). In autism films, particularly in *Mercury Rising*, both models are employed on the imaginative level, for example, when little Simon suddenly "goes wild."

From a biological perspective, the evolution of the male tool user, that is, the process of how (by which instance) the male ape became the male human, is a more appropriate analogy than that of the male brain and the computer. "Good systemizers are skilled at understanding, using and constructing tools, including mechanical systems and weapons" (Baron-Cohen 2004, 118). Tools are used by, for example, rats, owls, and many great apes for food processing and even as weapons, as biological anthropologists Jill D. Pruetz from Iowa State University (United States) and Paco Bertolani from the University of Cambridge (United Kingdom) recently observed in wild chimpanzees hunting in Senegal (Pruetz and Bertolani 2007). This finding was sensational not only because it, again, reduced the sphere of the uniquely human (this time: making weapons) but also because it reduced the sphere of the genuinely male, as it is primarily female chimpanzees who adopt this style of attack. One of the predominant tropes in autism films, the little boy and his computer, supports the predominant narrative in biological anthropology: the coevolution of "man," tool, "human" brain, and civilization (see Tanner 1981; Morbeck, Galloway, and Zihlman 1997; and Schmitz 2006b, for critique).

So, is the autist the model for being a man or male, or is the man or male the model for being an autist? Based on all the arguments gathered from various contexts—related to brains, behaviors, hormones, genes, and personal evaluations of what a woman is and what a man is—put forth by Baron-Cohen, this question cannot be definitively answered. Rather, asking the question makes the inconsistencies visible which are paradigmatic for the discourse on "essential" sex differences, said to be located in the brain.

However, one thing is eminently different: When using autists as scientific models for social cognition, scientists do not investigate how autists might possibly survive in more or less natural contexts (in which their brains were said to have evolved) but in highly industrialized, rationalized, and, above all, economic contexts. The ideas of natural order and social order obviously meet, and they are fused by means of systems theory, evolutionary biology, and evolutionary psychology. In Baron-Cohen's approach, the male savage's or male ape's aggression and struggle for status is transferred to social rank within societies and to leadership within corporations. Playing the *advocatus diaboli* and arguing from a Social Darwinist point of view that cultural selection and preadaptation exist, this selection is still based on sexual selection, and we will have to wait to see why hyperempathetic women might select HFAs as mates. Perhaps they are chosen for the money earned from their high-functional abilities as good systemizers—which would imply a female strategy rather than an innate empathy. Simon Baron-Cohen offers a clear answer: ". . . the higher the social rank, the higher your chances of survival. So if you are good at reading the group as a social hierarchy—a system—you could prosper. . . . Among monkeys, for example, a shocking 50 per cent of adolescent males are killed in conflicts over status. So the pressure is on to know your place, and monitor everyone else's place. Even though in this example we are talking about a *social* system, the same if–then (input–operation–output) conditionality rules are used. . . . The consequences of this for males is that higher social rank means more access to females. Males of higher social status are attractive because their ascent up the social hierarchy is evidence of both healthy genes and their potential as a provider and defender ... a good systemizer is likely to end up with a higher social status. Women may therefore find a man's systemizing abilities attractive" (Baron-Cohen 2004, 121f). However, these positions of male power, and a related female choice, are not represented in any of the films on autists.

12.2.2 Women Autists and Their Stereotyping in Films

Alongside a normalizing discourse for autism, we find the emergence of quite a number of sexual and gender stereotypes in the films dealing with autists as protagonists. Although men and women autists are portrayed similarly regarding elitist thinking—it is their special talents which makes them "useful" for society, or at least their way of being able to successfully cope with their "*dis*-ability"—the kind of talents portrayed differ based on their sex. Women autists are depicted as "pure." Because of their "natural abilities," they are brought into relation with pure nature, a nature which nevertheless seems extraordinary and almost extraterrestrial, like media star Temple Grandin (prominently portrayed in *An Anthropologist on Mars*, Oliver Sacks 1995). Note that it is Mars, not Venus. The Penguin 2004 edition (paperback) of Baron-Cohen's book, from which I am quoting here, is entitled: *The Essential Difference: Forget Mars and Venus and Discover the Truth about the Opposite Sex*. The original U.K. edition (Allen Lane: 2003) was subtitled *Men, Women, and the Extreme Male Brain*. The U.S. edition was subtitled *Male and Female Brains, and the Truth about Autism*. The German 2004 translation, with a very different title as well, is *Vom ersten Tag anders: Das weibliche und das männliche Gehirn* (translation: Different from the first day: The female and the male brain). This enumeration might serve to show how inhomogeneous linguistic markets (Bourdieu 2005a) are finely structured within what is often labeled as "Western culture."

Grandin is a woman biologist and professor at Colorado State University who suffers from Asperger's syndrome but is said to imagine and understand animals' feelings. Gifted with this sensitivity, for example, for how a cow feels before being slaughtered, she invented a new technique for killing cows which is now widely applied. As *Discover* magazine writes, "Say the words *cattle, autistic,* and *woman,* and a surprising number of Americans will come up with the name of Temple Grandin. . . . By designing chutes and alleys that respect a cow's sensibilities—reducing its fear and uncertainty—Grandin has done more to improve animal welfare than almost any human alive. Increasing a cow's comfort as it nears death may seem like a futile subtlety to many humans. But fear is one of the critical differences between humane and inhumane slaughter. It also happens to be one of the differences between good meat and bad" (*Discover*, January 5, 2005, article by Verlyn Klinkenborg).

Ironically, the hormones which are set free before slaughtering make the essential difference in taste. Grandin is portrayed as a woman autist who makes the world more humane. In Baron-Cohen's (2004) book, high morals and overwhelming empathy are typical characteristics of the female brain, or the E-type. Thus, also, a woman autist should, somehow, have them. Astonishingly, in the media Grandin's exceptional abilities in spatial thinking and architectural reconstruction—moreover of thinking as if she were inside a cow's head—are not described as systemizing but as empathizing capacities. Therefore her capacities are translated in terms of "imagination" and "understanding," that is, in aesthetic and empathetic emotional terms. This corresponds with Daniel Goleman's idea of "purely high-IQ women," who "have a wide range of intellectual and aesthetic interests" (Goleman 1995, 45). In the public media, Grandin's thinking capacities are rarely stressed, reducing her to a "real" woman with a "male" mind (see also the book by Grandin's mother, Cutler 2004). When she appears on TV, she is often shown next to cattle in the countryside, emphasizing a rural utopia which contradicts the urban utopia of computers and systems in which autistic men are prescriptively situated. The strong alliance between animals and women in cultural history seems to be extremely conservative, and in the history of biological systematics, for example, in those of eighteenth century scientist Charles Bonnet, the human woman was often an intermediary between the ape and the human man at the top of nature's ladder.

Temple Grandin is, of course, an exception, but a very prominent one. And, as in the case of railroad construction foreman Phineas Gage (1823–1860), whose extremely rare brain injury was highly relevant for the neuroscience of emotions (Damasio 1994; see also Wassmann 2007), one single case—a case study of the media—seems methodologically robust enough for the social actor to make social inferences on "her" brain's capacities (on gender in the media, see, e.g., Mathes 2006). By proclaiming an idealtype of a pathological state, a shortcut with a long tradition particularly in psychomedical research (see, e.g., Gelb and Goldstein 1920), the brains of all people alike, that is, all autists, all women, all men, then seem to share the same essence in the pathological sense as well. However, what if the essence of the brain—in the words of Baron-Cohen, its "brain-type"—contradicts the essence of the body? Thus, even if autists in general are said to lack empathy, a woman autist has to fit into the cultural gender prescriptions of what a "woman" is. If she has no empathy for humans, then she must at least have it for animals. This is "phenomenal grouping," which might be allowed in the public media, though the world of media is highly dependent on the authority of who's speaking to give "real" information about what a human being was, is, and can be.

12.2.3   Media Culture and the (Re-)Presentation of Science and Scientists

Researchers are preferably selected because they seem to be so close to the world of "real" knowledge. If you are a researcher and ever gave a TV interview, you might have noticed that the cameraperson always says before recording, "Please stand/sit in front of your bookshelf," supporting your authority with all the knowledge which is symbolized in the books. Preparing a setting for a researcher on TV follows strict rules, and they belong to an implicit media code for the way academic elites are presented to the public. Even if the fieldwork or laboratory work is recorded, the bookshelf is rarely missing. It is often missing in the case of Temple Grandin, though. Among researchers, preferably scientists and, in particular, those who are neuroscientists enter the public media. Thus a highly educated woman biologist like Temple Grandin who is an autist is worth a story, as is Stanford neurobiology professor Ben Barres, a female-to-male transgender person who, moreover, is courageous enough to confess in the scientific journal *Nature* that he suffered from sexual discrimination while he was still a woman (Barres 2006). His comment followed in the aftermath of the Larry Summers affair, in which the former president of Harvard University, inspired by psychologists' IQ test results (the same results which allow autists to become the idealtype of male genius), believed that women have lower innate abilities in science and mathematics. It would be worth discussing whether this statement would have been published if Barres had, in contrast, been a male to female transgender, and was experiencing this discrimination in the present rather than in the past. Though an exceptional story, it nevertheless fit into the established cultural codes of the heteronormativity of the sexes and the assumed need for refashioning the body, allowing the concept of a sexual "upgrade" within present male power structures (see the Introduction to this volume), which, moreover, easily corresponds with the idea of self-made progress. The point to be stressed here is that mainstream newspapers and scientific journals share the same structure which defines what is a story and who deserves what kind of attention. The same is true for the film industry. Thus we may say they both shape public opinion and make up a *media culture* in which not only is society inspired by science but also the other way around: Scientists are inspired by continually repeating cultural codes which are framed and reframed within different scientific contexts (one example is the concept of left-handedness and femininity, which is rediscovered in the context of autism research; see section 12.3.1). Therefore, in media cultures, it is, because of methodological constraints, not possible to fly the flag for the exclusive influence of either nature or "nurture," that is, the social world, as Paul Ekman rightly said with reference to established display rules (Ekman 2007, 4). Strictly speaking (and thinking of, e.g., Hegel's remarks on what scientific categories can explain about nature and what they cannot explain), a separation of a scientifically understood nature and culture was never possible because all science, done by humans for humans, belongs to the sphere of culture a priori. As Kant pointed out in his *Kritik der Urteilskraft*, scientists borrow models from technology to describe and explain nature *as if* it was made by humans, for example, some cognitive scientists currently describe the brain as if it was a computer. The nature–nurture divide is concealed in terms such as brain and body, on the one hand, and (social) environment and (social) universe, on the other. However, even if it is not possible to strictly separate nature from culture, it might be useful for scientists to use nature–nurture rhetoric within media culture, because modern people are obviously still interested in this divide, likewise in the division of woman and man, and, moreover, in scientific proofs of manifestations of this division.

In her new book *Animals in Translation: Using the Mysteries of Autism to Decode Animal Behavior* (Grandin and Johnson 2005), Grandin puts forward a provocative thesis, and thus there is a new turn in this old story of the closeness of animals and women: Women autists and animals do not *feel* alike, but they do *think* alike. Obviously, in this view, animals have become as intelligent as women, or the other way around. It is in this specific type of instinct-based, successful behavior—we may also call it emotional intelligence—where women seem to score higher than men, at least in the view of autism researcher Simon Baron-Cohen (2004). The resulting question of whether animals are thus more emotionally intelligent than men remains unanswered. And, is it possible that female animals of one species also "think" differently than do male animals of the same species? Or do all animals have a male brain and systemize their environment? These rhetorical questions should show the weakness of the idea that a sexualization of nature and their biological categories can provide a solid argument for the phenomena found in the human sphere, as nearly all scientists and philosophers agree that animals cannot think. Otherwise we would have to open the door to allow the human other in to become another part of ourselves, with regard to personhood and intelligence (a position advocated by philosopher Peter Singer; Singer 2005). Many animals feel, though, which we can infer particularly from how they express pain. We understand their pain when it is expressed similarly to ours, and we often feel sympathy (not empathy). We feel *for* the animal, not with it. If pain is not expressed similarly to ours, because of different anatomy like, for example, in fish or an octopus, we have less sympathy.

This is worth stressing because Simon Baron-Cohen (2004, 28f) defines *sympathy* as a subcategory of *empathy* (rather than the opposite, as it used to be). This is a strategy of trivialization of a crucial human feeling, and it takes place in the majority of brain studies on the empathic capacities of the female brain (e.g., Singer et al. 2004a, Singer et al. 2006). By means of this trivialization, the specific sociality of an emotion like sympathy, which can be addressed to more than just the heterosexual other, is narrowed.

These strategies of reduction and translation, related to the boundary objects of animal and computer/robot, have, first, an epistemological background, as they were supported by finding the functions of the newly detected mirror neuron system in the 1990s (see Gallese 2002, 2005), which is relevant for a sort of neural simulation of somebody else's behavior in which the amygdala is involved. The scientific context for discovering the functions of mirror neurons focused, in the very beginning, on action recognition but soon was transformed into social cognition (from the cognitive sciences; see Gallese et al. 2004) and defined "intersubjectivity" as its instance. Emotions are now found to be involved in instantiating this meta-instance, and the neuroscientific and the cognitive research on emotions constantly fuse their ideas of what determines behavior and the behavior of the other, including the emotions which give rise to a behavior. Moreover, intersubjectivity has been reduced to a relation in which only two persons are involved, thus purifying it of what is called sociality in philosophy, and relates to the life world (see, e.g., Schütz and Luckmann 2003). This predefined abstract human *couple* which shares intersubjectivity by means of mirror neurons has given rise to another important concept used in autism research: *mind reading.* To read another person's mind using feelings could easily be connected with the heteronomy of the sexes and the idea that the heterosexual couple is the origin of society (abstracting from society's instance, that is, sociality). Second, it relates to a strategic background, because when sympathy is redefined as a subcategory of empathy (and thus translated as "empathy") and the female brain is remodeled as solely adept at empathizing, then male autists and their extreme male brains are left with no feelings at all for others. Males become pure systemizers. In contrast, only against this background can the category of the pure male autist emerge. He is, for instance, unable to pass Baron-Cohen's reading-the-mind-in-the-eyes test.

Mind reading has become an object of knowledge in many ways and also in reference to a heterosexual couple and its emotional language capacities. In Daniel Goleman's best-selling book on EI (1995; published worldwide in more than 30 translations), which was published at the same time as the cognitive sciences and psychosciences were merging their concepts of mind reading, he introduced a concept entitled "emotional illiteracy." Goleman, at that time, had not yet mentioned autism. Nevertheless, the emotional illiterate, who, according to Goleman, has been proliferating in society, cannot read the emotions of others, and this is seen as the cause of a collective "emotional crisis." He addresses both sexes, nevertheless focusing on empirical psychological data concerning marriages, and explains why a husband's brain (not a *male* brain) cannot understand the emotional "flooding" of wives when they make their usual outbursts, and thus the man naturally comes to feel that he is losing control over the situation. In consequence, he rejects further communication (Goleman 1995, 139–142). Goleman redefines man as "the vulnerable sex" and advises the couple to train their EI before they get married and during marriage. Again, Hollywood is offered as a model of a specific type of manliness (see Mansfield 2006): "This suggests the possibility that the stoic, Clint Eastwood type of male imperturbability may represent a defense against feeling emotionally overwhelmed" (Goleman 1995, 140).

So, if women autists appear on the movie screen, do they also appear as overwhelmed by feelings, or do they overwhelm the men? Neither of the two. In autistic women as protagonists, the rare spontaneous[7] emotional expression nevertheless seems to provide direct access to the senses. Autistic women are imagined as having a special kind of sensitivity. Elisabeth Shue in *Molly* (United States, 1999) plays an autistic teenage girl with an exceptional sense of hearing. In one of the scenes, she is embarrassing her elder brother by naively taking her clothes off and walking naked into his business meeting. However, this is only half of the idealized autist woman. Idealtypically, autist women are thought to be both predictable and sensual, a combination rarely found. Sigourney Weaver in *Snow Cake* plays an autist woman living in the countryside who claims that eating snow feels like having an orgasm. She is not actually explaining her strange behavior in the winterly garden to the man who gazes at her (and whom she loves, if the cinema audience may allow her to have that feeling) but simply stating it while stuffing snow into her mouth. Somehow, contrary to gender-role-related expectations, this woman displays no emotions concerning her dead daughter (whom she lost in a car accident), revealing that she has none of the "natural" motherly instincts one would expect her to have. This shows that she is not a "normal woman." To make her resemble a "real" woman, she has a strange obsession with cleaning and control over her household: a purity and controlled femininity which the man who enters her life has to accept, and, to a great extent, is willing to accept. He not only accepts this behavior but even appreciates the controlled way in which she tells him to take the garbage out on time, so that the garden does not become messy, without any emotional flooding at all. She maintains control even though he is having an affair with the woman next door. She is an ideal wife, moreover, for a polygamous man (as Baron-Cohen envisions his general idealtypic concept of man). As Baron-Cohen (2004, 139) argues that people with autism "love to predict and control the world," this new female type constructed in the film seems to be a perfect match for the new idealtypic man: reproductive, predictable, future-oriented, and clean.

Somehow an exception is the dramatic comedy *Mozart and the Whale* (United States, 2005), where a man and a woman autist fall in love with each other after meeting in a self-help group. She has a disturbing outspokenness that he has to adjust to. However, he has the mathematical skills, and she the extreme sensual capacities (hearing). The film's title alludes to the opposition between a (male-encoded) genius and a (female-encoded) animal. This stereotype is successfully turned upside down, as it is the man who appears—at a party—dressed in a whale costume, and the woman who dresses as Wolfgang Amadeus Mozart's sister Nannerl (though, not as Mozart himself).

How do some features of this gender stereotyping come to light in science? In one of the tests of the Baron-Cohen group (the EQ test; note that here EQ refers to the empathy quotient, not Goleman's EQ [emotional quotient] concept), which determines whether you have a female brain or not, you rate how strongly you agree/disagree with the following statement: No. 2: "I prefer animals to humans" (Baron-Cohen 2004, 200ff). It is followed by statement No. 3: "I try to keep up with the current trends and fashions." Neither statement is scored, however, though they give the volunteer the idea that this questionnaire is focused on some sort of "woman stuff." As psycholinguists have emphasized, substantives and pronouns in specific compositions play a key role in word-specific gender stereotype information, even in languages like English where you do not put a gendered article in front of the substantive (Kennison and Trofe 2003). Baron-Cohen's questionnaires for determining the SQ and EQ direct people to accept or reject the general line of argument implied in the questionnaire, that is, to be feminine or masculine, thereby producing unintentional bias in the results which might not be detected. Femininity corresponds with culturally adopted emotional styles (see Reddy, this volume). An aversion to being what a specific society regards as feminine (or masculine) can outweigh the scientific aim of learning about a person's capacities for empathy. One of the next statements which reflects the social role of women (No. 6: "I really enjoy caring for other people") is definitely scored, as are No. 18 ("When I was a child, I enjoyed cutting up worms to see what would happen"—if you strongly disagree, your EQ increases) and No. 20 ("I tend to have very strong opinions about morality"—if you strongly disagree, your EQ decreases). In short, the questionnaire is rich in sex role stereotypes. That men (defined as such by biological sex) thus score lower on the EQ test than women does not turn out to be a surprise. More importantly, a scientific view of the world at an early age (remember the cut-up worm) seems to contradict moral engagement (a view which the author of this article, trained both in biology and philosophy, also personally objects to). Even if the EQ questionnaire is grammatically gender-neutral, it resorts to cultural codes which are explicitly feminine (see Vidal 2006), for example, in No. 28, the relation to hair, a cultural symbol of femininity (Stephan 2001): "If anyone asked me if I liked their haircut, I would reply truthfully, even if I didn't like it." If you disagree, you are said to have a higher level of empathy than people who agree. From a systematic point of view, this score architecture opposes No. 20, which asks for your self-judgment about morality. Lying or at least pretending, as it seems, is not included in this very special kind of morality (very Kantian, one might add).

Empathy is scored on the prescriptive sex or gender role (a differentiation is not really possible here, considering the newly established categories of male/female brains) that a woman has to read the wishes of her (autist) man in his eyes, including what he would like to hear. Moreover, the statement plays with a common Western cliché often seen on TV screens: the husband coming home from work and not noticing his wife's new haircut while she, bored in her private sphere, has waited all day to surprise him with the new look. At last, she forces herself to ask, "How do you like my new haircut?," and he, feeling guilty for having been so self-centered, has no other choice than to praise it.

Above all, cultural codes related to masculinity (Mosse 1996, Nye 1998), like sports, technology, and cars, are all absent from the EQ test. The SQ test for measuring the systemizing quotient (Baron-Cohen 2004, 206–211)—where high scores reflect the specific cognitive style of an extreme male brain—contains many questions concerning the functioning of machines (Nos. 7, 13, 18, 20, 33, 42, 43), cars and car driving (Nos. 5, 49), airplanes (No. 51), wireless communication (No. 57), an interest in science, technology, and mathematics (Nos. 11, 15, 32, 45), and life on other planets (No. 58). Only the final statement is not scored. Still, it tacitly underscores the "male" aura of science fiction, IT, and humanoid robots. Moreover, in a question which asks if the participant is drawn to tables of information while reading newspapers (No. 29; if you strongly agree, your SQ increases), the examples given are "football league scores" and "stock market indices"—addressing social domains which are almost exclusively dominated by men.

One thing is obvious: The more the alliance between the instincts of women and animals is scientifically cemented, the more men have to find their other self in machines and robots, or at least in other high-functional entities with increased power output and high performance ratings. As human beings are also concerned with morals, and the distribution of good and evil, a pertinent direction for the future modeling of autism could be to show how the autist man stays innocent even if the empathetic woman covers all areas of morality.

Rain Man (which was awarded four Oscars) was released in the cinema seven years before Daniel Goleman's first book on EI was published, which proved to be the first in a long series of publications on EI. In the film, the phone-book-memorizing genius, Raymond Babbitt (played by Dustin Hoffman), is presented as a character incapable of emotional development, and it is his brother Charlie Babbitt (played by Tom Cruise) who has to learn how to deal with the unpredictable situations arising from Raymond's eccentric behavior. Finally, he accepts the spontaneous chaos which Raymond, who is also organizing the world into a clear-cut structure, brings into both their lives. Moreover, this acceptance is based on an ethically motivated recognition of this "other" personality. And Charlie's girlfriend Susanna (Valeria Golino) even teaches Raymond how to kiss. Nevertheless, Raymond Babbitt has to return to his mental institution in the end. It was Dustin Hoffman himself who insisted on that "unhappy" ending. But this was back in the 1980s.

In the films of the 1990s and the early 2000s where "autists" play a leading role, they are typically portrayed as loveable from the very start and are more or less already socially integrated. For example, in *As Good as It Gets*, the famous author Melvin Udall (Jack Nicholson), the prototype of the male intellectual, is accepted from the very beginning by his gay neighbor Simon, a gifted artist, but not by Carol, the woman he eventually falls in love with. Here, two categories of male-encoded abnormality, with the genius idea of the still unknown artist lurking somewhere in the background, create an alliance against the normality of the female sphere. In contrast to waitress and single mother Carol Connelly (played by Helen Hunt; Jodie Foster in *Little Man*

Tate also plays a working-class single mother), the two men belong to the upper middle class, and they are both gifted with exceptional talents. On the other hand, Carol is a devoted mother caring for her disabled child (suffering from cystic fibrosis). At the beginning of the film, Carol dislikes Melvin because of his lack of charm and empathy, and Melvin dislikes Simon because of his "feminine" way of sympathizing with Carol. In one scene where they share a hotel room, she becomes Simon's muse when he is inspired merely by the beauty of her naked body and at once starts to sketch her. Nothing more than friendship develops between them. The outgoing Simon encourages Melvin to open up and leave his sphere of control, which he finally manages to do. Perhaps Melvin has only systemized how and when to say the "right" words—right according to social norms—to which the woman then positively reacts. However, the relationship, finally, seems to work. The happy ending is a heterosexual couple and a befriended homosexual artist who finally believes in his own personality and artistic spirit. Thus, either the autists portrayed in many films learn to overcome their lack of social skills or they have another ability which society can make use of. Empathy for others is depicted as learnable, and conventional social pathologies are transformed into something "normal."

Even if one argues that the films cited serve to establish social codes of "normal deviance," it is worth mentioning that rather than a small minority, we are talking about many, many diagnosed autists. Parents often make a tremendous effort to make their autistic child "sociable" and socially accepted, though. And, in a way, financial funding of these efforts (i.e., to get help from the health care system) is entirely based on the assumption that autists are not completely "normal" but are somehow disabled (as is stressed by the "pro-cure" autism rights movement). This is an important argument that should not be forgotten in the academic discourses which are framed around the idea of increasing public acceptance of autists by modeling their abnormality as genius-like and exceeding normality and which fail to take into consideration that a person does not necessarily have to be "normal" to be accepted. This idea of acceptance relates to marketing and social stigmatization, not reason. On the other hand, reasonable acceptance is based on toleration of difference. Although for societies limits to tolerance exist, these limits should be related to reason rather than to the idea of an unchangeable social stigma. The study by Anne Krendl and her colleagues shows the brain's capacity for controlling feelings of, for example, disgust related to stigma and models it neuroscientifically (Krendl et al. 2006; see the Introduction to this volume for details).

In Baron-Cohen's book (2004) on essential differences between the female and the male brain, the widely discussed environment hypothesis, which theorizes that autism might have spread broadly because of standard child vaccinations which contained a mercury compound (thiomersal, see endnote 3), is neglected and thereby trivialized. However, the insistence on the film title *Mercury Rising* (the film should have been titled *Little Simon*) politicized the scientific nonknowledge about autism even if the mercury hypothesis is not put forward in the film. The media's role can be a critical instance for the science policy level.

Why would it make sense for Baron-Cohen to insist on essential sex differences in the brain and then to omit the mercury hypothesis in scientific inquiry? Taking environmental factors into account would contradict a focus on the brain, hormones, and genes, and would also reveal that the majority of people with autism are *not* high functional. The psychopathological influence of mercury would manifest itself equally in both sexes, whereas the neuroendocrinological influence of imbalanced maternal gonadal hormones is sex stereotyped a priori.

12.3 Science Formations, and Gender in the Big Science of Autism

12.3.1 From the Sexualized Brain to the Sexualized Hand

Baron-Cohen's approach is interesting not only from a gender perspective but also from a philosophy of science perspective, as his research on autism covers a broad range of topics and represents some of the current transformations of (1) neuroscience and cognitive science, both of which have turned to emotions and society as epistemic objects during the last decade (highly inspired by sociobiology); (2) psychology, which is remodeling personality through the lens of neuroscience, psychobiology, and behavioral biology; (3) psychiatry, which is struggling with diagnostic criteria and treatments for "antisocial" behaviors (for related critique on biological psychiatry, see Ross and Pam 1995; see also Lilienfeld, Lynn, and Lohr 2004) and is inspired by the Human Genome Project (Cowan, Kapnisky, and Hyman 2002) and pharmacogenetics; and (4) genetics, which has moved into a new phase of proteomics since the Human Genome Project was completed in 2001 and insists on "using the map." It is greatly supported by computer science/bioinformatics, involving the model of random scale-free networks (Keller 2005, Karafyllis 2008c) for determining the so-called "interactome," a virtual model that helps to identify the structure–function relation between genes and proteins.

Therefore, much effort is currently being invested in finding genetic causes of autism and the different "autism risk loci" which are located on various chromosomes. Thus the media began to refer not to "autism" but to "autism risk," which implies, in the end, a statistical category of insurances. In the traditional clinical context, autism is still divided into "idiopathic autism" (where no specific cause is known), and (rarely diagnosed and not easily diagnosable) "secondary autism," which can comprise environmental factors or gene defects. Unfortunately for the science of genetics, there is no candidate gene for autism, and there are no hereditary studies of autists. In the view of genetics, autism is regarded as an "oligo gene defect" involving deletions, duplications, inversions, and many biochemical interactions in and between different chromosomes, each of which were found to also correlate with other diseases, disorders, and syndromes (e.g., Down's syndrome, epilepsy, ADHD; see Smalley et al. 2002). The first genome scan of autists and their family members took place in 1998 (International Molecular Genetic Study of Autism Consortium 1998). The suggestion that different regions on chromosomes 4, 7, 10, 16, 19, and 22 might be involved in developing autism was somehow disappointing. In 2004, the AGP was launched by the National Alliance for Autism Research (today known as Autism Speaks), supported by the U.S. National Institutes of Health and involving more than 50 other institutions. At that time, autism was already regarded as an "epidemic" in Western societies (the prevalence ratio changed from about 1 : 5,000 around 1990 to 1 : 150 around 2005; Hill and Frith 2003 mention a prevalence 0.6% of the general population; see Gillberg 1992 for a historical overview of prevalence rates and Byrd and Sage 2002 for a methodological discussion). The AGP used DNA array technology to scan the genomes of more than 1,100 Canadian, U.S., and European families with at least two affected members. Autism is also increasingly being diagnosed in Asia, particularly Japan, Hong Kong, and Taiwan (the Asian Autism Conference kicked off on August 13, 2006, at the Hong Kong Academy of Medicine). Due to studies of families, particularly siblings and twins, the main hypothesis for all genome scans is that *autism is heritable* (according to Skuse 2007, the estimated heritability is greater than 90%). In influential projects like the AGP, the word "genome" does not refer to the individual autist level but to a (inferred) global population of autists, thus othering the "normal" population and "the human" genome.

Results from the AGP include a newly found site on chromosome 11 that harbors genes for proteins which shuttle glutamate across the synapse (AGP Consortium 2007). Glutamate triggers the chemical messenger system of the brain. Other genetic dispositions for becoming autistic were already known, for example, related to fragile-X syndrome (referring to the sex chromosome X), Angelman syndrome (referring to chromosome 15), and an aberration in human chromosome 16 (Philippi et al. 2005). Though these syndromes occur in both sexes in various forms of genomic imprinting (an epigenetic phenomenon) which resist Mendelian genetics, the inclusion of the "X chromosome" pressed a stereotype button in some scientists' heads, resulting in the hypothesis that fragile-X syndrome should be more common in males (as the normal male diplotype only has one X chromosome) and that autism is probably transmitted by autist boys' mothers via a defective X chromosome (for an overview on this research area, see, e.g., Gillberg 1992, Reiss and Freund 1990). At present, a correlation with a defective maternal imprinting of chromosome 15 seems more correct, though there is at least one caveat: The maternal imprinting of genes has in general been far more an object of study than the paternal one. My suggestion for this disproportion is (to ignore, for the moment, the question of whether the father or the mother can be held accountable for a child's disorder, a question which is not so far-fetched) that genetic imprinting has historically been researched in the context of gynogenesis and parthenogenesis ("vegetative" forms of reproduction), thus most intensely in plant studies (see also Haig 2002). However, Kavita S. Reddy's (2005) genetic autism study reports no findings of structural anomalies in the X chromosomes in the investigated cohort of autists, whereas anomalies were found in other chromosomes. And Reiss and Freund's (1990) psychiatric study found that fragile-X males did not show abnormalities in reciprocal interaction with caretakers (a *DSM–III–R* criterion for autism) and that other features for autism were also lacking (though some were present).

In their publications (e.g., Piven 2001, Reddy 2005, Skuse 2007, to provide three examples of many), geneticists often complain to psychologists and psychiatrists that genetic scans on "autists" do not make sense due to the diffuse diagnostic criteria of autism; nevertheless, these are done, and they are financed. The heterogeneity of genotypes and phenotypes found in autistic persons does not allow researchers to draw conclusions about genetic *causes* of autism—and this is a thorn in the side for medical research programs (Piven 2001, Dawson et al. 2002). As geneticist David H. Skuse (2007) points out, autism's apparent association with mental retardation does not allow for inferences on common causes. It shows instead that the presence of both features greatly increases the probability of clinical ascertainment. These facts have led to the present scientific drive toward narrowing the range of the phenotype and toward characterizing behavioral skills and deficits. The diagnostic differentiation of Asperger's syndrome from the conventional form of autism can be interpreted in this way.

Genetic explanations have also been underestimated in Baron-Cohen's "brain-fashioned" pop-scientific writings (in contrast to his research), which concentrate on perinatal neurodevelopment and, with a rhetorical focus on the health care of babies, are thus targeted on mothers rather than women in general. The scientific explanations for why sexualized brains can be related to autism are threefold:

1. Maternal gonadal hormones influence the brain development of the fetus (developmental level).
2. Women and men behave differently, and this is said to relate back to their hormonal and neural outfitting (behavioral and social level).
3. Four out of five diagnosed autists are men (epidemiological level). The repeatedly recurring sex ratio of autism (4 men to 1 woman) in scientific literature (see also Baron-Cohen 2004), which has been expanded to the idea of male genius and an idealtypic male brain (see section 12.1 and below), was by no means introduced with this drive. In fact, the opposite is true. These sex ratios were mentioned in studies on mental retardation (Ritvo et al. 1989, Bolton et al. 1994), often related to observations of autistic features in individuals with Down's syndrome, Angelman syndrome, epilepsy, and fragile-X syndrome.

Seen from a time perspective of the last 30 years, the strikingly conservative approaches of constructing male and female brains are hormone research and intelligence testing. IQ tests are part of many autism diagnoses (and of many other mental disorders). Hormones mediate between brain and body and have organizing, signaling, and activating functions. Hormone research remained quite stable in its choice of hypotheses, objects, and methods because its paradigm of a triangular interdependence of gonads, emotions, and behaviors has never been seriously challenged (with the exception of questions about the contexts of its application; see, e.g., Oudshoorn 1994, Stoff 2004, Ebeling 2006). Above all, in both neurobiology and psychopathology there must always be a "third" to mediate between body and brain, which allows bridging dualism (and avoiding monopsychism).

Seen from a biologist's point of view, three important questions arise in relation to current research on male/female brains in reference to autism:

1. Where are the estrogen and progesterone studies for modeling the hyperfemale brain?
2. Since the child not only receives testosterone from the mother but also produces hormones with his own gonads, where are the studies (or even publications) on abnormal gonadal and genital development in hypermales (known from studies already undertaken on animals)?
3. As testosterone and estrogen occur in both sexes, where are the "gender studies" on how hormonal imbalances influence gender identity?

All three questions are related both theoretically and at the pragmatic level of experimental design. The easiest question to answer is the last: The studies are already there. Gonadal hormones were a necessary tool for developing successful operations for transsexuals, and this was accomplished by basic research. Studies on lesbian women and gay men (in the biological context it is still "homosexual," whereas "lesbian" has been adopted as a new category) now go beyond the medical context, or at least the medical aura of curing adults, and adopt the (genetic) imaginaries of intrauterine developmental and prenatal testing, as well as intelligence testing. However, then the studies are not "fashioned" by the sexualized brain but rather by another organ which is more politically correct regarding the issue of essential sex differences: the *hand*.

The digit ratio of ring finger and point index finger lengths of the right hand (4D:2D, sometimes calculated 2D:4D) is known to be different in both sexes, that is, it is a dysmorphic characteristic of the sexes. Women, in general, are found to have a relatively longer ring finger than men. Psychologist Mark Brosnan from the University of Bath (United Kingdom) has calculated how digit ratios (as the ratio of the length of the ring finger to the length of the point index finger) relate to (in a row) developmental disorders, homosexuality, and dyslexia. The hypothesis was developed, because, historically, digit ratios were found to be related to testosterone (in adults!) in studies on the causes of "left-handedness." And, as Brosnan mentions (Tay 2007), because testosterone is said to influence mathematical and other abilities in the brain, the digit ratios might correlate with intelligence tests (he found that they do). This implies sex-related intelligences, based on the hormonal outfit.

Digit ratios were also tested by Brosnan (2006) in relation to mathematical and spatial abilities (the classical domains in which men in IQ tests were found to score higher) and academic qualifications (part of the result: Senior Lecturers' "hands" are not "more intelligent" than those of the Juniors). Brosnan said in an interview with *Australian PC World* that he thinks finger ratio tests might also be used to indicate "technophobia" and "computer anxiety," and, though not very likely, might one day replace the Standard Assessment Tests for finding a child's ideal career path. These statements were circulating in the IT journals and Web sites in particular, because the association of computer brain, digit, and being digital (Negroponte 2000) was more than metaphorically suggestive.

Referring to methodology, asymmetries in the body can reveal asymmetries in the brain's hemispheres. As Doreen Kimura (1999) has shown, there are correlations between the size of the right/left hemisphere and the size of the right/left testis or breast and/or ovary. "Great-Lefters" perform better in language tests, regardless of sex (note that the scaling devices for volunteers used during fMRI image runs are almost exclusively made for right-handers). This better performance is attributed to early fetal androgen levels, which influence both brains and sexual organs. Baron-Cohen uses this argument to support the assertion that, in theory, a woman can have a male brain and a man can have a female brain (Baron-Cohen 2004, 107f). Studies on, for example, transsexuals or transgender persons (see Nye, this volume) are not mentioned. And, answering question 2 above ("Where are the studies on abnormal gonadal/genital development?"): Neither is any hypermaleness of autists' gonads mentioned, nor did I even find a scientific publication on the subject from other research groups working on autism. The autist is scientifically only modeled as abnormal/hyperintelligent regarding behavior, not anatomy or sexuality.

Yet, laws of statistics have determined that one has to search for "gradual" differences between the sexes, who are seen as opposite poles on an axis with graduated properties of how sex differences appear. And this is why Brosnan's studies and those of others (Baron-Cohen is also involved; see Lutchmaya et al. 2004) on how being gay or lesbian can be seen in the *hands* are already a preparation for turning in the direction that intrauterine hormone ratios predetermine your sexual preferences and intellectual abilities. Martin Voracek and Stefan G. Dressler (2006) have documented a respectable number of objections to the digit-ratio methodologies. Answering question 1 above ("Where are the hormone studies on modeling the hyperfemale brain?"), Lutchmaya et al. (2004) measured the fetal hormones (both testosterone and estradiol) in amniotic fluid (as a by-product of routine amniocentesis) and compared it with the digit ratio of the embryo visualized in ultrasonic tests. However, there are no explicit studies on the hyperfemale brain in the uterus. How could there be any? What would the abnormal phenotype of behavior be, determined by a hyperfemale structured brain? Women, it seems, are seen as "naturally" hyperfemale in general. If they have an extra capacity for empathy, this is not regarded as abnormal, although there are many documented disorders in which self-abnegation and overfulfillment play an important role.

One can also reverse the argument about the lack of a phenotype for the female brain, as it is mostly men with typically "female" illnesses who are ignored by medical science as—due to an occurrence in the "wrong" sex—there is no self-evident phenotype. When a phenomenon (e.g., breast cancer) and its category of well-known symptoms clashes with biological categories, it does not explain "itself" to the scientist, that is, it does not become *evident*. Scientists' perception is somehow captured by the created epistemic objects. One example of an illness in the "wrong" sex would be breast cancer in men, which is rarely detected, though it does occur (particularly in men above the age of 60). Like the male brain, the female body (and its reproductive capacities) has long been an exclusive boundary object for scientific scrutiny, and the public institutionalization of gynecological examinations of women is much older than comparable concepts of andrology (which developed in the 1950s; see also Dinges 2007).

Measuring implies assessment. It is important for a philosophy of science approach to relate these digit-ratio studies, inspired by hormone research on intelligent male brains, to experimental culture, visualization techniques, and background theories. As mentioned before, geneticists are already struggling with complex phenotypic phenomena at the population level. An individual risk assessment is not in sight, and intelligence, autism, and homosexuality belong to such complex phenomenal traits of an individual. The hand is a highly individualized organ, and its fingers were always an object of biometrical analysis (already in the late seventeenth century, when Nehemiah Grew discovered the "fingerprint" fine structures). In a culture of prenatal testing, where genetic testing of individual gene "abnormalities" of phenotypic traits is not (yet) possible, the hand might replace the gene as a new and old essence of "the human." Digit ratios could be calculated already in the womb by means of ultrasound examinations, and the quasi-ideology of "the wrong hormone in the womb" could help to encourage women to undergo this testing. Moreover, this testing is noninvasive.

Put in a historical perspective, first, the established aura of the weak, feminine, and sensitive left-hander will continue, and, second, women's wombs will continue to be measured and invaded by technology. With regard to future applications, the neuro-developmental studies on autism, involving psychobiological approaches, do make sense with regard to testing contexts rather than cure contexts.

12.3.2   Male Genius in Light of Autism: "Would You Have Allowed Bill Gates to Be Born?"

Not astonishingly, autism as a topic has entered bioethical discourses. Alongside the serious ethicists, who discuss the different medical treatments of autists and recognize the stressful life of parents with an autist child, there are also attempts to exploit HFAs to gain public attention in order to put other arguments forward. The idea of combining elitist thinking with a biologicalization of human potentials is obviously *en vogue* among critics of biopolitics. Arthur Caplan, director of the Center for Bioethics at the University of Pennsylvania and involved in the transhumanist movement, connects the idea of a male elite to geneticized abnormal behavior in his article entitled "Would You Have Allowed Bill Gates to Be Born?" (Caplan 2005), which argues against prenatal genetic testing of autism:

> But what if I told you it's possible that Gates has a medical condition that accounts, in part, for both his tremendous achievements and for his "nerdiness"? Gates is widely reported to display many personality traits characteristic of a condition known as Asperger's syndrome. Asperger's is a mild version of autism, a more serious condition that renders many children unable to talk, be touched, communicate or socialize. While I certainly do not know if Gates has Asperger's, his difficulties in social settings are nearly as legendary as his genius, so it's possible. (Caplan 2005)

Caplan asserts that with the possibility of prenatal testing for autism there will now be "fewer geniuses" in the world. It should be mentioned that in at least one place, he also claims that Lewis Carroll was one of the geniuses the world would have missed if genetic testing of unborn children had then been possible. However, no gene has been found which can be tested for in order to diagnose a disorder Caplan calls "advantageous." Although the humanist approach of accepting children the way they are may lurk behind this, the rhetorical strategy of encouraging parents to envision their unborn child a genius (boy), due moreover to a congenital disability, is particularly elitist. Where the same argument worked some years ago in the discourse on prenatal testing for cystic fibrosis in Europe with the famous composer Frédéric Chopin (though he may have suffered from it, he left the world his beautiful music), the resentment inspired by testing for autism in the United States is supported with reference to an icon of the economic elite. A turn from cultural to economic elites may work in Europe, too, but economic as well as cultural elites are still almost exclusively male today. In such a narrow cultural concept of elite, only the "natural" and "moral" elites can consist of women. Misogynous feminists like Camille Paglia, who wrote that "there is no female Mozart because there is no female Jack the Ripper" (Paglia 1990, 274), support the male genius thinking with reference to biological hypotheses concerning the nature of aggression, sexual violence, and mental creativity.

It is not surprising that in his latest book Daniel Goleman also turns to autists as difficult persons whose "mind-sight" is impaired (Goleman 2006, 138ff). In Goleman's reflection on autists, sexualization of the brain also plays a role. He reiterates the explanation that autism is a very special kind of behavior related to a typical version of a "male brain" (see also the Introduction, section 1.3, this volume), and he reformulates it as advice for talent scouts: "While those with the most 'male' brain have a high likelihood of exhibiting symptoms of Asperger's or autism, they can excel in many fields if . . . they find a congenial setting to apply their talents. Yet the ordinary social world seems an alien planet to them, so that the most basic rudiments of interaction have to be learned by rote, if at all" (Goleman 2006, 140). To sum up, outside the ordinary world there can exist a congenial setting which allows autistic geniuses to emerge. With reference to Baron-Cohen's neurodevelopmental approach to autism, one might conclude: The congenial setting meets the congenital setting.

The case of HFAs, who are prominent in the media while autists without any remarkable abilities are ignored, reflects a kind of *genius thinking* already familiar from cultural studies on schizophrenics and epileptics. Being a *genius* while simultaneously being physically or mentally disabled presents a combination which was admired in the ancient world and still is admired in modern cultures, from epileptic Gaius Julius Caesar to "locked-in" Stephen Hawking. Already Theophrast had asked why all people with exceptional intellects are melancholic (Greek: *perittoi*). The genius remains a symbol of exceptional human abilities in general, for exceeding the category of the human itself. In the bell-curve representation, the genius is situated in the right-end tail.

According to the basic works of Edgar Zilsel on the intellectual history of the idea of geniuses, modern notions of genius in Western thought are still related to religious thinking (Zilsel 1918, 1926; see also Woodmansee 1984). The genius introduces a new element into the intellectual and social world, something which was not there before and which, once it appears, receives approval. In a history of ideas perspective, genius is related to innovation and thus to the idea of progress. HFA geniuses, with their brains' tremendous capacity for systemizing, are thought to lead to (first of all: economic) progress, especially in the digital age (Negroponte 2000).

To select some humans as geniuses is, of course, antithetical to egalitarian beliefs (Stephan 2000). Thus, when autists are labeled as geniuses, their mental or physical disabilities are at the same time somehow comforting to the mass of ordinary people. As Nancy Bombaci (2005) puts it, "The fact remains that because of the cultural fascination with genius, it remains a supreme object of desire, despite its associations with tragic oddity. The current fascination with Asperger's syndrome is based on an attempt to resurrect and explain genius—an idea onto which people project their desire to be exceptional, Promethean, and immortal. While the 'Aspergian' genius may be a god among men, his flaws make him more human." The message is that there seems to be a moral justice in nature; you can never have it all. Here, the idea of nature shows its intimate relation to transcendence and the sphere of what is not known and, in general, not knowable. Moreover, assuming that geniuses exist gives the impression that everyone, potentially, could belong to this group of the exceptional. Like stardom, it helps others to envision upward mobility within social stratification. If, on the contrary, geniuses are portrayed, for example, in the films, as too eccentric and reveal socially destructive behavior, viewers will gain the impression that their own mediocre normality is preferable.

12.3.3   Autism and the Loss of Memory

Since it is situated in the clinical context of psychology and psychiatry, until recently the major methodologies used to diagnose autism in the individual relied on a variety of tests (appropriate for different developmental levels, starting with toddlers) on selected skills (e.g., sensorimotor skills), verbal ability, IQ, interviews, and question-naires, all involving statistics to calculate quotients and determine indices. Current diagnoses are defined by the Autism Diagnostic Interview—Revised, the Autism Diagnostic Observation Schedule, the AQ, or by clinical evaluation. Baron-Cohen developed a number of additional tests, for example, the previously mentioned EQ/SQ test and the "Reading the mind in the eyes" test, which includes photographs of eye pairs. Grouping variables are dependent on age, IQ, and severity of the observed phenomena. It goes without saying that methodological inconsistencies are involved which I cannot address in this chapter.

While it is often claimed that, in trying to become "more experimental," psychology and psychiatry have in the last decades been invaded by biological methods and were willing victims of "*anatomo*-politics" (e.g., Hacking 1998, 217, referring to Foucault 1980), I would like to emphasize the reciprocal process: Biology has been invaded by what Ian Hacking called *memoro*-politics. *Memoro*-politics relate to the cultural history of the concept of soul and are empowered by the introjectionistic idea that there is a deeper (and higher) knowledge of the self than is actually experienced in everyday life. Psychology, in particular, embraces the notion of a deeper knowledge which lurks in the self, as a dark or bright side of personality, as trauma, as a second person, or even as several persons. However, the therapeutic idea is holistic, that is, to make this other side visible with various kinds of psychotechniques in order to obtain "full" knowledge of oneself, primarily by remembering what has been forgotten. It relates to modern ideas of subject and society, as the feeling of being "complete" is dependent on social recognition and social norms. According to Hacking, one of the conse-quences of *memoro*-politics is that individuals have become more and more concerned with what they have hidden than with what they have forgotten. Being self-centered, at the same time they have become used to the increasing loss of information about the larger world, situated in a culture which constantly reminds them that remembering is important.

This invasion of biology by *memoro*-politics happened under the influence of the cognitive branches of psychology and computer science which engaged in neuroscience. Since the 1980s, the cognitive sciences have debated on neural networks and mind modules. They have their own understanding of "full" knowledge about the interior and exterior world, a calculable, systematic, and—concerning the exterior world—ahistorical view of the world. However, the interior world of the computational mind learns by memorizing objects. And it is against this background that high-functional autists are fascinating to those in the cognitive sciences: Autists systemize and calculate, but they resist the metaphorical language of psychotherapy and thus rarely find a second self hiding inside themselves. Situated in a culture of *memoro*-politics, they often feel they are situated in the wrong world, like "being on Mars," as Temple Grandin once said (Sacks 1995). Instead of a deeper knowledge, they seem to gain a "more complete" knowledge of the empirical world of objects. It seems they can systemize it "all," as if the world is a totality of objects which can be placed into natural categories. In fact, the brain's memory region is—funny, somehow—forgotten in Baron-Cohen's studies on autism. Memorizing is an ability in which women in particular score high in classical IQ tests. If the extreme male brain is a good systemizer, how is this capacity enabled without memorizing? As Doreen Kimura (1999) has shown in her studies on sex and cognition, women are more able to rapidly identify matching items (perceptual speed). Why does this not count for being better "systemizers" than men? Even in a conservative anthropological approach of man the hunter/woman the gatherer, one could argue that gathering especially requires a high perceptual speed in identifying what belongs together.

Less obvious elements invading biology are other strong influences from psychology. In a perspective of systems biology with the human brain and behavior at the very top, all biological subdisciplines have to deal with phenotyping and measurements of behaviors and emotions somehow. Psychology has influenced, for example, psychobiology and social neuroscience with its methods (e.g., the use of questionnaires, photographs, and emotion scales after the neuroimage run, asking, "How much pain/disgust/empathy/revenge did you feel while viewing X?"; see the Introduction to this volume), norms ("healing"), and values, related to what are "normal" and "typical" behaviors and emotions of humans in a social (and societal) dimension.

My first observation is that against this background, autism has recently been modeled more and more as a "lack-of-emotion" disorder, probably to fit into the new research field of social cognitive sciences. Autism researcher Christopher Gillberg (1992) reports that in the 1960s autism research pioneer Leo Kanner himself advocated a similar model and objected to neurological causes of autism. However, it comes as a surprise that Baron-Cohen (2004, 137) also refers to autism as an "empathy-disorder," a definition that is inspired by neuro-related behavior, hormone, and emotion research. Previously, central topics of autism research were more focused on the "self" rather than on society and included (still ongoing) research on repetitive and ritualist behavior, impaired verbal abilities, reduced executive functions, and atypical sensorimotor skills, or the lack thereof. In short, research on autism in the 1980s was more interested in the concepts of personality and mind than the brain.

The second observation I would like to share with my readers is that the new alliance of autism research and social cognitive neuroscience was assisted by the developmental branch of psychopathology, which focuses in part on intrauterine fetus development, searching for prenatal abnormalities resulting from above-normal testosterone levels in the maternal blood (Baron-Cohen 2004). Hormones and neurotransmitters are also the crucial media for locating sex-typed emotions in the brain's emotional system (particularly the amygdala and the hypothalamus; Geher and Miller 2007, Brizendine 2006) and for hypothesizing a causal relation between sex-specific emotions and behaviors (classic: testosterone-dependent feelings of revenge, resulting in aggression; new: OT-dependent feelings of "reward," resulting in happiness; see Ulshöfer, this volume). Before the neuroscientific idea of emotions "in" the brain and their somatic markers, which has been put forth by Antonio Damasio since the mid 1990s, behavioral science in the 1970s modeled the relation testosterone/aggression without the middle term "feeling of revenge." In the often-used animal models, reward or happiness as newly defined emotions were irrelevant. They were imported later, following a detour through cognitive psychology and AI research which focused on behavioral science's "black box" in which input and output were operative. When neurobiology adopted topics like feeling or not feeling rewarded, for example, in depression research, it became a victim of *memoro*-politics. Here "reward" does not refer to something like the fodder for Pavlov's dog. Under serious scrutiny, reward is a normative term which makes sense as a feeling only in the context of social ontology, based on an architecture in which the arising feeling can be understood *as* reward, whereas from a biological view there is no reward. Likewise, there is no guilt. Rather, there is survival. In a neuroscience approach, there is no questioning of which social norms allow for *deserving* the feeling of reward.

Again, a goal of *memoro*-politics is, according to Hacking (1998), to influence individuals in such a way that they are less concerned with their minds' forgetting something than with their minds' hiding something which can be unveiled and made visible. When analyzing a predefined antisocial behavior, the idea of forgetting the influence of social norms of a society, and the biography of the individual embedded within, is part of the outcome of that politics approach. This development can be seen in social neurosciences and their neuroimages of visible, "real" emotions which are, moreover, to be found in the newly defined *cognitive unconscious*. Psychology teaches social neurosciences which knowledge about the human mind is measurable and meaningful in relation to the real world of social relations (which Hacking calls the "larger" world). Reward feelings (or a lack thereof), depression, face recognition, stigmatization, and so forth—all these concepts which are currently entering social neurosciences derive from psychology and psychiatry, not from biology itself.

In the 1970s, a new discipline, which was named "psychobiology," emerged, largely based on neurochemistry and computer animations of the brain. It led to a close relationship between psychology, psychiatry, and biology. In addition to the psychologist's idea of a subject's own personality, which can be methodologically examined from top-down, that is, starting with the phenomena or symptoms in order to construct traits, psychobiology models personality in terms of "complex phenotypes." A typical bottom-up approach is behind this, seeking causes for the different personality types in a neuronal and/or genetic constitution. Variations in phenotypes are said to occur, for example, due to different modifier genes (genetic variants) or susceptibility genes (functional variants) (note the recent use of "susceptibility" for autism, related to geneticists seeking to find "autism susceptibility genes"; see, e.g., Dawson et al. 2002). As has happened in genetic findings since the 1970s, the application of psychobiological findings within the medical context has led to a biomedical normative background, bringing with it the moral obligation to relieve the suffering of the human individual (no matter whether the mentally disturbed individual is really suffering or not). The therapeutic cultures of psychology and psychiatry have eased the creation of a new identity for neurobiology, but psychologists have often ignored the fact that due to a biologicalization of the psyche their role has been reduced to providing phenotypic categories and therapeutic training methods. In contrast, biologists are often not aware that they have imported new, nonmaterial units of evolution, such as emotions, facial expressions, and social skills, which refer back to evolutionary psychology rather than evolutionary biology.

Let me give you one example for the shift which took place: Psychologists' main category of the self is personality, upon which Goleman's concept of EI is also based. Paul T. Costa and Robert R. McCrae (1992) developed the standard personality test the NEO Five-Factor Inventory (NEO-FFI), based on language (i.e., a lexical approach).[8] The acronym NEO stands for three of the five categories within which multidimensional personality traits fall: Neuroticism (emotional stability), Extraversion (concerning activity and interpersonal behavior), and Openness (to experiences). The other two categories are Agreeableness (how well you get along with others, related to altruism and sympathy) and Conscientiousness (control and regulation of impulses). Even when regarded as a descriptive approach, the criteria contain normative assumptions. Conscientiousness refers to factors which are relevant in most standard economic job contexts, like planning and impulse control (as opposed to jobs where creativity is required). When psychologists are interested in stress-and-coping techniques and adaptation success, the following question arises: what, exactly, does a person have to adapt to in order to be *regarded* as, for example, emotionally intelligent, or socially acceptable? Social norms remain important for any personality testing method.

In the biopsychological sense, personality-related extraversion potentials have been found to be connected with an increased sensitivity of the mesolimbic dopamine system to potentially rewarding stimuli (Depue and Collins 1999). According to psychobiologist C. Robert Cloninger, author of *Feeling Good: The Science of Well-Being* (2004), dopaminergic neurons regulate the dimension of novelty seeking, serotoninergic neurons regulate harm avoidance, and norepinephrinergic neurons regulate reward dependence. Comparable to hypotheses in hormone research on emotions, the body itself influences its mental condition by releasing endogenous, neuroactive chemicals. The outside world remains one influencing factor among many others. Some of these regulators are found to have a genetic basis. Neurotransmitters, hormones, and the genes which produce them are seen as biological causes of personality traits. In the pharmaceutical context, they represent key substances for designing antidepressants and stimulants. In fact, psychobiology was not very popular when it emerged in the 1970s, in the hippie days and in the days when mental depression was being called a public epidemic (like autism today). At the public level, psychobiology was instantly associated with the taming of deviant behavior in society and the oppression of those who were questioning authority. One well-known mirroring of this societal antipathy toward new psychoactive drugs is the renowned film *One Flew over the Cuckoo's Nest* (United States 1975), with the rebellious Randall Patrick McMurphy (Jack Nicholson) refusing to take them (saying: "But I don't like the idea of taking something if I don't know what it is . . . I don't want anyone to try and slip me salt-peter. You know what I mean?" "I'm a goddamn marvel of modern science."). As a consequence, he is initially treated with the "old" methods to calm him down: first, electroconvulsive therapy ("electroshock therapy") and, second, lobotomy. From a philosophy and history of science point of view, at that time a really "old" method, with regard to hormones/neurotransmitters as suspected causes of aggressive mood disorders, would have been visible in a scene showing the protagonist's castration. In addition, psychosurgery (particularly hypothalamotomy and amygdaloidotomy, both special forms of lobotomy) had been recommended since the 1940s for patients with aggressive or other kinds of abnormal behavior (Meier 2007, Freeman and Watts 1942). It was still practiced in the 1970s (Kiloh et al. 1974; see also El-Hai 2005, Egan 2007) and 1980s (Sano and Mayanagi 1988). In simple terms: The underlying idea of these surgical interventions was to cut the connections between the brain circuits involved in emotions and those necessary for intellectual capacities, that is, destroying the neural connection which Daniel Goleman ("EI") in 1995 considered crucial for healing social relationships. These operations had side effects which were severe (memory loss) and less severe (impotence and eating disorders), since the hypothalamus also regulates appetite and lust. Recent neuromedical interest in deep brain stimulation as a cure for various kinds of emotion-related "disturbances" (e.g., traumas and depressions) reveals some continuity of the lobotomists' ideas and methods, and the "healing" loss of the memory of a traumatizing incident is, as a therapeutic concept (see Roelcke 2004), part of *memoro*-politics. In the 1970s, the amygdala, which is currently being celebrated as the "organ of organs" of the brain's emotional system, was obviously thought to be dispensable.

The recent split of cognitive science in *developmental* and *social* cognitive science corresponds perfectly to the evolutionary hierarchies of ontogeny and phylogeny, and with genotype and phenotype of behavior in populations in sociobiology. At this point, *anatomo*-politics and *memoro*-politics meet *bio*-politics (Foucault 1980), a triangle of power that Ian Hacking (1998, 215ff) characterized as the modern "triangulation of the soul." With the new approach of social cognitive neuroscience, nothing less than *the* social world and *the* mental world is modeled. Both are modeled by means of the body, including the brain. The market for pharmacogenetics is in sight. In 2006, Psychology Press launched a new journal entitled *Social Neurosciences*, which opened with a special issue on *Theory of Mind* edited by Simon Baron-Cohen and Rebecca Saxe. Under the category "aims and scopes" on the Web page is the following: "The Articles published in Social Neuroscience cover all neuroscience techniques including neuro-imaging methods (e.g., fMRI, PET [positron emission tomography], ERP [event-related potential], TMS [transcranial magnetic stimulation]), as well as more traditional neuroscience techniques (e.g., animal studies, case studies, psychiatric populations, post-mortem studies, pharmaceutical agonist/antagonist). Social Neuroscience does not publish articles that report only behavioral data.... Abnormal behaviors and populations are focused on in terms of understanding social/brain relationships. Language, memory, attention and perception are appropriate topics if they relate to specific social behaviors or cognitions."[9]

Considering present autism research within this scope of big science, one major aim is to find distinct phenotypic categories for the complex and heterogeneous clinical symptoms of autism in order to connect these symptoms with genes which are relevant for expressing exactly this phenotype (and not so many others) and thus make the knowledge applicable to pharmacogenetics. The statement that "Social Neuroscience does not publish articles that report only behavioral data" is a reflection on both the autism rights movements' and *DSM* critics' complaint that the diagnostic categories of autism still exclusively depend on behavioral domains and behavioral data acquisition.

Autism, at present classified among the PDDs, faces a sort of taxonomy crisis. It is often misdiagnosed as a personality disorder (e.g., schizoid personality disorder, obsessive–compulsive personality disorder), schizophrenia, ADHD, or a mood disorder (e.g., bipolar disorder). The lack of concreteness in criteria appears in the history of the *DSM* classifications: In the first edition of the *DSM* (1952, 000-x28) it is referred to as "schizophrenic reaction before puberty," in *DSM–II* (American Psychiatric Association 1968, 295.8) autistic behavior is summarized under "schizophrenia, childhood type," *DSM–III* (American Psychiatric Association 1980, since this edition: 299.00) constructs the category of "infantile autism" (using one of Leo Kanner's terms) and differentiates it from schizophrenia, chiefly because of autists' lack of hallucinations, *DSM–III–R* (1987) classifies autism as "autistic disorder," and *DSM–IV* (American Psychiatric Association 1994) creates the subcategory of Asperger's disorder (Asperger's syndrome, 299.80), finally acknowledging Hans Asperger's findings on high-functional autism from the 1940s (Asperger 1944). This subcategory might be accompanied in future editions by crypto-sensitivity syndrome, in order to encompass not only the intellectual but also sensual extremeness (e.g., a keen sense of hearing) of high-functional autists.

The new Asperger category of autism resembles one of the narrowings of phenotypes which I have already mentioned. By the same token, one could, of course, suggest that autism was already a narrowing of schizophrenia and vote for defining schizophrenia as a spectrum in which autism falls (see, e.g., Parnas, Bovet, and Zahavi 2002). But what would that have solved? There is also no valid evidence for a genetic cause of schizophrenia. Obviously, other criteria for accepting the new Asperger's syndrome category were taken into consideration in the mid-1990s. The most important one was the high functionality and the high IQs of Asperger's syndrome persons who have become more and more prominent in a Western culture obsessed with IQ testing (in the United States more than in Europe, and within Europe, e.g., in the United Kingdom more than in Germany, in Germany more than in Poland). Thus, the more intelligent autists were separated from the others as elite autists, and, backed with a new diagnostic category, soon gathered into their own "anti-cure" autism movements. Again, taking gender issues into consideration, this new diagnostic category, with high-flyers in the fields of mathematics and science, shifted the sex ratio from 1 (woman) to 4 (man) being autistic to 1 (woman) to 9 (man) being Asperger autistic.

Another scientific problem is that the *DSM* criteria are not distinctly separated into necessary and sufficient criteria. The *DSM–IV* criteria for autism aggregate the following: (A) qualitative impairment in social interaction (manifested by at least two of four suggested symptoms, ranging from marked impairments in the use of multiple nonverbal behaviors—such as "eye-to-eye gaze and facial expression" to "lack of social or emotional reciprocity," (B) qualitative impairments in communication (manifested by at least one of four suggested symptoms, e.g., delay in, or total lack of, the development of spoken language; repetitive use of language; lack of varied, spontaneous make-believe play or social imitative play appropriate to developmental level), and (C) restricted repetitive and stereotyped patterns of behavior, interests, and activities, as manifested by at least two of four suggested abnormal behaviors: all-encompassing preoccupation with one or more stereotyped and restricted patterns of interest that is abnormal either in intensity or focus; apparently inflexible adherence to specific, nonfunctional routines or rituals; stereotyped and repetitive motor mannerisms; persistent preoccupation with parts of objects. In the neurosciences, this collection is condensed to one phenotypic characteristic of autism: *insistence on sameness*.

One of my predictions is that the public and academic discussions of EI will receive a new boost from the powerful autism movements gathering the "left-behinds," the many individuals who have "normal" IQs. The limits of classical IQ testing have become people's own personal limits within the diagnostic system, uniting both "normal" autists and normal nonautists.

12.4   Epilogue: Pop Science and Othering

12.4.1   Structure and Function of Pop Science

The purpose of this last section is to broaden the understanding of strategies of othering involved in pop science and its markets, particularly strategies that have been exemplified in this chapter. These strategies might sometimes appear far-fetched, however, as they are not always apparent at first sight. Public media play a key role in communicating science and shaping public acceptance of specific scientific theories, as sociologist Peter Wehling (2006, 254f) argues. Media convey and transform knowledge claims and ignorance claims of science. Thus, they model systemic knowns and unknowns at the public level by means of filtering what is, presumably for everybody, relevant to know and what is not. With reference to *memoro*-politics (Hacking 1998): They also model what has to be remembered and what can be forgotten. According to S. Holly Stocking (1998, 169), journalists' own *interests* are a crucial part of this filtering process. On the content level, the modern idea of the *public relevance* of scientific knowledge and nonknowledge is based on heterogeneous concepts such as progress and innovation, economic well-being, social justice, security, and human nature, all of which have to be mediated as particularly relevant for individuals in order to be read and "taken in." Scientific knowledge of the human brain seems to assemble all of the above-mentioned target concepts for public relevance. Connecting scientific propositions with terms traded in already existing "linguistic markets" (Bourdieu 2005a) and cultural stereotypes (as part of an act called "framing") eases public acceptance by upholding the notion that laypeople and experts do not differ substantially in their scientific knowledge capacities. Referring to the institutional dimension of science, this notion can be used for conveying the impression of existing participatory elements in political decision making concerning new (and old) research areas in science and technology ("scientific citizenship"; see Wehling 2006, 259). Since it itself already uses linguistic market terms (e.g., emotion and intelligence), symbolic images and graphs (neuroimages and bell curves), and stereotypes (man/woman, female/male, black/white), the mediating process only gains in efficiency and effectiveness, which is also necessary for successful science fundraising. However, this efficiency contains reactionary elements, and it functions at the cost of envisioning a normatively "better" society by means of scientific progress. Hence, it contradicts the idea of cultural progress. Public ignorance of science can be a social reflection of this contradiction and normative disillusion rather than merely exemplifying the "knowledge deficits" of society. Neuroscientists' critiques of their colleagues' science marketing styles (e.g., Hines 2004, Phelps and Thomas 2003) can have a corrective function within the scientific community.

The particular influence of pop-science literature—written by scientists (e.g., Simon Baron-Cohen) rather than journalists—on the mediating process of scientific knowledge has not yet been sufficiently scrutinized, and I can do nothing but offer a rough sketch here. The genre of pop science developed back in the middle of the nineteenth century, related to the new concept of public life (and its counterpart: private life), as well as to the ideas of publicity and civil society, and was instantiated by an enormously expanding newspaper and journal market for mass distribution (Daum 2002) and the building of museums (Chittenden, Farmelo, and Lewenstein 2004). From its very beginning, scientists trivialized pop science because of its simplifications and viewed pop science as an add-on within an imagined two-phase approach of scientific writing, which, nevertheless, was regarded as necessary for the advancement of science. In fact, science and pop-science literature offer complementary ways of understanding scientific knowledge. Pop science established unique transformations of knowledge (Daum 2002, 26), particularly related to holistic ideas of "nature" and "world," and it still does. According to historian of science Andreas Daum, European pop science started (at least in the German and French contexts) with Alexander von Humboldt's *Kosmos* (1845ff), at about the same time as the 1848 revolution was breaking out. Bruce V. Lewenstein (1992) regards pop science as a (French) *genre americain* (Lewenstein 1997) which emerged around 1820.

In the pop-science literature, the author speaks both as scientist and journalist. In so doing, he or she is able to perform a double filtering process of knowledge: First, the author speaks as scientist (backed by his or her personal authority), clearly describing what is known within his or her scientific community (and, implicitly, what is not known); second, the author gives voice to the lay reader, individually selecting what is important (according to the author's set of norms and values) to know and reframing this knowledge within the cultural perspective as to why it is worth knowing. Typical writing styles of pop science include a first-person perspective (singular: "I") in the introductory passages to stress scientific authority, a third-person perspective in the middle section as typical for classical science writing, implying an objective meta-level, and, again, a first-person perspective at the end (both singular and plural, and the "we" most often outweighs the "I"). As a result of this rhetorical strategy, both the "known unknowns" (disguised by generalizations and abstractions during scientific modeling) and the "unknown unknowns" of science (often related to scientific paradigms, in the tradition of Thomas S. Kuhn) are less likely to become part of public "ignorance claims" (Wehling 2006), compared to the mediating process instantiated by serious science journalists. It is important to remember that science, in general, is not only exporting terms and symbols from laboratories into the public sphere but is also importing them from public issues which crop up in society, for example, in social movements (e.g., the autism rights movement, the animal rights movement, or the women's rights movement). In the pop-science literature, both scientific knowledge and ignorance can actively be constructed in tacit accordance with features of existing social and political conditions—for instance, concerning gender issues and divisions of labor.

The presentation of science in popular culture media, for example, in popular films shown in cinema or on TV (see also Illouz 2008), is directly related to establishing a market value for pop-science literature. At the beginning of this essay, I examined cinema productions on autists as hidden mediators of scientific gender modeling, particularly related to the extreme male brain of HFAs. Referring to the TV contexts and their science sections, Claudia Wassmann (2007) analyzed the multi-episode TV series on the brain, all produced by the New York based Public Broadcasting Service station WNET: *The Brain* (1984), *The Mind* (1988), and *The Secret Life of the Brain* (2002). Lined up in a row, this concatenation mirrors the shift from viewing the brain as an organ within a person's body to viewing it as an entity with a life of its own. In the new millennium, this trend has not only persisted but expanded, particularly regarding its influence on the categorization of normality and abnormality. Moreover, this turn to the objectification of the self (Honneth 2005) currently makes it possible to hold the individual responsible for personal deviance. Previously, media focus had been on explaining why and how mental illnesses are physically based, that is, why there is no real chance of self-healing and why pharmaceutical drugs or brain surgery are needed to overcome the abnormal personal condition and to aid the patient's exhausting struggle for normality. As Claudia Wassmann puts it: "While brain imaging was used during the 1990s in order to excuse socially deviant behavior or underachievement in a society of success, at the turn of the twenty-first century the picture changed again. . . . In 2002, . . . [t]he brain's surprising power of renewal was the dominant trope. The use of brain images balanced back the burden of responsibility to the individual who can choose whether or not to train his or her brain and keep up high performance even in old age" (Wassmann 2007, 158f). At the same time as Antonio Damasio was arguing that "it is emotions that are at the heart of our thoughts" (in "The Adult Brain: To Think by Feeling" of the 2002 TV series *The Secret Life of the Brain*, quoted in Wassmann 2007, 160), the image of the brain was appearing on the television screen as a free-standing object. It was presented as an independent, living entity, with a personal essence: therefore a self and an icon.

Because of the new-found plasticity of the brain and its popularization by public media, it has become *obvious* that with training the brain can increase its capacity and renew its powers. However, it also became *relevant*, because the pop-scientific message, put forth in particular by Daniel Goleman in his best-selling books on EI since the mid 1990s, was this: The same is true for you—meaning: your brain—if you really want to. Though the neurosciences share common ground with genetics in shaping biological determinisms, the genetic discourse (except when related to eugenic thinking) never blamed the subject for being dysfunctional. Having bad genes still remains in the realm of fate; having a bad brain obviously does not. The effort to imbue societies with the idea that the individual is responsible for his or her brain condition still profits from the philosophical concept of free will, though there is no neuroscientific proof that free will actually exists. Therefore, the acceptability of neuroscientific research depends on anthropological convictions which still have to be confirmed in society, for example, that the human being is not only part of the highest form of mammalian life but also possesses special abilities which make her or him human. It is against this normative background that emotional (dis)abilities are the focus of both science and pop science.

Emotions have to appear as cultivated and civilized to construct the genuinely human sphere of the world, thus othering animal nature. The first step of cultivation was to scientifically model emotions as cognition laden by suggesting an emotional system in the brain that encompasses areas for decision making and memory. The second step was to model the brain as a living entity that is able to learn during all stages of its life (neuroplasticity). These two scientific approaches set the stage for the new, that is, emotion-laden, *intension* of the "brain." The third step, now, is to show the *extension* of the newly constructed object in question, that is, that all human beings (and not other mammals) are inhabited by such emotion-laden, rational, and fluid brains, and that "reeducating the emotional brain" (Goleman 1995, 208) represents a window of opportunity for society at present. Particularly on the level of this third step, science often crosses the border to pop science, suggesting concepts like EI, which are presented as applicable to everyone, with male autism (and the "emotional machine"; Minsky 2006) as its antithesis. Pop science offers unification strategies on the societal level of science, that is, it helps to bridge the differences between the model of the human in science and individual humans in society. Still, it is the overall idea of human nature, no matter how reduced by technomorphous labeling, that allows for the occurrence of intelligent emotions in all human individuals (equity). During scientific modeling within the previously mentioned scientific contexts of emotion and cognition research, the idea of the human being is, first, isolated from the social and personal contexts of everyday experience. He or she is sex-typed, mentalized, and biologicalized by psycho–bio–cogno–neuroscience. Secondly, the person is behavioralized, emotionalized, and reimported into "society" by sociobiology and social neuroscience, which model society as a (global or national) population with different groups. At the same time, society, its groups, and social actors are remodeled as normal, and thus the corresponding idea of exceptional brains and behaviors, for example, those of autists, crop up as abnormal, extreme, genius-like, and, at the same time, pathological. As often happens, a specific ontological *equity* ("every human has emotions"; "every human has a brain"; "every human belongs to nature") is normatively extended to *equality* in order to gain public attention and acceptance through ignorance of modal terms ("because of ubiquitous human emotionality, and its inherent rationality, everyone can reach the same social status by brain training"), though the real world of social conditions proves that the opposite is true. The modality hidden in the differences between emotionality/emotion, can/do, capacity/ability remains a blind spot.

The expression "human nature" is used in the life sciences as a rhetorical instrument for unification at the popular level of science communication, whereas within the scientific context of neurosciences this expression is rarely used. This special, rhetorical use of "human nature" is one reason why the high-functional male autist must, of necessity, appear as *not* completely human, rather than machine-like: He does not even have to train; he is high-functional from the very beginning of his existence. If he were completely human, then his exceptional abilities would seem to be guaranteed by a meta-instance over which humans do have no control. Given that uncontrollable instance, the normative impetus for individual brain training, for the sake of society, would not seem appealing. Thus, to encourage people to train their brains, the male autist has to appear as if he lacks emotions in general (though he does not). Because of existing gender role clichés, the pop-scientific image of the rational and HFA man (and his extreme male brain) is more acceptable than his female counterpart. Just as Ian Hacking (1998, 69ff) wondered why feminists of the 1970s did not object when the sex ratio of MPD was said to be 9 (women) to 1 (men), I wonder why the purported high-functional Asperger's syndrome sex ratio of 1 (women) to 9 (men) has not yet hit feminists' radar. Hacking's suggestion, written with a touch of irony, is that as MPD is related to sexual abuse, many women deliberately identified with the familiar role of the passive and the oppressed. At present, do women consider themselves less likely to be geniuses than men? Is their attention to the real power structure (intelligence and high functionality) distracted by the mass of sexual-arousal studies on the female brain (see Brizendine 2006)? Are they content to find their intellectual capacity located in the belly parts of the body, revealing a "female" way of integrating knowing and feeling—for instance, when Natalie Angier (2000) writes that the clitoris with its 8,000 nerve fibers almost resembles a small brain? Hopefully not. If men do not see that their intellectual upgrading, by means of the extreme male autist-brain idealtype, involves a painful loss of emotionality and the necessity of joining a capitalistic labor force working even more efficiently in competitive markets, then, maybe, there will be another turn in this sexualized brain story. The issue of women autists as no minority will hit the public radar when the discourse on sexual abuse and sexual harassment in the context of autism develops. In fact, the discourse has already begun (see below).

Looking at recent TV documentaries on the brain (and thus extending Wassmann's findings on the iconicity of the brain to the post-2002 years), essential sex differences have become a new topic. These differences restrict the idea of individual brain training, as the idea remains limited to the potentials assumed to be found in heterosexual people. In the famous German documentary trilogy *Expeditionen ins Gehirn* (by Petra Höfer and Freddie Röckenhaus, first broadcast on public TV in 2006; channels: ARD [Arbeitsgemeinschaft der öffentlich-rechtlichen Rundfunkanstalten der Bundesrepublik Deutschland (Cooperation of the public broadcasting stations of the Federal Republic of Germany)], 3Sat, and the German–French channel ARTE), which also appeared under the English title *Beautiful Minds: A Voyage into the Brain*, the three episodes closely examined autism and the neural "Einstein effect." The filmmakers present and interview long-known autistic media stars: Howard Potter, who loves counting football scores, Kim Peek, the "real" Rain Man who inspired Hollywood, and *wunderkind* musician Matt Savage. Not surprisingly, the only woman autist shown is Temple Grandin, who appears in episode III, which examines sex differences of brains (the original German title, *Der große Unterschied*, could be literally translated as "The Big Difference" but was toned down to *A Little Matter of Gender*). The narrator's voice in the documentary stresses that Grandin will probably never have a boyfriend, while Simon Baron-Cohen comments, "In Grandin's head is a male brain." In the same episode, German neuroscientist Gerhard Roth asserts that women are not less aggressive than men, rather they show their aggressions less physically, as "women are the typical poisoners" (on the pathologization of women as poisoners back in nineteenth century brain science, see Hagner 2004, 104). In 2005, two years after Baron-Cohen published his *The Essential Difference* and one year before neuroendocrinologist Louann Brizendine reinvented *The Female Brain*, a U.K. TV trilogy (a British Broadcasting Corporation [BBC] production) entitled *Secrets of the Sexes* was broadcast. The first episode dealt with *Brainsex*, and examined hormones as mediators of emotions in the brain. During the episode, the viewer became witness to how, under the influence of monthly testosterone injections, 20-year-old Max turns from a woman into a man. The second episode (*Attraction*) dealt with sexual chemistry, hormones, and, naturally, finding Mr. Right, while the third one (*Love*) asked how new insights into psychobiology can prevent divorces. Of course, the BBC also produced a more psychology-oriented trilogy, *The Human Mind* (2003; episode I: *Get Smart*, II: *Personality*, III: *Making Friends*).

The *Psychology Today* article about a teenage girl with Asperger's syndrome, entitled "The Girl with a Boy's Brain" (Flora 2006), demonstrates how effectively the concepts of sexualized brains and male genius have been communicated to the public. As a consequence, whenever a woman is high-functional, she must have a man's brain. In the *Psychology Today* article, psychologist Shona Nichols, who works on the special needs of Asperger's syndrome women, reports that "girls have been neglected" by science. Therefore, they have also been neglected by pop science.

To sum up: The emotions-and-brain-related approaches of Goleman and Baron-Cohen which are supported by public media productions operate on the surface with arguments for healing, social inclusion, and respect for the currently disadvantaged (Goleman: for the "unsuccessful" ones in society; Baron-Cohen: for autists), whereas upon closer inspection they appear to be arguments for economic and social exclusion, concerning both heterosexually oriented and lesbian women and gays. At the explanatory level, Goleman focuses on heterosexual, married couples and overall leadership, while Baron-Cohen, much more aggressively, points out how HFA men will "naturally" become the leaders of the future IT society.

For many reasons—some of which have been outlined in this chapter and in this book—the idea that EI is a conceptual *alternative* to cognitive intelligence(s) is a pop-scientific myth. As long as a functional rationality underlies the scientific concepts of world and its static entities, there is no chance to even model another, more processual type of intelligence. On the contrary, under present political and socioeconomic conditions in the Western hemisphere, it is more likely that emotions will be more and more modeled as rational and static and include sexual and gender role stereotyping. Outside the laboratory, that is, in the real world of lived experience, there is no other way to advocate "another" form of typified intelligence than appealing to people's interests, values, needs, and desires and encouraging them to adopt the suggested testing and training techniques more or less voluntarily. This quasi-voluntary act relates to what Michel Foucault has called *governmentality* and *power-knowledge* (Foucault 1979, 1980; see also Lemke 2001). Pop science presents effective strategies for making people believe that the application of scientific findings to their own life worlds will make their lives better. In fact, this works out as long as the general idea persists that science and—both true and "good," that is, normatively wishful—knowledge about the world and the human being belong together.

There are different relationships and markets concerned, related to different ideas about where and how empathizing and altruism, systemizing and "egoism" (or, better, self-centeredness), are effective strategies. The general concepts of EI and sexualized brains (empathizing female and systemizing male ones), demarcating two heteronormative approaches to the idea of an alternative superior intelligence, do not necessarily depend on having real feelings. Rather, they use the category of emotions for a collection of neural representations, behaviors, and performative actions which can be a useful addition to a functional rationality in some situations, particularly combat, rivalry, and competition.

The pop-scientific mixture of accumulating decontextualized scientific findings (including terms and images), declarations of social inequalities and the existence of unhappy individuals, the suggestion of personality-based solutions, and visions of a better future for everyone is persuasive: Your body is society's body; your brain is society's brain. Therefore, try to train it! Thinking about the brain–body divide in relation to organism-like society, Goleman, in his latest book (Goleman 2006), stresses the feedback mechanism of emotions. Reactions to others have a biological impact. They regulate the heart and the immune system via hormones. Establishing good relationships will lengthen lives. Moreover, the ability to form relationships guarantees, according to Goleman, a nourishing marriage, successful leadership, happy children, and peace on earth. We can relate this again to autism. In the media, HFAs are often thought to comprise an "abnormal elite" of geniuses. As such they can be understood as the latest icons of the functional human in individualistic societies. As innate high performers in special fields, HFAs function as "the other" to the argumentative strategies upon which the concept of EI is based: the human being as an empathic, socially responsible, charismatic leader, who can improve his or her high scores on the emotional quotient (EQ) tests (Goleman, Boyatzis, and McKee 2002), thus qualifying for success in different areas. Autists have to undergo a very different type of training, that is, therapy, to express emotions, and if they do manage to let them out, then the emotions are considered original and pure. As autists have difficulties in understanding someone who pretends, they also rarely pretend themselves. They are unable to manage their emotions as means for strategic ends as in EI concepts regarding the business world.

In competitive circumstances, showing emotions can function as an appeasement strategy. That some autists lack this strategic ability somehow makes their minds beautiful, as opposed to those who communicate their real feelings openly and for their honesty face the consequences—isolation. However, neither has anything to do with altruism (Nagel 1970) or empathy, which in pop-scientific discourses on sexualized brains both remain empty categories. As far as I can see, the idea that subjective feelings generally make sense, for the individual and for society, and thus scientific attention should be devoted to them, has only survived in a few branches of psychology, particularly those with a humanist tradition. However, in pop science it is generally women who are placed in this empty category. That the category is in fact hollow can be demonstrated by the fact that there is no existing human idealtype suggested for the extreme female brain by Baron-Cohen or Brizendine, not even Mother Teresa or the Virgin Mary. The HFA man is left alone in future society. However, looking at the previously outlined attributes of the female brain suggested by Baron-Cohen, the idea that Baron-Cohen's othering of the extreme male brain is in fact a (m)othering of the male brain becomes obvious. The increase in the number of single mothers in Western societies within the last decades seems to correspond with Baron-Cohen's modeling of the polygamous man as someone who also naturally lacks a moral framework. Thanks to the study of Van Bourgondien, Reichle, and Palmer (1997) on the sexual behavior of adults with autism, the scientific community knows that 68% of a sample of autists (representing all levels of autism, including 72 men and 17 women, ages 16–59) in North Carolina were reported to masturbate at least weekly—according to the questionnaires completed by group home staff. A high percentage of the "person-oriented" group (which represented about one third of the entire sample) showed a same-sex orientation. An Australian study documented a high rate of "inappropriate" sexual behavior (e.g., public masturbation) in particular HFAs as reported by their parents and measured on a sexual behavior scale, a result which seems "consistent with the nature of the disorder" (Stokes and Kaur 2005, 281). One gets the impression that it is inappropriate for systemizers to feel attracted to systemizers or to focus on experiencing their own desire. Apparently, the HFA is in desperate need of sexual education, for different reasons: first, to avoid victimization, second, to avoid becoming a sexual offender, and, last but not least, to learn how to reproduce. And he is in desperate need of an empathetic and flexible woman. The sexual education of autists would also benefit genetic research on autism, which is still faced with the problem that the bloodline for autism (in reference to the new diagnostic category) is short and that autists have low reproduction rates.

Obviously, the high sales of pop science literature on EI and high-functional, heterosexualized brains profit from the fears of some technocrats and conservatives that biological reproductive rates in highly industrialized Western nations are currently decreasing (excluding, among other groups, many of the immigrants), while at the same time highly educated women compete with men in the limited labor market. In addition, the concept of labor is undergoing an increasing subjectivation, which means that the flexible employee is becoming ever more responsible for his or her economic fitness within the labor market (Arbeitsgruppe SubArO 2005). In this context, the pop-scientific conceptualization of sexualized brains and EI types makes sense, suggesting male concepts of leadership for job areas already dominated by men (IT, finance, science) and no concept at all of leadership for jobs in the "female" sector of emotional labor (Hochschild 1983) or in the private sector of emotional work. Regarding HFAs, Baron-Cohen redefines the categories of disability and leadership: "Indeed, if autism involves an intact or superior systemizing ability, and if systemizing requires an ability to predict that input X causes output Y in a system, then this suggests that those with autism are capable of some executive function (planning)." Following this statement, Baron-Cohen provides an example of a male mathematician, who "has terrific systemizing skills . . . , considerable difficulties in empathizing, but not a trace of any executive dysfunction" (Baron-Cohen 2004, 176). This person would make an ideal leader, it seems (though not in Goleman's view, as the empathic commitment to society is lacking). Obviously, among all individuals, only a special class of autists

(HFAs) seems to truly "understand" the world (system) if the world is a machine. The LFAs are left behind in pop science, though they constitute the majority of diagnosed autists. As the niche for the empathizing female brain remains the familiar private realm of biological reproduction, where altruism and empathy make sense in the context of child care, it becomes quite obvious that, in the end, the EQ/SQ divide is dealing with stereotyped biological concepts in complicity with the binary-coded gender roles of women and men. Both the brain as interior system and society as an exterior system are interpreted teleologically by Baron-Cohen (in sharp contrast to Charles Darwin): "When we find someone with the extreme female brain, my guess is that we will also find that society has made it easy for them to find a niche and a value, without that person having to feel that they must in some way hide their systemblindness" (Baron-Cohen 2004, 184).

This leads to another exclusion related to same-sex sexuality, for as previously mentioned gay men have at least a genetic chance of having a male brain (Baron-Cohen) or of acquiring the habitus of being masculine (Goleman), while lesbian women may have neither a genetic constitution for a male brain nor the will to biological reproduction or feminine self-fashioning. They appear to have no ecological niche in society.

The general concern with health, technology, and the pursuit of happiness circumscribes the cultural mentality in which the seed of EI and essential differences of men's and women's brains has been planted. The pop-science strategy functions by *inviting readers to give a self-report of their status* in society, including the access to and management of their emotions. And this provocation succeeds because of the competitive structure it is built upon. On the other hand, if you do not voluntarily do a self-report, perhaps you do not do so because you are an autist whose mindsight is impaired, in which case brain research, it seems, can do the self-report for you.

12.4.2 Activists of Pop Science

The last part of my chapter will deal with the profane question of who, besides the authors of pop-science books, stands behind these best-sellers, organizes scientists and scientific opinions, and dissolves the borders between science, pseudoscience, and pop science. What we are going to turn to now are the disclosure strategies and in-group discourses by means of which this chimera is able to proliferate. It is handled within a marketing discourse on two central questions, principally put forth by literary agent and media activist John Brockman: First, what is reality? Second, what is science?

Daniel Goleman and John Brockman, his literary agent, both market the American Dream by advertising their own personal, economic success, leading to biographical success, on their own home pages.[10] John Brockman is also Simon Baron-Cohen's literary agent, as well as the agent of many others involved in discourses on the new genetics, neurosciences, and cognitive sciences. Steven Pinker, Daniel C. Dennett,

Richard Dawkins, Jared Diamond, Francisco Varela (before he died in 2001), and many other "big names" belong to the A-list of Brockman's clients. Their books have also become very influential in European discourses, and this influence has increased since Frank Schirrmacher, editor in chief of the highly respected German daily newspaper *Frankfurter Allgemeine Zeitung*, confessed to being "brockmaned" in 2001 and, consequently opened the newspaper's feuilletons to neuroscientist authors. Brockman is a well-connected media activist, who uses the Internet in particular for opinion making. In U.S. print media, he has been both criticized and envied for his economic success and provocative behavior in the literary business. Astonishingly, however, his critics neither touch on the highly selective topics Brockman has been marketing and editing since the 1990s (for an overview, see John 1999) nor do they mention the fact that his clients marketed as elite thinkers are almost exclusively white males, most of them based in the United States. This selection may be by chance, though, and the British Baron-Cohen represents at least a sort of exception. John Brockman is also the editor of best-selling books like *The Third Culture: Beyond the Scientific Revolution*, published in the same year as Goleman's *Emotional Intelligence* (1995), *Curious Minds: How a Child Becomes a Scientist* (2004b), and, most recently, *What Is Your Dangerous Idea? Today's Leading Thinkers on the Unthinkable* (2006; with an introduction by Steven Pinker and an afterword by Richard Dawkins). This last book title in particular shows how not only the scientific knowns but also the (known) unknowns are publicly shaped by pop science activists. Readers of these books may observe that the "leading thinkers" gathered in these follow-up editions have many things in common and that the topics and disciplines involved always reflect similarities: scientific leadership, the emergence of mind and universe, Alife, AI, evolution, and transhumanism.

In addition, Brockman founded the not-for-profit Edge Foundation. "Edge Foundation, Inc., was established in 1988 as an outgrowth of a group known as The Reality Club. Its informal membership includes some of the most interesting minds in the world."[11] "Edge" stands for both a marketing company and a sort of intellectual *in-group* of some of the best-known scientists in the Western hemisphere. The disciplines involved (biology, biomedicine, neuro- and cognitive science, theoretical physics, computer science) all model the world of consciousness, behavior, and cosmos with empirical data analysis based on a theoretical background that deals with evolution, "emergence," and self-organization. Their words for world are *universe*, *computer*, *mind*, and *brain*. Philosophers, for example, only join if they refer to these topics, while sociologists and historians (and economists) are not represented at all. The Gaia hypothesis (Lovelock 1988) of the superorganismic earth—another world concept, in addition to universe, system, cyberspace, and environment—is quoted excessively in many of the texts from the Brockman club. Lovelock hypothesized that the earth is a living (highly feminized) entity which continually stabilizes itself and is involved in biota and abiota processes. Lovelock's idea, reminiscent of the ancient concept of cosmic harmony, is strongly related to the ecology movement, which however is not a topic of interest for the Reality Club. Stefan Helmreich points out why the Gaia hypothesis was adopted by Alife scientists in particular, a group of scientists who, since the early 1990s, have stood paradigmatically for a research program that seeks to overcome the phenomenological concept of the body's primary world of experience: "Defining life as a process of continual self-maintenance promised to include a wide range of processes in life's cycles of origin, existence and demise. Life could be seen to arise from and return to inert materials. Biota and abiota would become different stages of the same stuff, the distinction between life and nonlife, organism and environment, would become blurred . . ." (Helmreich 2000, 206; regarding gender arguments, 276, endnote 7).

In the publications edited and marketed by Brockman, the word "reality" is often used in the infusion strategy of pop science, as is "science" and "emergence." For instance, Goleman (1995) introduced his concept of EI as an "emerging new science" and provided a "self science curriculum" for training EI (Goleman 1995, 303), though without providing suggestions for how this "new" science might be structured. However, we can all, apparently, take part in the emergence of "the new" in our "social universe," obtaining both a deeper insight into the meaning of the world and finally *becoming* scientists. Simon Baron Cohen uses the same argument about the union of the male human being with science by means of systemizing capacities, but he turns the argument around, asserting that we *have always already been* scientists: "Although academic science is relatively recent—a mere few hundred years old—'folk' science is as old as humans themselves. Tribal peoples have been developing their own understandings of natural systems, building their own technologies, formulating their own medical systems and establishing systems to govern their social groups, for tens of thousands of years" (Baron-Cohen 2004, 118).

On his *Edge* home page, John Brockman writes what he thinks academic elites have to think about nowadays and why we need a "third culture":

The third culture consists of those scientists and other thinkers in the empirical world who, through their work and expository writing, are taking the place of the traditional intellectual in rendering visible the deeper meanings of our lives, redefining who and what we are. . . . A 1950s education in Freud, Marx, and modernism is not a sufficient qualification for a thinking person in the 1990s. Indeed, the traditional American intellectuals are, in a sense, increasingly reactionary, and quite often proudly (and perversely) ignorant of many of the truly significant intellectual accomplishments of our time. Their culture, which dismisses science, is often nonempirical. . . . It is chiefly characterized by comment on comments, the swelling spiral of commentary eventually reaching the point where the real world gets lost.[12]

This is a clear vote in favor of empiricism and ahistoricism, while ignoring that Freud was a trained neurologist and Marx was highly inspired by soil chemistry and cell biology. Some intellectuals might nod in agreement while reading this passage. Most, however, will probably just shrug their shoulders and return to their books (including those by Freud and Marx) and their colleagues again and do a good job in finding out what modernity actually is built upon. This noble ignorance of effective disclosure and marginalization strategies can be quite dangerous, particularly with regard to the role of pop science in society, and it touches on more than the issues of "Who is the real intellectual?" or "Who is really intellectual?" It is concerned with "Who is allowed to speak with authority about what is real?"

Many people on both sides of the Atlantic have no idea that there is a Reality Club aggressively shaping discourses and discursive practices in fields of pop science which have an impact on science.[13] For the sake of producing a best-seller, authors supervised by Brockman have adjusted their texts to well-established stereotypes and linguistic markets.

In this particular process of pop-science production, European science policy differs significantly from U.S. policy. Finding out that a scientist or philosopher is being promoted by a paid literary agent, specialized in establishing elitist circles in which extensive cross-referencing is practiced in the publications, would ruin her or his reputation. One cannot predict whether, under the present political and economic climate, with the middle class shrinking, this gap will increase or decrease.

Let us examine the relation of gender issues and Brockman's marketing strategy of pop science. For example, if you look in the index in *The Third Culture*, you will not find "gender," but you will find "sex and evolution" and "sexual reproduction." Only one of the 23 authors in *The Third Culture* is a woman (the evolutionary biologist Lynn Margulis), and her article on the organismic view of the earth is entitled "Gaia is a Tough Bitch." Whoever is interested in the misogynous structure of the Edge experts' public but closed "mailing list journal" (note: it is not a list to which everyone can subscribe; it is by invitation only) should take a look at the questions posted by Carl Djerassi and Natalie Angier in *Edge* 22 (July 17, 1997).[14] They ask Brockman why there are so few women scientists both writing and being mentioned in *Edge*. Brockman does not really provide an answer. Instead, he invites more female contributors to join (though one has to be invited). The most recent publications and postings submitted by Brockman include more women scientists, and there was even a sort of gender issue of *Edge* in 2005—but the gender topic itself is never discussed as a crucial and necessary part of a science on the edge, comprising the "third culture" or a club of realists. Instead, in this special topic issue, Brockman offers video and audio streams of the public debate between two renowned Harvard professors (Steven Pinker and Elizabeth Spelke) a few months after Harvard president Larry Summers' public comment about men's and women's innate sex differences, which seemed to appear in average test scores, and the presumably related differences in qualifications and career opportunities (see also Hagner, this volume). The issue is entitled "The Science of Gender and

Science: Pinker vs. Spelke." Again, science is envisioned as the only way to gain knowledge of the world, and, again, academics in the humanities are also ridiculed: "It's interesting to note that since the controversy surrounding Summers' remarks began, there has been an astonishing absence of discussion of the relevant science." He continues: "Scientists debate continually, and reality is the check. They may have egos as large as those possessed by the iconic figures of the academic humanities, but they handle their hubris in a very different way. They can be moved by arguments, because they work in an empirical world of facts, a world based on reality."[15]

Moreover, Brockman has also founded a virtual club called "Digerati" (meaning: computer and Internet experts). They are introduced as "cyber-elite," the doers, writers, and thinkers who have "tremendous influence on the emerging communication revolution." And: "The digerati evangelize, connect people, adapt quickly."[16] This sounds like the description of a virus or a sect, but it refers to a group of people who contribute to the mass communication capacities of the Internet.

So why does the Reality Club not directly address religion if the club is on a mission for supraintelligence and the emergence of the world? It comes as no surprise that under the pressure of the spreading movements of Intelligent Design and Creationism, some members of the Brockman club have turned to this topic, the most prominent ones being philosophers Daniel C. Dennett and Richard Dawkins. There are, however, two different approaches to dealing with the topic of science and religion among Brockman's authors. Both strategies seek to integrate religion into science, though into different kinds of science, and thereby transform the idea of what the aim of science is: either to explain "all" phenomena in the universe by means of objective knowledge or to heal the subjective self from its immanent crisis by self-transcendence.

The first approach is exemplified by philosopher Daniel Dennett. Dennett avoids the question of *why* these movements (Creationism, Intelligent Design) crop up; instead, they are simply labeled as wrong. Dennett's strategy is to argue that religion does not belong to a sphere of transcendence, and, moreover, to claim that religious thought can be proven by evolutionary theory. His argument is that religion as "an inert idea, if it were designed just right, might have a beneficial effect on a brain without having to know it was doing so" (Dennett 2006, 6). It is a user illusion. This way of turning feelings into epiphenomena was established before, as they are, in the words of Dennett, "an artifact of our immersion in human culture" (Dennett 1998, 346). Thus it also works with religious feelings. Note that the same argument regarding "an inert idea"—here: immortality—could be used to criticize the transhumanistic idea of uploading your self into the Internet to gain eternal life as is discussed in some discourses on AI and nanotechnology (Coenen 2006). Religious "over-tones" related to eternal life are also found in the rhetoric of Alife research (Helmreich 2000, 84–88). That the argument presented above is not applied to the contexts of technofuturism and transhumanism might be due to the fact that creationism questions Darwinism and argues backwards, whereas transhumanism extends the idea of environment and technical survival of the fittest on a temporal and spatial scale. Technofuturism seems to be progressive. More noteworthy, confessed atheist Dennett has a reductive understanding of religion(s), with regard to the social and historical origins of religion(s) and to the differences between how and where religion is currently practiced (on the discursive relations of naturalism and religion, see Habermas 2004). Therefore, the religious qualities of science itself remain a blind spot in Dennett's book (since, by definition, there is no such thing as transcendence) as does the posture of cultural dominance in which it is immersed (e.g., regarding Islamic cultures).[17]

In the second approach to the discourse field of neuroscience and religion, some scientists search for neural correlations with spiritual phenomena, that is, they try to find a neuroscience of religious feelings—rather than to explain religious thought scientifically. Amusingly, this alternative strategy, on the part of some members of the Brockman club, to bringing science and religion together excludes Muslims, in particular, for technical reasons, as well as people of other religions who move while praying—because brain-imaging does not function then. In a new research field called "neurotheology," the aim of brain-imaging is to detect religious feelings in the brain, and it is the nonmoving Christians and Buddhists who make perfect research objects while praying or meditating (Newberg et al. 2001, Newberg and Lee 2005, Wallace 2003). Buddhism is especially favored by neuroscientists working on spiritual feelings because it includes the idea of self-transposal and the *no-self*.

Daniel Goleman is particularly engaged in research in this area of neuroscience and Buddhism. Since his time at the University of California, Berkeley, in the United States, Goleman has practiced meditation. He was keen on studying it in Asia, which he was later able to do (in India). Goleman's first book was on meditation, but, compared to *Emotional Intelligence*, it was hardly read. Some of his later books contained interviews with the (XIVth) Dalai Lama. As one of the spiritual leaders of Buddhism, the Dalai Lama is popular both for his religious ideas on peace and his peaceful fight for Tibet's political freedom. One might say he is the icon (in the terms used by Goleman: the purest male EQ type) of an emotionally intelligent leader. Female Buddhist masters are quite rare. Goleman is engaged in the Mind & Life Institute in Boulder, Colorado. The institute's aim is "[t]o establish mutually respectful working collaboration and research partnerships between modern science and Buddhism—two of the world's most fruitful traditions for understanding the nature of reality and promoting human well-being."[18] A series of cross-cultural dialogues on science and Buddhism were established, under the influence of Goleman and the famous neuroscientist and biosemiotician Francisco J. Varela, a Buddhist practitioner since 1974, aiming at some sort of "healing" of society. Varela and the U.S. businessman Adam P. Engle, also a Buddhist, founded the Mind & Life Institute in 1990. Varela envisioned a form of brain research which could understand some spheres of the human mind that are important for meditation, as, for example, emptiness. In the meantime, his vision has "materialized." In contrast to Dennett's book, where transcendence is merged with evolutionary biology, transcendence here becomes the new scientific objective, embodied in meditating brains and emerging in unlimited minds.

This new discourse field of neurotheology leads back to the political dimension of brain research, or, in other words, *neuropolitics*. The social and political conditions which hinder altruism seem to be negligible compared to the potentially huge capacities of the human brain. When Goleman (1995, 34) speaks of EI as being able to "delay gratification" (a diagnostic core symptom of many personality disorders), one is reminded of rhetoric in the Middle Ages by which the Catholic Church kept the masses under control. Goleman links EI very closely to the search for meaning and transcendence, and the promises of "self-healing" and self-redemption add to the attractiveness of EI. Within this established "emotional-spiritual" market, pop science on ubiquitous autistic brains nourishes public fears of possibly being "lost" also in the transcendental sense.

12.4.3   The End: Existential Feelings under Neuroscientific Scrutiny

Neurotheology is an important new focus for pop science due to its transcendental premises and implications, which remain blind spots in classical neuroresearch. Now we come full circle to thoughts on essence and existence, and the idea of oneself as another, at the beginning of this chapter. In a way, when modeling the world and the "I," neuroscience had to arrive at neurotheology if the modeling was to be consequent. However, this poses an old question of ontology again: What is being? Being itself (Latin: *esse*) exceeds explanatory contexts of science and resides in the sphere of metaphysics (Heidegger 1929). Both ontic categories, essence and existence, are challenged by the idea of essential differences in the idea of the human being, when this idea is discussed within the context of contemporary cognitive neurosciences, as their ontology is based upon the idea that the brain is the essence of the human being, shaping and carrying the all-inclusive category "embodied mind." Because the world, in the cognitive science approach, is also regarded as an all-inclusive category of kinds of entities and properties, individual (and cultural) differences in perceiving the world are left behind.

There is a difference between having a world and being in it (Heidegger 2005, 229–231). The latter is also known as *conditio humana* (Plessner 1968, 143). It is ontologically determined by the eccentricity and elusiveness of the human being and by an existential gap which relates to the public importance of nonknowledge. Only when the idea of *what the human is* (essence) is not fixed and systemized can the human be sure *that* she or he is (existence). This implies the ability to be self-distant, that is, to continuously reflect on one's own position in the world and to *thereby* make the world. "World" will thus be a category as open as the mind of the human being is, his or her *Weltoffenheit*. Therefore, the task of the human being is a self-task, to find out what it means to be human. In other words, the human is a task unto the human himself or herself, who still has to face the important (Middle Ages) question of the *homo duplex* (i.e., why was the human being created in the form of two sexes, or why do we assume that there *is* something like this divide in being human).[19]

Of course, if a being's essence is reduced to the mental construction of its systems, then the systemizing capacity of "the male brain" is what living beings (also seen as systems) primarily need, and empathizing is just a nice addition, primarily relevant for reproduction (seen both economically and biologically). This popular view, as we have seen, involves a confusion of categories and a reduction of the existential relations between "being," "I," and "world": Male brains are relevant for maintaining the proposed high-functional individual (prototype of the *ideal* of "human"), and female brains are needed for maintaining the human species (prototype of the *idea* of "human"). Society, then, is modeled on a social-Darwinistic environment, in which the functions' ends are already determined.

Once emotions are no longer mediators between the "I" and the world, and thought is embodied in the mind, that is, if the temporal process of instantiating the relation between selfhood and mineness is regarded as irrelevant, the question crops up as to whether this implies a special kind of biological holism, or social holism, or possibly both. Most likely, it implies both and is reminiscent of a functionalist and objectivist version of the ancient microcosm/macrocosm analogy.

Martin Heidegger (1929) suggested that the constituency of a human being is characterized by an existential gap between two metaphysical poles: *Anxiety* and *Nothing*. Though it might seem counterintuitive, this concept genuinely does refer to the human as a practitioner or a technician in the broadest sense, a being who exceeds both the sphere of nature's boundaries and, occasionally, the anxiety that there might be nothing which manifests his or her own existence, while at the same time being assured of the own existence through attaining intentionality and agency. In this view, emotions are existential for being human. In contrast: The categories of cognition and behavior in the cognitive neurosciences simply refer to the concept that there is a world, not that one is *in* it, and this touches the shaping of emotions within the related scientific ontologies. Anxiety is narrowed and reduced to fear, and one of its indicators, pain; and the idea of Nothing is replaced by a static world that is empirical.

Probably there is a lot to learn from autists regarding the transcendental sphere of being human if science would ask the relevant questions and turn unknown unknowns, at least, into known unknowns. For instance, I would like to know how autists feel anxiety and how they imagine their own death. Not only autists, but also nonautists have limits in creating, and thus, understanding metaphors. In fact, the mechanisms of pop science make strategic use of this existential incompetence when they help to imagine "totalities" and "beyonds." Philosopher Hans Blumenberg (1997, 50), who worked intensively on the existential role of metaphors, pointed out that "the own world" has no name which we explicitly refer to as being our own. We also do not have a name for our own death, which we normally expect to happen but still cannot experience in advance.

It is Anxiety (German: *Angst*) related to Nothing (German: *Nichts*) which the individual has to face in his or her own existence. Angst and individual world constitution belong inseparably together and make the human being a being on the edge of immanence and transcendence, opposed to the idea that the world is an external and internal system. The phrase "German angst" has often been employed, particularly regarding the cliché of the economic risk aversion of German entrepreneurs, without knowing what this phrase really means in philosophical terms. In phenomenology, angst is the emotion that, while feeling unpleasant, enables humans to take the risk of leading their own life, of making decisions according to ends rather than avoiding decisions altogether. However, the phenomenon of angst resists biological scrutiny. At the same time, the concept of pop science benefits from existential feelings deriving from angst.

Thus, after uncountable neuroimaging studies of different versions of pain (financial, physical, psychical, social; see the Introduction to this book) have been carried out, that is, studies which were at least trying to indicate neural processes related to fear (still not angst), *Angst*'s existential other is now under scrutiny in Neurotheology. At last, neuroscientists want to have a representation of *Nothing*.

Acknowledgments

I want to thank my friend and co-editor Gotlind Ulshöfer for making valuable comments on the final version of this chapter. Anne C. Krendl was very helpful in supplying important literature, and Stephen L. Starck took care of the final English version. Last but not least, I would like to dedicate this chapter to transgender diseur/chansonette Georgette Dee, whose music and philosophical lyrics inspired my academic life, and particularly my work on this project.

Filmography

A Beautiful Mind. United States, 2001. Director: Ron Howard. Writer: Akiva Goldsman. Starring: Jennifer Connelly (Alicia Larde), Russell Crowe (John F. Nash), Ed Harris (William Parcher). Universal Studios and Dreamwork.
As Good as It Gets. United States, 1997. Director: James L. Brooks. Writer: Markus Andrus. Starring: Helen Hunt (Carol Connelly), Jack Nicholson (Melvin Udall), Greg Kinnear (Simon Bishop). Sony Pictures.

Backstreet Dreams. United States, 1990. Director: Rupert Hitzig. Writer: Jason O'Malley. Starring: Joseph Viezzi (Shane Costello), Brooke Shields (Stephanie Bloom), Anthony Franciosa (Angelo), Jason O'Malley (Dean Costello). Vidmark Entertainment.

Boy Who Could Fly. United States, 1986. Director: Nick Castle. Writer: Nick Castle. Starring: Lucy Deakins (Milly Michaelson), Jay Underwood (Eric Gibb). 20th Century Fox Studios.

L'Enfant Sauvage. France, 1969. Director: François Truffaut. Writers (screenplay): François Truffaut and Jean Gruault. Starring: François Truffaut (Dr. Jean Itard), Jean Dasté (Professor Philippe Pinel), Jean-Pierre Cargol (Victor, l'enfant sauvage). United Artists.

Invasion of the Body Snatchers. United States, 1956. Director: Don Siegel. Writers: Jack Finney and Daniel Mainwaring. Starring: Kevin McCarthy (Dr. Miles Bennel), Dana Wynter (Becky Driscoll), Larry Gates (Dr. Dan Kauffman). Allied Artists Pictures Corporation.

Invasion of the Body Snatchers. United States, 1978. Director: Philip Kaufman. Writers: Jack Finney and W. D. Richter. Starring: Donald Sutherland (Matthew Bennell), Brooke Adams (Elizabeth Driscoll), Leonard Nimoy (Dr. David Kibner). United Artists.

Little Man Tate. United States, 1991. Director: Jodie Foster. Writer: Scott Frank. Starring: Jodie Foster (Dede Tate), Dianne Wiest (Jane Grierson), Adam Hann-Byrd (Fred Tate). Orion Pictures Corporation.

Mercury Rising. United States, 1998. Based on the novel *Simple Simon* by Ryne Douglas Pearson. Director: Harold Becker. Writers: Lawrence Konner and Marc Rosenthal. Starring: Bruce Willis (Art Jeffries), Alec Baldwin (Lt. Colonel Nicolas Kudrow), Miko Hughes (Simon), Kim Dickens (Stacey). Universal Pictures.

Molly. United States, 1999. Director: John Duigan. Writer: Dick Christie. Starring: Elizabeth Shue (Molly), Aaron Eckhart (Buck McKay), Jill Hennessy (Susan Brookes). Metro-Goldwyn-Mayer.

Mozart and the Whale. United States, 2005. Director: Peter Naess. Writer: Ronald Bass. Starring: Radha Mitchell (Isabel Sorenson), Josh Hartnett (Donald Morton). Equity Pictures Mediafonds/Robert Lawrence Production.

Nell. United States, 1994. Based on the drama *Idioglossia* by Mark Handley. Director: Michael Apted. Writer: William Nicholson. Starring: Jodie Foster (Nell Kellty), Liam Neeson (Dr. Jerome Lovell). 20th Century Fox.

One Flew over the Cuckoo's Nest. United States, 1975. Based on the novel by Ken Kesey. Director: Miloš Forman. Writers (screenplay): Lawrence Hauben and Bo Goldman. Starring: Jack Nicholson (Randle Patrick McMurphy), Louise Fletcher (Nurse Mildred Ratched), Will Sampson (Chief Bromden). United Artists.

Rain Man. United States, 1988. Director: Berry Levinson. Writers (screenplay): Ronald Bass and Barry Morrow. Starring: Tom Cruise (Charlie Babbitt), Dustin Hoffman (Raymond Babbitt). United Artists.

Snow Cake. United Kingdom, 2006. Director: Marc Evans. Writer: Angela Pell. Starring: Alan Rickman (Alex Hughes), Sigourney Weaver (Linda Freeman). Revolution Films.

The Wizard. United States, 1989. Director: Todd Holland. Writer: David Chisholm. Starring: Luke Edward (Jimmy Woods/The Wizard), Fred Savage (Corey Woods), Beau Bridges (Sam Woods), Christian Slater (Nick Woods), Wendy Philips (Christine Bateman). Universal Pictures.

Notes

1. Autism belongs to the diagnostic category of the pervasive developmental disorders (PDDs), together with Asperger's syndrome (and three others). Baron-Cohen points out that "[a]bnormalities in understanding other minds is not the only cognitive feature of autism spectrum disorders—two other prominent ones being weak central coherence and executive dysfunction," though "it seems to be a core and possibly universal abnormality among such individuals" (Baron-Cohen 2000, 3).

2. Stefan Helmreich (2007) stressed this point for Alife research, in the scientific culture tradition of the brain in the tank.

3. Thiomersal (also known as thimerosal) is an organomercury compound used as an antiseptic agent in vaccinations since 1931. Because of its high mercury content, it is vehemently debated whether it is neurotoxic when given children under the age of 6. Proponents of causal links between child vaccinations including the preservative thiomersal and the increased occurrence of PDDs (and attention-deficit/hyperactivity disorder, ADHD) use control groups like children in Amish communities in the United States (who are not vaccinated and have lower rates of autism) or children from European countries like Denmark or Germany, where thiomersal was used in lower concentrations in the vaccine during the 1990s (Mutter et al. 2005), and where the epidemiological rate of child autism is lower (although, since the 1980s, it has also increased there, but less so than in the United States). Up to now, the European Union has not had robust data for providing figures on the prevalence of the autistic spectrum disorders among its members, due to, for example, different definitions of autism used in different countries. See http://ec. europa.eu/health/ph_information/dissemination/diseases/autism_1.pdf (accessed 27 July 2007). M. F. Blaxill (2004), among others, pointed out that the argument of a diagnostic substitute can not be established as a factor in the increased rate of autism. Starting in 1999, the U.S. Food and Drug Administration (FDA) continuously has licensed new pediatric formulations for vaccines, first in vaccines against hepatitis B. According to the FDA, at present all routine vaccinations to U.S. infants are thimerosal-free (except inactivated influenza vaccine) (see U.S. Food and Drug Administration, Center for Biologics Evaluation and Research: Thimerosal in Vaccines. http://www.fda.gov/cber/vaccine/thimerosal.htm#intro; accessed 28 July, 2007). A new study conducted by the State Public Health Department (CA), published in January 2008, reports California's autism rate rises despite vaccine change ("Study Finds Vaccine Preservative Is not Linked to Risks of Autism." *The New York Times*, 8 Jan. 2008. http://www.nytimes.com/2008/01/

08/health/08autism.html, accessed 2 February, 2008). However, for example, in Argentina, the old vaccines are still used, and in many African countries the thimerosal-containing vaccines are recommended by the World Health Organization.

4. http://en.wikipedia.org/wiki/People_speculated_to_have_been_autistic (accessed September 4, 2007).

5. In the original: "Denn auch die Soziologie, die vom Verhalten der Menschen in der Gesellschaft handelt, kann nichts anderes sein als angewandte Psychologie. Streng genommen gibt es ja nur zwei Wissenschaften, Psychologie, reine und angewandte, und Naturkunde" (Freud 1999, volume 15, 194).

6. Sometimes feminalists are incorrectly labeled "new feminists."

7. One statement on Baron-Cohen's autism spectrum quotient (AQ) test is: "I enjoy doing things spontaneously" (No. 34; Baron-Cohen 2004, 212). If you disagree, this increases your chances of falling into a category in the autistic spectrum.

8. This lexical approach was already in use in the 1930s (Allport and Odbert 1936).

9. http://www.psypress.com/socialneuroscience/aims.asp (accessed July 22, 2007).

10. Goleman himself personifies this winning strategy of becoming successful with the help of emotions and an upper-middle-class background, as a brief glance at his personal home page shows (http://www.danielgoleman.info; accessed June 26, 2006).

11. http://www.edge.org/about_edge.html (accessed November 4, 2006).

12. http://www.edge.org/about_edge.html (accessed November 4, 2006).

13. For the German debate on Brockman's reality issues' infecting the European feuilletons, see the article "Der Geist zu Geld macht" by Jochen Wegner, FOCUS No. 41, 8 Oct. 2001.

14. If you have a very strong stomach, you can also read the response "Men, Women, and the Talk Show Effect" by the neurobiologist and psychologist Robert Provine (Edge 26, Oct. 6, 1997).

15. http://www.edge.org/3rd_culture/debate05/debate05_index.html (accessed November 4, 2006).

16. http://www.edge.org/about_edge.html (accessed November 4, 2006).

17. Academics engaged in political philosophy cannot discard pluralism as easily as neurophilosophers, because they have to deal with the real-world issues of injustice, war, and violations of human rights, which is why they are currently debating how the idea of a nationally constructed self can be overcome, if only for the sake of an intercultural dialogue. For instance, a national self could be overcome with the idea of cosmopolitic virtues, as the Chicago-based philosopher Jason Hill recently argued (Hill 2000). Rather than focusing on static cultures, societies, and nations with fixed identities, Hill's understanding of cosmopolitic virtues is based on the humanist idea that every human being shares a common ground of both rationality and

emotionality, enabling her or him to socialize. Society is then addressed as a process, not an entity. Consequently, cultural identities are fluid, but this fluidity corresponds to the socialization process of the self and thus remains consistent. There is much to learn from this argument for neuro- and cognitive sciences.

18. http://www.mindandlife.org/mission.org_section.html (accessed September 15, 2007).

19. "Miteingeschlossen in diese Harmonie ist . . .—und das ist das Einzigartige des Lebewesens Mensch—ihre Durchbrechung, womit wir das Vermögen des Menschen meinen, von sich Abstand nehmen zu können, seine Weltoffenheit, seine Exzentrizität" (Plessner 1968, 143).

13 Social Emotions and Brain Research: From Neurophilosophy to a Neurosociology of Law

Malte-Christian Gruber

13.1 Introduction

From a neuroscientific point of view, we are living in the age of the brain, and, at the same time, this also seems to be the dawning of the era of emotions. Though this popular characterization mainly refers to recent developments in the area of the life sciences, it nevertheless embraces the humanities: morals, politics, law, and, finally, social life in general.

In the following essay, I will examine recent developments in neuroscientific research with regard to affective or emotional aspects of the individual and social life. In this respect, neurophilosophers like Antonio Damasio emphasize the close relationship between emotions and social capacities. They want to show that *social cognition* has a neural basis, evolutionary developed over time from early forms of affective self-evaluations. Even though they might originate from the nonrational and nonhuman living, self-referential emotions appear to provide a rudimentary basis for both high-level self-representations and human social competencies.

In this respect, it can be considered a remarkable sign of progress that the "irrational"—that is, those kinds of minds, thoughts, ideas, and actions that cannot be completely understood by means of modern rationality—may no longer be isolated as extraneous and, so to speak, as a nonhuman part of different human beings but instead will become a subject of rational consideration. Actually, with the recovery of the concept of "emotion," modern people have built a rational bridge to the world of irrationality. Even so, they still do not immediately understand irrational behavior. However, they create indirect access to the irrational by searching for functional explanations. Different behavior, then, is no longer seen as incomprehensible, especially when it appears socially successful. Moreover, deviant behavior is becoming less objectionable morally. From now on, almost every kind of extraordinary behavior is merely supposed to form part of an "irrational" or "emotional" act of volition. As such, it ought to be principally explicable on the basis of rational methods. Emotions and their mental counterparts—referred to as "feelings"—therefore are ascribed to fulfill cognitive functions and to subserve consciousness. Both of them are based on the well-known dichotomy of subject and object. In short, they comprise an element in the mind–body problem.

In addition, this step could include a critical presupposition: Rational explanations of emotions and feelings strongly depend on the preceding definitions of what it means to experience such mental states. This remains one of the fundamental challenges of neurophilosophy. However, neurophilosophy may also generate popular concepts of emotionality. In 1995, Daniel Goleman, with his well-known book *Emotional Intelligence*, who led such popular interpretations of neurophilosophy into the mentioned age of emotions, wrote as follows:

The emotions, then, matter for rationality. In the dance of feeling and thought the emotional faculty guides our moment-to-moment decisions, working hand-in-hand with the rational mind, enabling—or disabling—thought itself. Likewise, the thinking brain plays an executive role in our emotions—except in those moments when emotions surge out of control and the emotional brain runs rampant. In a sense we have two brains, two minds—and two different kinds of intelligence: rational and emotional. How we do in life is determined by both—it is not just IQ, but *emotional* intelligence that matters. Indeed, intellect cannot work at its best without emotional intelligence. Ordinarily the complementarity of limbic system and neocortex, amygdala and prefrontal lobes, means each is a full partner in mental life. When these partners interact well, emotional intelligence rises—as does intellectual ability (Goleman 1996, 28).

As striking as Goleman's analysis of emotional relevance seems to be, it is actually the special vocabulary of physical and mental states, with their abilities to possess intelligence, to control decision making, to think purposively, or to act in a target-oriented fashion, which should be given attention. When parts of bodies and brains are associated with those particular abilities that usually only human persons are supposed to possess—that is, when the brain is imagined as some form of an actor, in short, when it is personified, this has anthropological consequences. Then, strictly speaking, it is no longer human beings by themselves who are planning and initiating their actions. Instead, it is their brain "who" is *acting* as a (partly) personal entity, solely determined by physical mechanisms, and—as might be expected—excluding any form of mental interference with the so-called free will.

13.2 Between the Biology and a Sociology of Emotions

While Goleman told his story about acting brains, there were exceptional authors who attempted to give a deliberate account of emotions and feelings and what it means to be in or to experience these mental states. One of these authors, Antonio Damasio, developed his insights into the affective aspects of human living and made them clear for a broader audience in his three famous books: *Descartes' Error* (1994), *The Feeling of What Happens* (1999), and *Looking for Spinoza* (2003).

What is new about such neuroscientifically inspired theories of emotion? In the first place, their source material offers further empirical information: Their study of emotions and feelings is no longer limited to the well-known aspects of scientific findings, the combination of theory, observation of behavior, and subjective experience. Instead, neurophilosophers like Damasio are searching for additional technological access, based on the material substrates of the affective aspects of human as well as nonhuman living. This interest explains why human beings are not the only objects of neuroscientific research. Neuroscientists, therefore, are not interested solely in human brains of "normal" persons nor in patients with lesions in certain neural areas. They also utilize nonhuman animals in their experiments. In contrast, though, they rarely distinguish between matters of sex and gender (Wild, Erb, and Bartels 2001, 109ff; Singer et al. 2006, 466ff; see also Brizendine 2006).

What many neuroscientists have in common, however, is the increasing application of techniques of neuroimaging, which has recently branched out into so-called functional brain imaging (see Hüsing, this volume). Since then, so it seems, there have been many new developments in the field of neuroscientific research: Insights into the human brain, including its affective basis, have even influenced many different fields of research, such as artificial intelligence (AI), robotics (e.g., Chrisley 1995, 141ff, Holland and Goodman 2003, 77ff), and—recently from a more sociological point of view—socionics (Fischer, Florian, and Malsch 2005; see also Fellous and Arbib 2005). Today, the idea seems to have become commonly accepted that artificial, autonomous agents cannot merely stick to the increasing efforts to implement a barely logical calculus but rather must be extended to a development of "simulated emotions" and "self-motivational tools." The objectives of all these advances in AI are the construction of future robots and electronic agents as affective systems with "emotion-inspired mechanisms." Henceforth, these artifacts should be able to act under the contingent conditions of human environments, and even more: They should learn to interact with human beings in a sociable way (Breazeal and Brooks 2005, 271ff).

However, most attention remains focused on the neuroscientific view of emotions and the feelings of living beings, placing emphasis on human concerns. As a consequence, special fields of research have recently been established, especially the disciplines of affective neuroscience (Panksepp 1998) and social neuroscience (Cacioppo 2002, Cacioppo and Berntson 2004; see also Adolphs 2003, 165f). Both of these fields are focused on crossing the boundaries of the neural substrates of an individual by extending their research focus to the social correlates of mental processing and interactions between humans.

All these efforts originate from authors such as Damasio—authors who, in the presence of striking neuroscientific phenomena, are working on emotions, feelings, and their role in social context, based on a former philosophy of emotion (Spinoza). As one might expect, Damasio's concept of emotions and feelings could have remarkable consequences for our treatment of mental and social issues. In his own words, "elucidating the neurobiology of feelings and their antecedent emotions contributes to our views on the mind–body problem." He argues that "emotions and related reactions are aligned with the body, feelings with the mind" (Damasio 2003, 7).

Referring to Spinoza, Damasio draws a distinction between (1) the "process of feeling" and (2) the "process of having an idea about an object that can cause an emotion" (Damasio 2003, 11). Damasio's word choice is problematic, because process (1) is not yet identical to a genuine feeling by itself. It primarily denotes a bodily emotion. Beyond those kinds of bodily processing, process (2) stems from another basis to get initiated: In order to develop a "real" feeling, one has to form an "idea," that is, a mental representation of what an object means to her. In short, Damasio holds that (bodily) emotions precede feelings as mental representations of emotionally relevant phenomena. They do so in two ways—first, as described above, in consideration of a current bodily or mental processing of an individual organism, and second, with regard to evolutionary approaches: They are antecedent to feelings even from an ontogenetic as well as from a phylogenetic perspective. To make these assumptions clear, Damasio uses the image of a branched tree (Damasio 2003, 29ff).

This tree, as if it were some sort of an *emotional* tree, bears several levels of automated mechanisms for life regulation. All of them—from basic reflexes and metabolic regulation to full-fledged emotions and feelings—are, as Damasio suggests, "built from simple reactions that easily promote the survival of an organism and thus could easily prevail in evolution" (Damasio 2003, 30). More precisely, Damasio refers to the entire ensemble of these life-serving devices as *homeostasis* (Damasio 2003, 30). In this context, however, "life-serving" does not simply mean "useful for survival." It also embraces "a better than neutral life state," such as "wellness" or "*well-being*" (Damasio 2003, 35).

Taken as a whole, emotions and feelings seem to be closely related to the lower "branches" of homeostatic regulation, to emotions in the broadest sense—to "drives and motivations," to "pain and pleasure behaviors," to "immune responses," to "basic reflexes," and to "metabolic regulation" as well. Near the treetop, Damasio finally locates all the rest of the emotions in the narrow sense of the term, that is to say, "emotions-proper," such as "joy," "sorrow," "fear," "pride," "shame," and "sympathy" (Damasio 2003, 34). Above these emotions, at the very top of Damasio's tree, there are only those mental states which represent all the aforementioned lower levels of homeostatic regulation: Feelings come into being when information about the life process is represented in certain "maps" generated by certain circuits of nerve cells in the brain. They are somehow part of what other authors would call a *self-representation* or a *self-model* (Metzinger 2004, 299). As a consequence, Damasio defines "feelings" as "*the idea of the body being in a certain way*" (Damasio 2003, 85).

The Damasian emotional being, after all, seems to react rather than to respond: "Even the emotions-proper," he writes, ". . . aim directly at life regulation by staving off dangers or helping the organism take advantage of an opportunity, or indirectly by facilitating social relations" (Damasio 2003, 39).

Damasio points out that the success of an emotion depends in large part on "context" as well as on "current human circumstances." From this it obviously follows that—at least in human concerns—life has more meaningful aspects than the aim of bare survival. Of course, biological existence and physical well-being remain necessary, but they are accompanied by another important aspect: the interest in survival within human society. *Social survival* requires more than regulatory reactions; it also demands responses. Although Damasio seems to realize this further aspect, invoking both the "biology of emotions and the fact that the value of each emotion differs so much in our current human environment" (Damasio 2003, 40), he does not give precise criteria for an understanding of human behavior with all its complex facets of mind, sociality, and culture (see Reddy, this volume). Apparently, Damasio faces a completely new issue which exceeds all those evolutionary questions of biological mechanisms and survival, the so-called "biology of emotions," and comes up with the *sociology of emotions*: "I am thinking, for example, that reactions that lead to racial and cultural prejudices are based in part on the automatic deployment of social emotions evolutionarily meant to detect difference in others because difference may signal risk or danger, and promote withdrawal or aggression" (Damasio 2003, 40).

Damasio interprets *social emotions* in evolutionary terms, that is, as formerly useful mechanisms in tribal societies which, nowadays, may be considered socially inappropriate reactions to otherness, to difference, and to uncertainty. At last, he obviously obeys his intuition when he appeals for disregard of such reactions (Damasio 2003, 40).

In another respect, *social emotions* are of a similar type as all those aforementioned abilities which Goleman has in mind. They also seem to be essential for social success and to provide a basis for *emotional intelligence*. By contrast, the absence of an inner experience of emotions would lead to social isolation or *autistic aloneness* (Frith 2003, 98ff; see also Karafyllis, this volume).

Now, Damasio tells us that *social emotions* such as "sympathy, embarrassment, shame, guilt, pride, jealousy, envy, gratitude, admiration, indignation, and contempt" are not confined to humans. Even nonhuman beings are capable of being socially emotive (Damasio 2003, 45f). However, if Damasio is right, should we then picture the emotional being as an emotional (nonhuman) animal rather than as a tree?

13.3   Emotions, Animals, and Self-Consciousness

One may find oneself immediately recalling an article from Konrad Lorenz with a catchy title: "Tiere sind Gefühlsmenschen"—"animals are emotional people" (Lorenz

1980, 251; my translation). In support of this hunch, Damasio enumerates several indices for the specific socioemotional competence of various nonhuman species, such as "the proud ambulations of a dominant monkey; the literally regal deportment of a dominant great ape or wolf that commands the respect of the group; the humiliated behavior of the animal that does not dominate and must yield space and precedence at mealtimes; the sympathy an elephant shows toward another that is injured and ailing; or the embarrassment the dog shows after doing what he should not" (Damasio 2003, 46).

Although they might certainly entail describing animal behavior in an anthropomorphic way, these examples nevertheless appear to be plausible indices for socially relevant emotional capabilities in nonhuman animals, particularly in mammals. Communication abilities especially—the tactile and visual as well as olfactory signals of many animal species (Zeller 1987, 433ff), the grunts of vervet monkeys (Cheney and Seyfarth 1982, 739ff; 1988, 477ff), the language trained in the well-known ape-language projects (Gardner and Gardner 1969, 664ff; 1975, 752f; Premack 1971, 808ff; Savage-Rumbaugh et al. 1993; for an overview, see Seyfarth 1987, 440ff; Radner and Radner 1989, 149ff; for ethical and legal consequences of communication abilities, see Gruber 2006, 75ff, 128ff)—demonstrate that communication in a rudimentary sense—at least in its nonverbal, emotional shape—is not unique to humans. Applying emotional communication to a social context, using nonverbal expressions for instrumental purposes, reporting inner representations and mental states—even nonhumans do it. However, this behavior is precisely what people tend to call emotionally intelligent behavior. In fact, nonverbal communication appears to be a precondition for emotionally intelligent behavior and for social intelligence. It obviously serves as a basis for the ability to detect other individuals' intentions and to deceive them by means of miming, gestures, and nonverbal utterances, and, as Damasio argues, it is a way of displaying *social dominance and dependence* (Damasio 2003, 48). Here, evolutionary theorists would emphasize the role of emotionally intelligent behavior for (social) problem solving and, in brief, they would interpret it as synonymous with "Machiavellian intelligence" (Byrne and Whiten 1988; Whiten and Byrne 1997). According to this view, emotionally intelligent individuals are "natural psychologists" who have some sort of an "inner eye" (Humphrey 2002, 32, 65ff). This might also serve as a basis for consciousness: "By consciousness I mean the inner picture we each have of what it is like to be ourselves—self-awareness: the presence in each of us of a spirit, (self, soul . . .) which we call 'I.' It's 'I' who have thoughts and feelings, sensations, memories, desires. It's 'I' who am conscious of my own existence and my continuity in time. 'I' who am, in short, the very essence of a human being" (Humphrey 2002, 52).

In neuroscientific terms, as an ability to read the minds of others, emotional intelligence means to form a *theory of mind*, referring to the capacity of constructing a meta-representation of the mental states of another individual. With regard to the neural processes underlying the ability to see through other minds, some social neuroscientists assume that this kind of emotional intelligence originally is based upon *implicit* self-involvement in contingent situations, but it also relies on *explicit* meta-representations of mental states (Frith and Frith 2003, 459ff). Others hold that a single *mentalizing system* implicitly enables humans to imitate and to feel being imitated as well as to create a representation of both self and other minds (Gopnik and Meltzoff 1994, 166ff; Meltzoff and Decety 2003, 491ff). Since imitation and its neural correlates—*mirror neurons*—are therefore supposed to be an essential part of emotional and social intelligence, at first glance many species may seem to fulfill these requirements formerly believed to be limited to humans (Premack and Woodruff 1978, 515ff).

However, several studies draw a distinction between the human ability for genuine imitation and all the rest of (nonhuman) reproducing behavior (e.g., Tomasello 1990, 274ff; see also Meltzoff and Decety 2003, 491ff). In this sense, imitation relies on the capacity to construct a mental model, which is crucial for learning behavior. Imitating individuals, therefore, do not require any immediate stimulus for learning. Instead, they learn from their mental representations.

Nevertheless, animals might partly appear to be *emotional persons* (for an overview of research on animal emotion, see Paul, Harding, and Mendl 2005, 469ff). But should we then define humans likewise as some sort of *emotional animals* (*locus classicus*; Darwin 1872/1998; see also Nussbaum 2001/2003, 89ff)? Or is there an alternative criterion for human personality, some peculiarity which is beyond the mere instrumental ability of social intelligence? In other words: Does a more complex human capacity for mentalizing exist, assisting more than simple deception and cheating, dedicated to another end beyond mere survival?

This appears to be the reason why many studies prefer young children to nonhumans as test objects (e.g., Meltzoff 1996, 347ff; Frith and Frith 2003, 459ff): They obviously intend to find qualitative differences between humans and nonhuman animals, as well as to explore the thresholds in between. And in the long run, they apparently succeed: They discover specific differences between humans and nonhumans, and, moreover, they detect neural differences between human children and adults (Kobayashi, Glover, and Temple 2007, 1522ff). By contrast, studies of gender-related differences are still rare (for a rare counterexample, see Wild, Erb, and Bartels 2001, 109ff; see also Singer et al. 2006, 466ff). Neuroscientists seem to presume that there are no relevant discrepancies, while their work is usually bound to a limited number of test persons who display the same characteristics: They are in the same age group, they are of the same gender, and they all use the same hand. However, in any case, they could still find differences in the level of neural activation at most. Is that difference important? Is there a risk of political incorrectness? Even monkeys' brains have mirror neurons, even though they lack a theory of mind or a capacity for genuine imitation. Thus, on a neural level, they are similar to humans. However, the question remains whether they are similar to humans in other respects.

Perhaps we should take a step forward and assume that emotions are more than evolutionary mechanisms for survival. Here, Damasio's concept, mentioned above, of *feeling* as "*the idea of the body being in a certain way*" (Damasio 2003, 85) could be of some help. What Damasio has in mind is a sort of ontological self-representation or self-mapping of bodily states. Many philosophers, however, refer to other conceptualizing metaphors: An *idea* or a *thought*, for example, is also interpreted as "a mental state with a specifiable content" (Davidson 1989, 193), alternatively as "inner speech" (for a famous example, see Plato 1961, *Theaetetus*, 189e–190a; *Sophist*, 263d), or—as mentioned above—as an "inner picture" (Humphrey 2002, 52; from a neuroscientific view, see Kosslyn 1994).

All these concepts have in common that they are essential elements of cognitive consciousness, generally better known as *thinking*. Strictly speaking, *thinking* goes beyond the scope of imagining or having something in mind. Moreover, *thinking subjects* have the ability to take part in determining the content of their mental states. For this reason, *thinking subjects* are capable of disengaging themselves from the contingencies of the environment, likewise getting rid of temporal modi. In its relation to the past, *thinking* means what we used to characterize as *remembrance*. Regarding the future, it is usually called *anticipation*. Both memory and anticipation are elements of human consciousness and, thus, form part of a full-fledged personality by constituting mental continuity. That is one of the origins of autonomy: Pushing the boundaries of passive *reactions*, autonomous human persons are actively searching for *responses* (Cassirer 1944/1972, 27ff). At this stage, they construct and impart novel contents (or images) within their mental spheres. Finally, they are even capable of constituting a mental *self-representation*, in particular—referring to Thomas Metzinger (2004) and others—a *phenomenal self-model* as a pivotal fundament of self-consciousness (Ricœur 1992).

All of these newly created mental representations can only be understood by symbolic intelligent individuals who, in addition, require a certain motivation to comprehend their meaning. This leads to another affective aspect of consciousness: *emotional intelligence* as motivation to create sense.

13.4   Neurosociology: Emotions as Elements of the Social and Legal World

With the discovery of the motivational aspects of symbolic intelligence, we likewise come into reach of a higher level of *emotional intelligence* which notably relates to the social interactions of humans. Survival, well-being, and homeostasis are now of less importance—rather, when we think about emotional intelligence, we should attend to the symbolic intelligent being, the Cassirerian "animal symbolicum" (Cassirer 1944/1972), that is, the proper *emotional human person*. From this it follows that emotions are not—as Damasio says—"beautiful and amazingly intelligent" by themselves (Damasio 2003, 54), instead, the focus is on their carriers. Damasio touches on this matter by considering the "neurobiological wisdom" of the brain as well as humans' abilities to control their emotions and, thus, the life process in general by maintaining a self: "When the consequences of such natural wisdom are mapped back in the central nervous system, . . . the result is feelings, the foundational component of our minds" (Damasio 2003, 79). "Feelings," Damasio writes, "can guide a deliberate endeavor of self-preservation and assist with making choices regarding the manner in which self-preservation should take place." From his point of view, they "open the door for some measure of willful control of the automated emotions" (Damasio 2003, 79f).

Damasio surely knows that his discussion of the "natural intelligence" of emotions is just metaphoric. He also recognizes that human beings at least partly have a free will, enabling them to control emotions and life processes. Furthermore, he sees clearly that humans are capable of modulating the execution of emotions in order to adapt to individual circumstances, particularly the social context (Damasio 2003, 56). However—and this is the crucial point—he seems to overemphasize the "natural" objective of survival.

Even though Damasio must concede that many human emotions are by no means "useful," he adheres to the single principle of self-preservation: Somewhere along the way, from an objective point of view, each of those useless emotions must have been advantageous. Taking this view, Damasio runs the risk of neglecting the role of affective processing in other respects, for example, in cultural terms, in relation to unconscious imagination, and particularly regarding generation or regeneration of self-esteem (Benecke and Dammann 2003, 147).

Self-esteem means an individual's subjective appraisal of herself or himself in the broadest sense, and that is the reason why it is different from self-preservation in barely biological terms. Rather, it is considerably influenced by both social and cultural circumstances. The feeling of self-worth arises from an emotionally based, biographically developed, and mentally fixed self-representation which can only be understood on the grounds of a meaningfully constituted social and cultural context. The emotional experience of an individual, therefore, does not depend solely on the biological configuration. Moreover, since people are subjected to the surrounding society and culture, the phenomenal perspective of individuals constantly evolves in connection with a common *emotional knowledge* within a certain collective (Deighton and Traue 2003, 240ff). Although this affective kind of knowledge is essential for social life, certain group- and gender-specific elements—particularly the knowledge of women— are left out of many areas of the economy and science, especially of neuro- and information technologies (Adam 1998). Therefore, these participants of a collective emotionality are permanently underrepresented in highly regarded social and professional sectors.

With regard to the emergence of various circles of such a kind of collective emotionality, it now seems plausible to suggest that the existing multiplicity of different collective identities has its seeds in different emotional communities. For this reason, collective identity is not simply a matter of living within a certain cultural context, it also derives from social affiliation to subgroups which sometimes may be subordinate and disrespected, sometimes dominant or elitist, and seemingly always dependent on sex, gender, and their corresponding role attribution in society. Indeed, self-preservation is a striking incentive for social action and decision making on an individual level (Damasio 2003, 166). However, first and foremost, human beings appear to preserve social systems—in other words, they unwittingly stabilize an existing collective differentiation by acting with intent to gain an individual advantage.

As a matter of fact, women and men play different roles in preserving and stabilizing social systems. Most societies apparently continue to follow the evolutionary principles of variation, selection, transmission—and retention: From a biologist's point of view, women are still primarily expected to fulfill domestic functions. At best, they are allowed to play their biologically defined role of gatherers, but men are still the hunters. However, this does not have to be the way societies are arranged. Despite all seemingly natural differences of sex, gender, and brains, social systems are capable of overcoming traditional roles, ancient attributions, and quasi-tribal structures as well. They regularly do so when they are confronted with changing external expectations from other social actors: Irritated by the social environment, individuals, as well as groups, modify their own concepts of knowledge, rationality, and subjectivity. Under certain circumstances, they might deny the old assumption that human brains are functionally equivalent to ("male") computers. They might, likewise, contradict associations of the rational mind with masculinity and reject biases about the irrational body as a female characteristic (Adam 1998, 99ff). And, as a consequence, they might admit women into formerly "masculine" professions and vice versa (accept men who are doing traditionally "feminine" jobs).

From this point of view, social groups might also be seen as sort of *collective selves* and, under several particular conditions, they might constitute *juridical persons*, embedded in a legally regulated organizational frame (Teubner 1988, 130ff). Such a process of personification is especially caused by a legal characteristic: Responding to the extrinsic expectations which derive from the social environment, law reconstructs individuals and groups as legal persons. Thus, in a legal context, collective selves can play the social role of persons. They are, then, in a sense, collectively neural-based, socially constructed, personified meta-subjects.

The process of personification even applies to individuals, whose legal personality likewise results from communicatory social processes, ascribing legal personhood and rights to different kinds of social systems. In fact, there is no individual self per se—no one with an intrinsic identity. The self is—as mentioned—a *self-model*, in both senses: phenomenally and socially as well. Primarily, identities are constituted by surrounding social systems. Individuals, as well as collectives, gain their subjectivity from social ascriptions based on a socially binding self-model as well as on a cyclical coupling of identity and action attribution (Luhmann 1995, chapter 5 VI; Teubner 2006, 497ff).

At least one blind spot, however, still remains: Focusing on the social role of emotions and on forms of emotional knowledge as well as on individual and collective emotionality, we run the risk of failing to acknowledge that emotions are exceptional internal states in living beings. Although they always mean something to their owners, it sometimes happens to us that we are not willing or even are unable to talk about emotions. From time to time, emotions and feelings are not communicable because of their intimate character. However, the internal aspect of emotions similarly affects the law (Kiesow and Korte 2005). It could explain, for instance, why criminal courts in Germany do not admit lie detectors: In fact, they formerly prohibited lie detectors on the grounds that they violate the personal integrity by delivering insight into the soul (*Bundesgerichtshof BGHSt* 5, 332; for further examples, see Tancredi 2004, 103ff; Greely 2004, 128ff). In another high court decision, polygraph evidence was judged as "completely unsuitable" for answering the question of whether a test person is telling the truth (*BGHSt* 44, 308; for further reference, see Fiedler, Schmid, and Stahl 2002, 313ff).

In some respects, humans seem to require legal protection against technological processes in neuroscience. Although neuroscientific insights into brain differences and (bodily) emotional states might improve patient care and medication, there is a serious risk of abusing insights into the emotional states of individuals in a socially unacceptable manner: Advances in predicting behavior, as well as in detecting neural ab*norm*alities, could jeopardize people's freedom and, based on neuroscientific information, discriminate against them as a kind of "neurological underclass" (Garland 2004, 32ff). On the other hand, there is the question of detecting bias, that is, strong emotional reactions to certain groups (Richeson et al. 2003, 1323ff): These reactions might be evidence of manifest racism or chauvinism. And, finally, in moral as well as in legal discourse, we are forced to decide whether we want to treat all these neuroscientific methods restrictively, or if we—for example—should allow the use of all sorts of cognitive enhancers, knowing for certain that this would mean the achievement of a new standard of social "*norm*ality" and human health.

What does all this mean with respect to debates about elites, sex, gender, and brain? Far from providing an answer to all those open-ended questions—particularly in social as well as cultural respects—neuroscience will continue to need advice from the humanities. Human biographies and collective histories cannot be understood by neuroscientific methods alone. Later on, there will be a need for critical reflection on patterns of social expectations referring to elites and gender. However, it must be conceded that social neuroscience as well as legal neuroscience will have a significant impact on genuine humanities issues which are suitable objects of empirical research. Finally, we can apparently agree with Damasio when he states that "in the absence of social emotions and subsequent feelings, even on the unlikely assumption that other intellectual abilities could remain intact, the cultural instruments we know as ethical behaviors, religious beliefs, laws, justice, and political organization either would not have emerged, or would have been a very different sort of intelligent construction" (Damasio 2003, 159). Of course, Damasio knows that such cultural instruments are based upon "complex autobiographies" as well as upon the process of "extended consciousness" which makes neurobiological explanations difficult. Nevertheless, he believes that someday neurobiology could explain cultural phenomena such as ethics, religion, law, and justice. "But," as Damasio further writes, "in order to comprehend these cultural phenomena satisfactorily we need to factor in ideas from anthropology, sociology, psychoanalysis, and evolutionary psychology, as well as findings from studies in the fields of ethics, law, and religion" (Damasio 2003, 159f).

Taking seriously the Damasian aim of integrated knowledge, neurosciences should pay attention to critical comments and responses from all of these other disciplines.

Assuming sex and gender differences as given, accepting the formation of elites as a fact—in short, taking a current social situation for granted—will no longer suffice. It is a simple truth that *survival of the fittest* bears another meaning than *preference for the most valuable*. Damasio's second principle, the objective of *well-being*, thus should be construed broadly, that is to say, as a *normative* principle. As such, it partly leaves the sphere of neurobiology and touches on both ethical and socioeconomic debates.

Research into individual brains will never displace the search for reasons for social success and disadvantage. Otherwise, this brain research would only become a justification for an already established social status quo. If neuroscientists want to be accurate, they need to bargain for dynamics evolved by a long-lasting historic chain of social interactions of individuals and collectives as well. In particular, they will have to take into account that every mental phenomenon allows for different levels of description, each combined with another explanatory claim. And, finally, they must keep in mind that emotions are identifying social attributes of both individuals and personified collectives.

Acknowledgments

I am in debt to Claudia Scott for her invaluable help. I would also like to thank the editors of this volume for their considerable comments on an earlier version of this chapter.

References

Abbott, Andrew. 1988. *The System of Professions: An Essay on the Division of Expert Labor*. Chicago: University of Chicago Press.

Abu-Lughod, Lila. 1986. *Veiled Sentiments: Honor and Poetry in a Bedouin Society*. Berkeley: University of California Press.

Abu-Lughod, Lila. 1990. Shifting politics in Bedouin love poetry. In *Language and the Politics of Emotion*, ed. Catherine A. Lutz and Lila Abu-Lughod, 24–45. Cambridge: Cambridge University Press.

Acker, Joan. 1989. *Doing Comparable Worth: Gender, Class and Pay Equity*. Philadelphia: Temple University Press.

Acker, Joan. 1990. Hierarchies, jobs, bodies: A theory of gendered organizations. *Gender and Society* 4, no. 2: 139–158.

Acker, Joan. 1998. The future of "gender and organizations": Connections and boundaries. *Gender, Work and Organization* 5, no. 4: 195–206.

Ackerman, Phillip L., Kristie R. Bowen, Margaret E. Beier, and Ruth Kanfer. 2001. Determinants of individual differences and gender differences in knowledge. *Journal of Educational Psychology* 93, no. 4: 797–825.

Adam, Alison. 1998. *Artificial Knowing: Gender and the Thinking Machine*. London and New York: Routledge.

Addison, Joseph. 1713. *Cato: A Tragedy*. London: J. Tonson.

Adolphs, Ralph. 2003. Cognitive neuroscience of human social behaviour. *Nature Reviews Neuroscience* 4, no. 3: 165–178.

Agassi, Joseph, and Nathaniel Laor. 2000. How ignoring repeatability leads to magic. *Philosophy of the Social Sciences* 30: 528–586.

Aharon, Itzhak, Nancy Etcoff, Dan Ariely, Christopher F. Chabris, Ethan Oçonner, and Hans C. Breiter. 2001. Beautiful faces have variable reward value: fMRI and behavioral evidence. *Neuron* 32: 537–551.

Ahearn, Laura M. 2001. *Invitations to Love: Literacy, Love Letters, and Social Change in Nepal*. Ann Arbor: University of Michigan Press.

Ahlert, Dieter, and Peter Kenning. 2006. Neuroökonomik. *Zeitschrift für Management* 1, no. 1: 24–47.

Alcoff, Linda Martin. 1996. *Real Knowing: New Versions of the Coherence Theory*. Ithaca: Cornell University Press.

Allen, Ann Taylor. 2005. *Feminism and Motherhood in Western Europe, 1890–1970: The Maternal Dilemma*. New York: Palgrave Macmillan.

Allman, John, Hakeem Atiya, and Karli Watson. 2002. Two phylogenetic specializations in the human brain. *The Neuroscientist* 8, no. 4: 335–346.

Allport, Gordon W., and Henry S. Odbert. 1936. Trait-names: A psycho-lexical study. *Psychological Monographs* 47, no. 1.

American Psychiatric Association. 1952. *Diagnostic and Statistical Manual of Mental Disorders*, 1st ed. (*DSM–I*). Washington, DC: American Psychiatric Association.

American Psychiatric Association. 1968. *Diagnostic and Statistical Manual of Mental Disorders*, 2nd ed. (*DSM–II*). Washington, DC: American Psychiatric Association.

American Psychiatric Association. 1980. *Diagnostic and Statistical Manual of Mental Disorders*, 3rd ed. (*DSM–III*). Washington, DC: American Psychiatric Association.

American Psychiatric Association. 1987. *Diagnostic and Statistical Manual of Mental Disorders*, 3rd ed., revised (*DSM–III–R*). Washington, DC: American Psychiatric Association.

American Psychiatric Association. 1994. *Diagnostic and Statistical Manual of Mental Disorders*, 4th ed. (*DSM–IV*). Washington, DC: American Psychiatric Association.

American Psychological Association. 1996. Intelligence: Knowns and unknowns. *American Psychologist* 51, no. 2: 77–101.

Anderson, Joseph D. 1996. *The Reality of Illusion: An Ecological Approach to Cognitive Film Theory*. Carbondale: Southern Illinois University Press.

Andrejevic, Mark. 2005. Nothing comes between me and my CPU: Smart clothes and "ubiquitous" computing. *Theory, Culture & Society* 22, no. 3: 101–119.

Andrews, Kristin. 2002. Interpreting autism: A critique of Davidson on thought and language. *Philosophical Psychology* 15, no. 3: 317–332.

Angier, Natalie. 2000. *Woman: An Intimate Geography*. New York: Anchor Books.

Antonakis, John. 2004. On why "emotional intelligence" will not predict leadership effectiveness beyond IQ or the "Big Five": An extension and rejoinder. *Organizational Analysis* 12, no 2: 171–182.

Antonakis, John, Anna T. Cianciolo, and Robert J. Sternberg. 2004. Leadership: Past, present, and future. In *The Nature of Leadership*, ed. John Antonakis, Anna T. Cianciolo, and Robert J. Sternberg, 3–15. Thousand Oaks: Sage.

Arbeitsgruppe SubArO (Ed.). 2005. *Ökonomie der Subjektivität—Subjektivität der Ökonomie*. Berlin: Edition sigma.

Arbeitskreis Postautistische Ökonomik. 2006. Bundesdeutsches Positionspapier. In *Die Scheuklappen der Wirtschaftswissenschaften: Postautistische Ökonomik für eine plurale Wirtschaftslehre*, ed. Thomas Dürmeier, Tanja von Egan-Krieger, and Helge Peukert, 29–30. Marburg: Metropolis.

Aristoteles (Aristotle). 1995. *Gesammelte Schriften*. 6 vols. Hamburg: Meiner.

Arnold, Arthur P., Jun Xu, William Grisham, Xuqi Chen, Yong Hwan Kim, and Yuichiro Itoh. 2004. Minireview: Sex chromosomes and brain sexual differentiation. *Endocrinology* 145, no. 3: 1057–1062.

Asperger, Hans. 1944. Die "Autistischen Psychopathen" im Kindesalter. *Archiv für Psychiatrie und Nervenkrankheiten* 117: 76–136.

Autism Genome Project (AGP) Consortium. 2007. Mapping autism risk loci using genetic linkage and chromosomal rearrangements. *Nature Genetics* 39: 319–328.

Baasner, Frank. 1988. *Der Begriff "sensibilité" im 18. Jahrhundert: Aufstieg und Niedergang eines Ideals*. Heidelberg: Carl Winter.

Bailyn, Sarah J. 2002. Who makes the rules? Using Wittgenstein in social theory. *Journal for the Theory of Social Behavior* 32: 311–329.

Baker, Monya. 2007. Making money and opening minds. *Nature Biotechnology* 25, no. 4: 377–379.

Bandura, Albert. 2003. *Self-Efficacy: The Exercise of Control*. 8th ed. New York: Freeman.

Bannister, Robert C. 1979. *Social Darwinism: Science and Myth in Anglo-American Social Thought*. Philadelphia: Temple University Press.

Barchard, Kimberly A., and Michelle M. Christensen. 2007. Dimensionality and higher-order factor structure of self-reported emotional intelligence. *Personality and Individual Differences* 42, no. 6: 971–985.

Barker-Benfield, G.J. 1992. *The Culture of Sensibility: Sex and Society in Eighteenth-Century Britain*. Chicago: University of Chicago Press.

Barnett, Douglas, and Hilary Horn Ratner. 1997. Introduction: The organization and integration of cognition and emotion in development. *Journal of Experimental Child Psychology* 67: 303–316.

Bar-On, Reuven. 1997. *Bar-On Emotional Quotient Inventory (EQ-i): Technical Manual*. Toronto: Multi-Health Systems.

Bar-On, Reuven. 2000. Emotional and social intelligence: Insights from the Emotional Quotient Inventory. In *The Handbook of Emotional Intelligence*, ed. Reuven Bar-On and James D.A. Parker, 363–388. San Francisco: Jossey-Bass.

Baron-Cohen, Simon. 1988. Social and pragmatic deficits in autism: Cognitive or affective? *Journal of Autism and Developmental Disorders* 18: 379–402.

Baron-Cohen, Simon. 1999. The extreme-male-brain theory of autism. In *Neurodevelopmental Disorders*, ed. Helen Tager-Flusberg, 401–430. Cambridge: MIT Press.

Baron-Cohen, Simon. 2000. Theory of mind and autism: A 15 year review. In *Understanding Other Minds: Perspectives from Developmental Cognitive Neuroscience*, ed. Simon Baron-Cohen, Helen Tager-Flusberg, and Donald J. Cohen, 3–20. 2nd ed. New York: Oxford University Press.

Baron-Cohen, Simon. 2003. *The Essential Difference: The Truth about the Male and Female Brain.* (Hardcover ed.) (Sold also with the subtitle *Male and Female Brains, and the Truth about Autism.* Paperback ed.) New York: Basic Books. (In the United Kingdom sold with the subtitle: *Men, Women and the Extreme Male Brain.* London: Allen Lane).

Baron-Cohen, Simon. 2004. *The Essential Difference: Forget Mars and Venus and Discover the Truth about the Opposite Sex.* London: Penguin Books. (In Germany sold with the title and subtitle *Vom ersten Tag an anders. Das weibliche und das männliche Gehirn.* Düsseldorf and Zurich: Walter).

Baron-Cohen, Simon, and Jessica Hammer. 1997. Is autism an extreme form of the "male brain"? *Advances in Infancy Research* 11: 193–217.

Baron-Cohen, Simon, Rebecca C. Knickemeyer, and Matthew K. Belmonte. 2005. Sex differences in the brain: Implications for explaining autism. *Science* 310: 819–823.

Barres, Ben. 2006. Does gender matter? *Nature* 442: 133–135.

Bartsch, Anne, and Reinhold Viehoff. 2003. Meta-emotion: In search of a meta-account for entertainment by negative emotions. *Siegener Periodikum zur Internationalen Empirischen Literaturwissenschaft* 22: 309–328.

Bartsch, Anne, and Susanne Hübner. 2005. Towards a theory of emotional communication. *Comparative Literature and Culture* 7, no. 4. http://clcwebjournal.lib.purdue.edu/clcweb05-4/bartsch&hubner05.html (accessed April 11, 2007).

Bartsch, Anne, and Susanne Hübner. 2006. Emotionale Kommunikation—Ein integratives Modell. [Emotional communication—An integrative model.] PhD diss., Martin-Luther-University Halle-Wittenberg. http://sundoc.bibliothek.uni-halle.de/diss-online/04/07H050/index.htm (accessed April 11, 2007).

Bartsch, Anne, Jens Eder, and Kathrin Fahlenbrach (Eds.). 2007. *Audiovisuelle Emotionen: Emotionsdarstellung und Emotionsvermittlung durch audiovisuelle Medienangebote.* Cologne: Herbert von Halem-Verlag.

Bartsch, Anne, Roland Mangold, Reinhold Viehoff, and Peter Vorderer. 2006. Emotional gratifications during media use—An integrative approach. *Communications* 31: 261–278.

Bass, Bernhard M., and Bruce J. Avolio. 1997. Shatter the glass ceiling: Women may make better managers. In *Leadership: Classical, Contemporary and Critical Approaches*, ed. Keith Grint, 199–210. Oxford: Oxford University Press.

Bass, Bernard M., and Bruce J. Avolio. 2000. *Multifactor Leadership Questionnaire*. 2nd ed. Redwood City: Mind Garden.

Bastian, Veneta A., Nicholas R. Burns, and Ted Nettelbeck. 2005. Emotional intelligence predicts life skills, but not as well as personality and cognitive abilities. *Personality and Individual Differences* 39, no. 6: 1135–1145.

Baumeler, Carmen. 2005. *Von kleidsamen Computern und unternehmerischen Universitäten: Eine ethnographische Organisationsstudie*. Münster: LIT.

Beaufaÿs, Sandra. 2007. Alltag der Exzellenz. Konstruktion von Leistung und Geschlecht in der Förderung wissenschaftlichen Nachwuchses. In *Willkommen im Club? Frauen und Männer in Eliten*, ed. Regina M. Dackweiler, 145–168. Münster: Westfälisches Dampfboot.

Bechara, Antoine, Daniel Tranel, and Antonio R. Damasio. 2000. Poor judgment in spite of high intellect: Neurological evidence for emotional intelligence. In *The Handbook of Emotional Intelligence*, ed. Reuven Bar-On and James D. A. Parker, 192–214. San Francisco: Jossey-Bass.

Beck, Ulrich. 1999. *Risk Society Revisited*. Cambridge: Blackwell.

Becker, Gary S. 1991. *A Treatise on the Family*. Cambridge: Harvard University Press.

Becker, Jill B., Arthur P. Arnold, Karen J. Berkley, Jeffrey D. Blaustein, Lisa A. Eckel, Elizabeth Hampson, James P. Herman, Sherry Marts, Wolfgang Sadee, Meir Steiner, Jane Taylor, and Elizabeth Young. 2005. Strategies and methods for research on sex differences in brain and behavior. *Endocrinology* 146, no. 4: 1650–1673.

Beckmann, Nicolau, Didier Laurent, Bruno Tigani, Rogerio Panizzutti, and Markus Rudin. 2004. Magnetic resonance imaging in drug discovery: Lessons from disease areas. *Drug Discovery Today* 9, no. 1: 35–42.

Bedford-Strohm, Heinrich. 1999. *Gemeinschaft aus kommunikativer Freiheit: Sozialer Zusammenhalt in der modernen Gesellschaft: Ein theologischer Beitrag*. Gütersloh: Kaiser, Gütersloher Verlagshaus.

Bendelow, Gillian, and Simon J. Williams (Eds.). 1997. *Emotions in Social Life: Critical Themes and Contemporary Issues*. London and New York: Routledge.

Benecke, Cord, and Gerhard Dammann. 2003. Unbewußte Emotionen. In *Natur und Theorie der Emotion*, ed. Achim Stephan and Henrik Walter, 139–163. Paderborn: Mentis.

Bentin, Shlomo, and Raphiq Ibrahim. 1996. New evidence for phonological processing during visual word recognition: The case of Arabic. *Journal of Experimental Psychology: Learning, Memory, and Cognition* 22: 309–323.

Berger, Maurice. 1999. *White Lies: Race and the Myths of Whiteness*. New York: Farrar, Straus & Giroux.

Bernard, Jessie. 1981. *The Female World*. London and New York: MacMillan.

Besnier, Niko. 1990. Conflict management, gossip, and affective meaning on Nukulaelae. In *Disentangling: Conflict Discourse in Pacific Societies*, ed. Karen Ann Watson-Gegeo and Geoffrey M. White, 290–334. Stanford: Stanford University Press.

Besnier, Niko. 1995. *Literacy, Emotion, and Authority: Reading and Writing on a Polynesian Atoll*. Cambridge: Cambridge University Press.

Billacois, François. 1986. *Le duel dans la société française des XVIe–XVIIe siècles: Essai de psychosociologie historique*. Paris: Editions de l'EHESS.

Binet, Alfred. 1905/1916. Méthodes nouvelles pour le diagnostic du niveau intellectuel des anormaux. *L'Année Psychologique* 12: 191–244 (1905, coauthored with Théodore Simon). New methods for the diagnosis of the intellectual level of subnormals, transl. Elizabeth S. Kite. In *The Development of Intelligence in Children* (1916). Vineland: Publications of the Training School at Vineland.

Bischoff, Theodor Ludwig Wilhelm. 1872. *Das Studium und die Ausübung der Medizin durch Frauen*. Munich: Literarisch-Artistische Anstalt.

Blaug, Mark. 1993. *The Methodology of Economics: Or How Economists Explain*. 2nd ed. Cambridge: Cambridge University Press.

Blaxill, Mark F. 2004. Study fails to establish diagnostic substitute as a factor in increased rate of autism. *Pharmacology* 24: 812–813.

Bleuler, Eugen. 1911. Dementia Praecox oder Gruppe der Schizophrenien. In *Handbuch der Psychiatrie*, ed. Gustav Aschaffenburg, special part, division 4.1. Leipzig: Deuticke (English transl. 1950. *Dementia Praecox, or the Group of Schizophrenias*, transl. Joseph Zinkin. New York: International University Press).

Block, Jack. 1995. On the relation between IQ, impulsivity, and delinquency. *Journal of Abnormal Psychology* 104, no. 2: 399–401.

Blum, Deborah. 2007. *Sex on the Brain: The Biological Differences between Men and Women*. New York: Viking (revised reprint of 1997: Penguin Books).

Blumenberg, Hans. 1997. *Ein mögliches Selbstverständnis*. Stuttgart: Reclam.

Boehm, Gottfried. 1994. Die Wiederkehr der Bilder. In *Was ist ein Bild?*, ed. Gottfried Boehm, 11–38. Munich: Fink.

Böhnisch, Tomke. 1999. *Gattinnen. Die Frauen der Elite*. Münster: Westfälisches Dampfboot.

Böhnisch, Tomke. 2003. Karriereressource Ehefrau—Statusressource Ehemann. Oder warum Frauen von Topmanagern keine berufliche Karriere machen. In *Karrierepolitik: Beiträge zur*

Rekonstruktion erfolgsorientierten Handelns, ed. Ronald Hitzler and Michaela Pfadenhauer, 173–187. Opladen: Leske + Budrich.

Bolin, Anne. 1988. *In Search of Eve: Transsexual Rites of Passage.* New York: Bergin and Garvey.

Bollnow, Otto Friedrich. 1995. *Das Wesen der Stimmungen.* 8th ed. Frankfurt am Main: Vittorio Klostermann.

Boltanski, Luc, and Ève Chiapello. 2003. *Der neue Geist des Kapitalismus,* transl. Michael Tillmann. Konstanz: UVK (2006. Paperback ed.) (Orig. 1999. *Le nouvel Ésprit du Capitalism.* Paris: Edition Gallimard).

Bolton, Patrick, Hope Macdonald, A. Pickles, et al. 1994. A case-control family history study of autism. *Journal of Child Psychology and Psychiatry, and Allied Disciplines* 35: 877–900.

Bombaci, Nancy. 2005. Gods among Men: Asperger's Syndrome and the Gender of Genius. Paper presented at the conference *Autism and Representation.* Case Western Reserve University, Cleveland, Ohio, 28–30, October 2005. http://www.case.edu/affil/sce/Texts_2005/Autism%20and%20 Representation%20Bombaci.htm (accessed September 4, 2007).

Bonnell, Victoria E., and Lynn Hunt. 1999. Introduction. In *Beyond the Cultural Turn,* ed. Victoria E. Bonnell and Lynn Hunt, 1–34. Berkeley: University of California Press.

Borck, Cornelius. 2005. *Hirnströme: Eine Kulturgeschichte der Elektroenzephalographie.* Göttingen: Wallstein.

Bornstein, Kate. 1994. *Gender Outlaw: On Men, Women and the Rest of Us.* New York: Routledge.

Bougerol, Christiane. 1997. *Une ethnographie des conflits aux Antilles: Jalousie, commérages, sorcellerie.* Paris: Presses Universitaires de France.

Bourdieu, Pierre. 1977. *Outline of a Theory of Practice.* Cambridge: Cambridge University Press.

Bourdieu, Pierre. 1979. *La Distinction: Critique Sociale du Jugement.* Paris: Editions de Minuit (1984. Distinction: A Social Critique of the Judgement of Taste, transl. Richard Nice. Cambridge: Harvard University Press; 1987. *Der feine Unterschied: Kritik der gesellschaftlichen Urteilskraft,* transl. Bernd Schwibs and Achim Russer. Frankfurt am Main: Suhrkamp).

Bourdieu, Pierre. 1986. The forms of capital. In *Handbook of Theory and Research for the Sociology of Education,* ed. John G. Richardson, 241–258. New York: Greenwood Press.

Bourdieu, Pierre. 2000. *Pascalian Meditations,* transl. Richard Nice. Cambridge: Polity Press.

Bourdieu, Pierre. 2005a. *Language and Symbolic Power,* transl. Gino Raymond and Matthew Adamson. Cambridge: Harvard University Press (reprint).

Bourdieu, Pierre. 2005b. *Die männliche Herrschaft,* transl. Jürgen Bolder. Frankfurt am Main: Suhrkamp (Orig. 1998. *La domination masculine.* Paris: Seuil).

Bourdieu, Pierre, and Loïc Wacquant. 1992. *An Invitation to Reflexive Sociology,* transl. Loïc Wacquant. Chicago: University of Chicago Press (2006. *Reflexive Anthropologie,* transl. Hella Beister. Frankfurt am Main: Suhrkamp).

Brackett, Marc A., John D. Mayer, and Rebecca M. Warner. 2004. Emotional intelligence and its relation to everyday behavior. *Personality and Individual Differences* 36, no. 6: 1387–1402.

Brackett, Marc A., Rebecca M. Warner, and Jennifer S. Bosco. 2005. Emotional intelligence and relationship quality among couples. *Personal Relationships* 12, no. 2: 197–212.

Brackett, Marc A., Susan E. Rivers, Sara Shiffman, Nicole Lerner, and Peter Salovey. 2006. Relating emotional abilities to social functioning: A comparison of self-report and performance measures of emotional intelligence. *Journal of Personality and Social Psychology* 91, no. 4: 780–795.

Bradberry, Travis, and Jean Greaves. 2005. *The Emotional Intelligence Quick Book. Everything You Need to Know to Put your EQ to Work.* New York: Simon & Schuster.

Braun von, Christina, and Inge Stephan (Eds.). 2005. *Gender@Wissen.* Cologne, Weimar, and Vienna: UTB.

Breazeal, Cynthia, and Rodney Brooks. 2005. "Robot emotion": A functional perspective. In *Who Needs Emotions? The Brain Meets the Robot,* ed. Jean-Marc Fellous and Michael A. Arbib, 271–310. Oxford and New York: Oxford University Press.

Bredekamp, Horst. 1995. *The Lure of Antiquity, and the Cult of the Machine: The Kunstkammer and the Evolution of Nature, Art, and Technology.* Princeton: M. Wiener.

Bredekamp, Horst. 2005. *Darwins Korallen: Frühe Evolutionsmodelle und die Tradition der Naturge-schichte.* Berlin: Wagenbach.

Breidbach, Olaf. 1997. *Die Materialisierung des Ichs. Zur Geschichte der Hirnforschung im 19. und 20. Jahrhundert.* Frankfurt am Main: Suhrkamp.

Breiter, Hans C., Itzhak Aharon, Daniel Kahneman, Anders Dale, and Peter Shizgal. 2001. Functional imaging of neural responses to expectancy and experience of monetary gains and losses. *Neuron* 30, no. 2: 619–639.

Brenneis, Donald. 1990a. Dramatic gestures: The Fiji Indian Pancayat as therapeutic event. In *Disentangling: Conflict Discourse in Pacific Societies,* ed. Karen Ann Watson-Gegeo and Geoffrey M. White, 214–238. Stanford: Stanford University Press.

Brenneis, Donald. 1990b. Shared and solitary sentiments: The discourse of friendship, play, and anger in Bhatgaon. In *Language and the Politics of Emotion,* ed. Catherine A. Lutz and Lila Abu-Lughod, 113–125. Cambridge: Cambridge University Press.

Briggs, Jean L. 1970. *Never in Anger: Portrait of an Eskimo Family.* Cambridge: Harvard University Press.

Briggs, Katherine C., and Isabel Myers. 1976. *Myers-Briggs Type Indicator.* Palo Alto: Consulting Psychologists Press.

Brizendine, Louann. 2006. *The Female Brain.* New York: Morgan Road Books.

Brockman, John (Ed.). 1995. *The Third Culture: Beyond the Scientific Revolution.* New York: Simon & Schuster.

Brockman, John (Ed.). 1996. *Digerati: Encounters with the Cyber Elite*. San Francisco: HardWired.

Brockman, John (Ed.). 2004a. *Science at the Edge*. London: Weidenfeld & Nicolson.

Brockman, John (Ed.). 2004b. *Curious Minds: How a Child Becomes a Scientist*. New York: Pantheon Books.

Brockman, John (Ed.). 2006. *What Is Your Dangerous Idea? Today's Leading Thinkers on the Unthinkable*. With an introduction by Steven Pinker and an afterword by Richard Dawkins. London: Simon & Schuster.

Brody, Nathan 2006. Beyond g. In *A Critique of Emotional Intelligence,* ed. Kevin R. Murphy, 161–185. London: Lawrence Erlbaum Associates.

Brosnan, Mark. 2006. Digit ratio and faculty membership: Implications for the relationship between prenatal testosterone and academia. *British Journal of Psychology* 97, no. 4: 455–466.

Brothers, Leslie. 1997. *Friday's Footprint: How Society Shapes the Human Mind*. Oxford: Oxford University Press.

Brown, Peter M. 2000. *Closet Space: Geographies of Metaphor from the Body to the Globe*. London and New York: Routledge.

Buck, Ross. 1984. *The Communication of Emotion*. New York: Guilford.

Burns, James M. 1978. *Leadership*. New York: Harper and Row.

Burns, Robert M. 2002. Language, tradition, and the self in the generation of meaning. *Journal of European Ideas* 28: 58–75.

Butler, Judith. 1990. *Gender Trouble: Feminism and the Subversion of Identity*. New York: Routledge.

Butler, Judith. 1993. *Bodies that Matter: On the Discursive Limits of "Sex."* New York: Routledge.

Butler, Judith. 2004. *Undoing Gender*. New York: Routledge.

Byrd, Robert S., and Allison C. Sage (Eds.). 2002. *Report to the Legislature on the Principal Findings from the Epidemiology of Autism in California: A Comprehensive Pilot Study*. University of California, Davis. M.I.N.D. Institute.

Byrne, Richard W., and Andrew Whiten (Eds.). 1988. *Machiavellian Intelligence: Social Expertise and the Evolution of Intellect in Monkeys, Apes, and Humans*. Oxford and New York: Oxford University Press.

Byrne, William, and Bruce Parsons. 1993. Human sexual orientation: The biologic theories. *Archives of General Psychiatry* 50: 228–239.

Cacioppo, John T. (Ed.). 2002. *Foundations in Social Neuroscience*. Cambridge: MIT Press.

Cacioppo, John T., Gary G. Berntson, and David J. Klein. 1992. What is an emotion? The role of somatovisceral afference, with special emphasis on somatovisceral "illusion." In *Emotion and Social Behavior*, ed. Margaret S. Clark, 63–98. Newbury Park: Sage.

Cacioppo, John T., and Gary G. Berntson (Eds.). 2004. *Social Neuroscience: Key Readings*. New York: Ohio State University Psychology Press.

Califia, Pat. 1997. *Sex Changes: The Politics of Transgenderism*. San Francisco: Cleis.

Camerer, Colin F. 1999. Behavioral economics: Reunifying psychology and economics. *Proceedings of the National Academy of Sciences* 96, no. 19: 10575–10577.

Camerer, Colin F. 2003. *Behavioral Game Theory: Experiments in Strategic Interactions*. Princeton: Princeton University Press.

Camerer, Colin F., George Loewenstein, and Drazen Prelec. 2005. Neuroeconomics: How neuroscience can inform economics. *Journal of Economic Literature* XLIII: 9–64.

Camus, Jean-François. 1996. *La Psychologie Cognitive de l'Attention*. Paris: Armand Colin.

Canli, Turhan, and John D. E. Gabrieli. 2004. Imaging gender differences in sexual arousal. *Nature Neuroscience* 7, no. 4: 325–326.

Caplan, Arthur. 2005. *Would you have allowed Bill Gates to be born?* Commentary on MSN, 31 May 2005, http://www.msnbc.msn.com/id/7899821/ (accessed June 24, 2007).

Carless, Sally A. 1998. Gender differences in transformational leadership: An examination of superior, leader, and subordinate perspectives. *Sex Roles* 39, no. 11–12: 887–902.

Carroll, Noël. 1990. *The Philosophy of Horror, or Paradoxes of the Heart*. New York: Routledge.

Carus, Carl Gustav. 1814. *Versuch einer Darstellung des Nervensystems und insbesondere des Gehirns nach ihrer Bedeutung, Entwicklung und Vollendung im thierischen Organismus*. Leipzig: Breitkopf & Härtel.

Carus, Carl Gustav. 1841. *Grundzüge einer neuen und wissenschaftlich begründeten Cranioscopie (Schädellehre)*. Stuttgart: Balz'sche Buchhandlung.

Carus, Carl Gustav. 1843–45. *Atlas der Cranioscopie oder Abbildungen der Schaedel- und Antlitzformen beruehmter oder sonst merkwürdiger Personen*. 2 vols. Leipzig: Weichardt.

Cassirer, Ernst. [1944] 1972. *An Essay on Man: An Introduction to a Philosophy of Human Culture*. New Haven and London: Yale University Press.

Castiglione, Baldasar. [1528] 1967. *The Book of the Courtier*, transl. George Bull. Harmondsworth: Penguin.

Cattell, Raymond B. 1937. *The Fight for Our National Intelligence*. London: P. S. King.

Cattell, Raymond B. 1971. *Abilities: Their Structure, Growth, and Action*: Houghton Mifflin.

Cernovsky, Zack. 1995. On the similarities of American blacks and whites: A reply to J. P. Rushton. *Journal of Black Studies* 25: 672.

Chalela, Julio A., Chelsea S. Kidwell, Lauren M. Nentwich, Marie Luby, John A. Butman, Andrew M. Demchuk, Michael D. Hill, Nicholas Patronas, Lawrence Latour, and Steven Warach. 2007.

Magnetic resonance imaging and computed tomography in emergency assessment of patients with suspected acute stroke: A prospective comparison. *The Lancet* 369, no. 9558: 293–298.

Chapin, Francis S. 1942. Preliminary standardization of a social impact scale. *American Sociological Review* 7: 214–225.

Chapin, Francis S. 1968. *The Social Insight Test*. Palo Alto, CA: Consulting Psychologists Press.

Chartrand, Tanya L., and John A. Bargh. 1999. The chameleon effect: The perception–behavior link and social interaction. *Journal of Personality and Social Psychology* 76: 893–910.

Cheney, Dorothy L., and Robert M. Seyfarth. 1982. How vervet monkeys perceive their grunts. *Animal Behaviour* 30: 739–751.

Cheney, Dorothy L., and Robert M. Seyfarth. 1988. Assessment of meaning and the detection of unreliable signals by vervet monkeys. *Animal Behaviour* 36: 477–486.

Cherniss, Cary, and Daniel Goleman (Eds.). 2001. *The Emotionally Intelligent Workplace: How to Select for, Measure, and Improve Emotional Intelligence in Individuals, Groups, and Organizations*. San Francisco: Jossey-Bass.

Chess, Stella, Sam J. Korn, and Paulina B. Fernandez. 1971. *Psychiatric Disorders of Children with Congenital Rubella*. New York: Brunner/Mazel.

Chion, Michel. 1994. *Audio-Vision: Sound on Screen*. New York: Columbia University Press.

Chittenden, Dave, Graham Farmelo, and Bruce V. Lewenstein (Eds.). 2004. *Creating Connections: Museums and the Public Understanding of Current Research*. Walnut Creek: Altamira Press.

Chorover, Stephan L. 1980. *From Genesis to Genocide: The Meaning of Human Nature and the Power of Behavior Control*. New ed. Cambridge: MIT Press.

Chrisley, Ronald J. 1995. "Taking embodiment seriously": Nonconceptual content and robotics. In *Android Epistemology*, ed. Kenneth M. Ford, Clark Glymour, and Patrick J. Hayes, 141–166. Menlo Park and Cambridge: The Association for the Advancement of Artificial Intelligence Press/ MIT Press.

Ciarrochi, Joseph V., Amy Y. C. Chan, and Peter Caputi. 2000. A critical evaluation of the emotional intelligence construct. *Personality and Individual Differences* 28, no. 3: 539–561.

Ciarrochi, Joseph, Frank P. Deane, and Stephen Anderson. 2002. Emotional intelligence moderates the relationship between stress and mental health. *Personality and Individual Differences* 32, no. 2: 197–209.

Clark, Andy. 2003. *Natural-Born Cyborgs: Minds, Technologies, and the Future of Human Intelligence*. New York: Oxford University Press.

Clark, Margaret S. 1989. "Historical emotionology": From a social psychologist's perspective. In *Social History and Issues in Human Consciousness: Some Interdisciplinary Connections*, ed. Andrew E. Barnes and Peter N. Stearns, 262–269. New York: New York University Press.

Clarke Associates, Walter V. 1996. *Activity Vector Analysis: Some Applications to the Concept of Emotional Intelligence.* Pittsburgh: Walter V. Clarke Associates.

Cloninger, C. Robert. 2004. *Feeling Good: The Science of Well-Being.* New York: Oxford University Press.

Cockburn, Cynthia, and Susan Ormrod. 1993. *Gender and Technology in the Making.* London: Sage.

Coenen, Christopher. 2006. Der posthumanistische Technofuturismus in den Debatten über Nanotechnologie und Converging Technologies. In *Nanotechnologien im Kontext*, ed. Alfred Nordmann, Joachim Schummer, and Astrid Schwarz, 195–222. Berlin: AKA Verlag.

Cohen, Annabel J. 2001. Music as a source of emotion in film. In *Music and Emotion: Theory and Research*, ed. Patrik N. Juslin and John A. Sloboda, 249–275. Oxford: Oxford University Press.

Cohen, David. 2004. Men, empathy, and autism. *Chronicle of Higher Education* 50, Issue 26: A12 (issued March 5, 2004). http://chronicle.com/free/v50/i26/26a01201.htm (accessed August 8, 2007).

Cohen, Jacob. 1988. *Statistical Power Analysis for the Behavioral Sciences.* 2nd ed. Hillsdale: Lawrence Erlbaum Associates.

Cole, Diana. 2005. Rethinking agency: A phenomenological approach to embodiment and agentic capacities. *Political Studies* 53: 124–142.

Colley, Helen. 2003. Learning to do emotional labour: Class, gender and the reform of habitus in the training of nursery nurses. http://www.education.ex.ac.uk/tlc/docs/publications/LE_HC _PUB_CONF_06.03.htm (accessed June 5, 2007).

Collins, Randall. 1990. Stratification, emotional energy and transient emotions. In *Research Agendas in the Sociology of Emotions,* ed. T. Kempner, 27–57. Albany: State University of New York.

Collins, Randall. 2004. *Interaction Ritual Chains.* Princeton: Princeton University Press.

Colom, Roberto, Sergio Escorial, and Irene Rebollo. 2004. Sex differences on the Progressive Matrices are influenced by sex differences on spatial ability. *Personality and Individual Differences* 37, no. 6: 1289–1293.

Connell, Robert W. 1995. *Masculinities.* Berkeley: University of California Press.

Connellan, Jennifer, Simon Baron-Cohen, Sally Wheelwright, Anna Batki, and Jag Ahluwalia. 2001. Sex differences in human neonatal social perception. *Infant Behavior and Development* 23, no. 1: 113–118.

Cooper, Anthony Ashley, Third Earl of Shaftesbury. [1711] 1999. *Characteristics of Men, Manners, Opinions, Times*, ed. Lawrence E. Klein. Cambridge: Cambridge University Press.

Costa, Paul T., Jr., and Robert R. McCrae. 1992. *Revised NEO Personality Inventory (NEO-PI-R) and NEO Five-Factor Inventory (NEO-FFI) Professional Manual.* Odessa, FL: Psychological Assessment Resources.

Costa, Paul T., Jr., Antonio Terracciano, and Robert R. McCrae. 2001. Gender differences in personality traits across cultures: Robust and surprising findings. *Journal of Personality and Social Psychology* 81, no. 2: 322–331.

Côté, Stephane, and Christoph T. H. Miners. 2006. Emotional intelligence, cognitive intelligence, and job performance. *Administrative Science Quarterly* 51, no. 1: 1–28.

Coulter, Jeff. 1997. "Neural Cartesianism": Comments on the epistemology of the cognitive sciences. In *The Future of the Cognitive Revolution*, ed. David Martel Johnson and Christina E. Erneling, 293–301. Oxford: Oxford University Press.

Cowan, Maxwell W., Kathy L. Kopnisky, and Steven E. Hyman. 2002. The Humane Genome Project and its impact on psychiatry. *Annual Review of Neuroscience* 25: 1–50.

Crary, Jonathan. 1999. *Suspensions of Perception: Attention, Spectacle, and Modern Culture.* Cambridge: MIT Press.

Cronbach, Lee J. 1960. *Essentials in Psychological Testing.* New York: Harper & Brothers.

Cunningham, Andrew, and Perry Williams (Eds.). 1992. *The Laboratory Revolution in Medicine.* Cambridge: Cambridge University Press.

Cutler, Eustacia. 2004. *A Thorn in My Pocket: Temple Grandin's Mother Tells the Family Story.* Arlington: Future Horizons.

Dackweiler, Regina M. 2007. Elite, Exzellen, Exklusion? Elite und Eliten: Konjunktur eines politisch-rhetorischen Begriffs und einer analytischen Kategorie. In *Willkommen im Club? Frauen und Männer in Eliten,* ed. Regina M. Dackweiler, 9–28. Münster: Westfälisches Dampfboot.

DaCosta, Beatriz, and Kavita Philip (Eds.). 2008. *Tactical Biopolitics. Art, Activism, and Technoscience.* Cambridge: MIT Press.

Dahrendorf, Ralf. 1992. *Society and Democracy in Germany.* Aldershot: Gregg Revivals (reprint of 1967. London: Weidenfeld and Nicolson).

Dalai Lama XIV. 1999. *Consciousness at the Crossroads: Conversations with the Dalai Lama on Brain-science and Buddhism,* ed. Zara Hashmound, Robert B. Livingston, and B. Alan Wallace. Ithaca: Snow Lion.

Damasio, Antonio R. 1994. *Descartes' Error: Emotion, Reason and the Human Brain.* New York: Grosset/Putnam.

Damasio, Antonio R. 1999. *The Feeling of What Happens: Body and Emotions in the Making of Consciousness.* New York: Harcourt, Brace and Co.

Damasio, Antonio R. 2003. *Looking for Spinoza: Joy, Sorrow, and the Feeling Brain.* New York: Harcourt, Brace and Co.

Damrad-Frye, Robin, and James D. Laird. 1989. The experience of boredom: The role of the self-perception of attention. *Journal of Personality and Social Psychology* 57: 315–320.

Darwin, Charles. 1859. *On the Origin of Species by Means of Natural Selection, or the Preservation of Favoured Races in the Struggle for Life*. London: John Murray.

Darwin, Charles. 1874. *The Descent of Man and Selection in Relation to Sex*. 2nd ed. London: John Murray.

Darwin, Charles. [1872] 1998. *The Expression of the Emotions in Man and Animals*, ed. Paul Ekman. 3rd ed. London: HarperCollins.

Das, Veena. 1998. Wittgenstein and anthropology. *Annual Review of Anthropology* 27: 171–195.

Daston, Lorraine, and Katharine Park. 1998. *Wonders and the Order of Nature, 1150–1750*. Cambridge: Zone Books/MIT Press.

Daum, Andreas. 2002. *Wissenschaftspopularisierung im 19. Jahrhundert. Bürgerliche Kultur, naturwissenschaftliche Bildung und die deutsche Öffentlichkeit, 1848–1919*. 2nd ed. München: Oldenbourg.

Davidson, Donald. 1984. *Inquiries into Truth and Interpretation*. Oxford: Oxford University Press.

Davidson, Donald. 1989. The conditions of thought. In *The Mind of Donald Davidson*, ed. Johannes Brandl and Wolfgang L. Gombocz. *Grazer Philosophische Studien* 36, 193–200. Amsterdam and Atlanta, GA: Rodopi.

Davies, Michaela, Lazar Stankov, and Richard D. Roberts. 1998. Emotional intelligence: In search of an elusive construct. *Journal of Personality and Social Psychology* 75, no. 4: 989–1015.

Davis, Bernard. 1983. Neo-Lysenkoism, IQ, and the press. *The Public Interest* 74: 41–59.

Davis, Penelope J. 1999. Personality processes and individual differences: Gender differences in autobiographical memory for childhood emotional experiences. *Journal of Personality and Social Psychology* 76, no. 3: 498–510.

Dawda, Darek, and Stephan D. Hart. 2000. Assessing emotional intelligence: Reliability and validity of the Bar-On Emotional Quotient Inventory (EQ-i) in university students. *Personality and Individual Differences* 28, no. 4: 797–812.

Dawson, Geraldine, Sara Webb, et al. 2002. Defining the broader phenotype of autism: Genetic, brain, and behavioral development and perspectives. *Psychopathology* 14: 581–611.

Day, Aria L., and Sarah A. Carroll. 2004. Using an ability-based measure of emotional intelligence to predict individual performance, group performance, and group citizenship behaviours. *Personality and Individual Differences* 36, no. 6: 1443–1458.

Deeley, Quinton, Eileen M. Daly, Simon Surguladze, et al. 2007. An event related functional magnetic resonance imaging study of facial emotion processing in Asperger syndrome. *Biological Psychiatry* 62, no. 3: 207–217.

Deighton, Russell M., and Harald C. Traue. 2003. Emotion und Kultur im Spiegel emotionalen Wissens. In *Natur und Theorie der Emotion*, ed. Achim Stephan and Henrik Walter, 240–261. Paderborn: Mentis.

DeJean, Joan. 1991. *Tender Geographies: Women and the Origins of the Novel in France*. New York: Columbia University Press.

Deleuze, Gilles, and Félix Guattari. 1983. *Anti-Oedipus: Capitalism and Schizophrenia*. Minneapolis: University of Minnesota Press.

Dennett, Daniel C. 1998. *Brainchildren: Essays on Designing Minds*. Cambridge: MIT Press.

Dennett, Daniel C. 2006. *Breaking the Spell: Religion as a Natural Phenomenon*. New York: Viking.

Depue, Richard A., and Paul F. Collins. 1999. Neurobiology of the structure of personality: Dopamine, facilitation of incentive motivation, and extraversion. *Behavioral and Brain Sciences* 22, no. 3: 491–517.

Deruelle, Christine, Cécilie Rondan, Xavier Salle-Collemiche, Delphine Bastard-Rosset, and David DaFonseca. 2007. Attention to low- and high-spatial frequencies in categorizing facial identities, emotions and gender in children with autism. *Brain and Cognition* (online publication August 9, 2007).

Descola, Philippe. 1993. *Les lances du crépuscule: Relations Jivaros, Haute Amazonie*. Paris: Plon (1996. *The Spears of Twilight: Life and Death in the Amazon Jungle*, transl. Janet Lloyd. New York: New Press).

DeSousa, Ronald. 1987. *The Rationality of Emotion*. Cambridge: MIT Press.

Deuser, Hermann. 2004. Ist *Gemeinschaft* ein metaphysischer Begriff? In *Gottesinstinkt. Semiotische Religionstheorie und Pragmatismus*, ed. Hermann Deuser, 215–234. Tübingen: Mohr Siebeck.

Devine, James. 2002. Psychological autism, institutional autism and economics. *Post-autistic Economics Review* 16. http://www.peacon.net/PAEReview/issue16/Devine16.htm (accessed July 10, 2007).

Devor, Holly. 1997. *FTM: Female-To-Male Transsexuals in Society*. Bloomington: Indiana University Press.

Dewey, John. 1909. *Moral Principles in Education*. New York: Houghton Mifflin.

Diamond, Milton. 2000. Sex and gender: Same or different? *Feminism and Psychology* 10, no. 1: 46–54.

Dickenson, Donna. 2007. *Property in the Body: Feminist Perspectives*. Cambridge: Cambridge University Press.

Dickson, Lynda. 1993. The future of marriage and family in black America. *Journal of Black Studies* 4: 472–491.

Dimock, Edward C., Jr., Edwin Gerow, C. M. Naim, A. K. Ramanujan, Gordon Roadarmel, and J. A. B. van Buitenen. 1974. *The Literatures of India: An Introduction*. Chicago: University of Chicago Press.

Dinges, Martin (Ed.). 2007. *Männlichkeit und Gesundheit im historischen Wandel, ca. 1800–ca. 2000.* Stuttgart: Franz Steiner.

Dobzhansky, Theodosius. 1966. A geneticist's view of human equality. *The Pharos,* January: 12–16.

Dobzhansky, Theodosius, and Ashley Montagu. 1947. Natural selection and the mental capacities of mankind. In *Race and IQ,* ed. Ashley Montagu, 104 113. New York: Oxford University Press.

Doi, Takeo. 1973. *The Anatomy of Dependence.* Tokyo: Kodansha.

Doll, Edgar A. 1935. *Vineland Social Maturity Scale: Manual of Directions.* Minneapolis: Educational Test Bureau.

Domes, Gregor, Markus Heinrichs, Andre Michel, Christoph Berger, and Sabine C. Herpertz. 2007. Oxytocin improves "mind-reading" in humans. *Biological Psychiatry* 62, no. 6: 731–733.

Dopfer, Karl (Ed.). 2005. *The Evolutionary Foundations of Economics.* Cambridge: Cambridge University Press.

Dreger, Alice. 1998. *Hermaphrodites and the Medical Invention of Sex.* Cambridge: Harvard University Press.

Dreitzel, Hans P. 1962. *Elitebegriff und Sozialstruktur: Eine soziologische Begriffsanalyse.* Stuttgart: Enke.

Drevets, Wayne C., and Marcus E. Raichle. 1998. Reciprocal suppression of regional cerebral blood flow during emotional versus higher cognitive processes: Implications for interactions between emotion and cognition. *Cognition and Emotion* 12: 353–385.

Duclos, Sandra E., James D. Laird, Eric Schneider, Melissa Sexter, Lisa Stern, and Oliver Van Lighten. 1989. Emotion-specific effects of facial expressions and postures on emotional experience. *Journal of Personality and Social Psychology* 57: 100–108.

Duclos, Sandra E., and James D. Laird. 2001. The deliberate control of emotional experience through control of expressions. *Cognition and Emotion* 15: 27–56.

Duran, Jane. 2002. Wittgenstein, feminism and theory. *Philosophy & Social Criticism* 28: 321–336.

Dürmeier, Thomas. 2006. Post-autistic Economics: Eine studentische Intervention für plurale Ökonomik. In *Die Scheuklappen der Wirtschaftswissenschaften: Postautistische Ökonomik für eine plurale Wirtschaftslehre,* ed. Thomas Dürmeier, Tanja von Egan-Krieger, and Helge Peukert, 13–28. Marburg: Metropolis.

Düwell, Marcus. 2004. Research as a challenge for ethical reflection. In *Ethics of Life Scientists,* ed. M. Korthals and R. Borgers, 147–155. Dordrecht: Kluwer.

Eagly, Alice H., and Steven J. Karau. 2002. Role congruity theory of prejudice toward female leaders. *Psychological Review* 109: 573–598.

Eastman, Nigel, and Colin Campbell. 2006. Neuroscience and legal determination of criminal responsibility. *Nature Reviews Neuroscience* 7, no. 4: 311–318.

Eaton, Margaret L., and Judy Illes. 2007. Commercializing cognitive neurotechnology—The ethical terrain. *Nature Biotechnology* 25, no. 4: 393–397.

Ebeling, Smilla. 2006. Wenn ich meine Hormone nehme, werde ich zum Tier. Zur Geschichte der "Geschlechtshormone." In *Geschlechterforschung und Naturwissenschaften: Einführung in ein komplexes Wechselspiel,* ed. Smilla Ebeling and Sigrid Schmitz, 235–246. Wiesbaden: VS-Verlag.

Ebeling, Smilla, and Sigrid Schmitz (Eds.). 2006. *Geschlechterforschung und Naturwissenschaften: Einführung in ein komplexes Wechselspiel.* Wiesbaden: VS-Verlag.

Egan, Danielle. 2007. Brain surgery "Frankenstein" tells his story. *THE TYEE* (Canada), May 2, 2007.

Eisenberger, Naomi I., Matthew D. Lieberman, and Kipling D. Williams. 2003. Does rejection hurt? A fMRI study on social exclusion. *Science* 302: 290–292.

Ekman, Paul (Ed.). 2006. *Darwin and Facial Expression: A Century of Research in Review.* Cambridge: Malor Books.

Ekman, Paul. 2007. *Emotions Revealed: Recognizing Emotions and Feelings to Improve Communication and Emotional Life.* 2nd ed. New York: Owl Books.

Ekman, Paul, Wallace V. Friesen, and Phoebe Ellsworth. 1972. *Emotion in the Human Face: Guidelines for Research and an Integration of Findings.* Pergamon General Psychology Series, PGPS-11. New York: Pergamon Press.

El-Hai, Jack. 2005. *The Lobotomist: A Maverick Medical Genius and His Tragic Quest to Rid the World of Mental Illness.* New York: Wiley.

Elster, Jon. 1999. *Alchemies of the Mind: Rationality and the Emotions.* Cambridge: Cambridge University Press.

England, Paula. 1993. The separative self: Androcentric bias in Neoclassical assumptions. In *Beyond Economic Man: Feminist Theory and Economics,* ed. Marianne A. Ferber and Julie A. Nelson, 37–53. Chicago: University of Chicago Press.

Erk, Susanne, Manfred Spitzer, Arthur P. Wunderlich, Lars Galley, and Henrik Walter. 2002. Cultural objects modulate reward circuitry. *Neuroreport* 13, no. 18: 2499–2503.

Espeland, Wendy, and Mitchell Stevens. 1998. Commensuration as a social process. *Annual Review of Sociology* 24: 313–343.

European Commission. 2006. Communication from the Commission to the Council, the European Parliament, the European Economic and Social Committee and the Council of the Regions. *Tackling the Pay Gap between Women and Men.* Brussels: Commission of the European Communities. http://ec.europa.eu/employment_social/news/2007/jul/genderpaygap _en.pdf (accessed July 25, 2007).

European Commission. 2007. Group of experts on gender, social inclusion, and employment. *The Gender Pay Gap—Origins and Policy Responses: A Comparative Review of 30 European Countries*, ed. Janneke Plantenga and Chantal Remery. Brussels: European Commission. Unit G1. http://ec.europa.eu/employment_social/publications/2006/ke7606200_en.pdf (accessed July 25, 2007).

Eurostat. 2007. *Living Conditions in Europe: Data 2002–2005*. Luxembourg: Office for Official Publications of the European Communities. http://epp.eurostat.ec.europa.eu/portal/page?_pageid=1073,46587259&_dad=portal&_schema=Portal&p_product_codeKS-76-06-390 (accessed March 3, 2007).

Eysenck, Hans Jürgen. 1982. The sociology of psychological knowledge, the genetic interpretation of IQ, and Marxist–Leninist ideology. *Bulletin of British Psychological Society* 35: 449–451.

Faber, Malte, and John L. R. Proops. 1997. *Evolution, Time, Production and the Environment*. 3rd ed. Berlin: Springer.

Fahlenbrach, Kathrin. 2005. The emotional design of music videos: Approaches to audiovisual metaphors. *Journal of Moving Image Studies* 3, no. 1: 22–28.

Fahlenbrach, Kathrin. 2006. Aesthetics and audiovisual metaphors in media perception. *Formamente. Rivista Trimistrale*, no. 1–2: 63–77.

Fahlenbrach, Kathrin. 2007. Audiovisuelle Metaphern und Emotionen im Sound Design. In *Audiovisuelle Emotionen: Emotionsdarstellung und Emotionsvermittlung durch audiovisuelle Medienangebote*, ed. Anne Bartsch, Jens Eder, and Kathrin Fahlenbrach, 330–349. Cologne: Herbert von Halem-Verlag.

Fajans, Jane. 1997. *They Make Themselves: Work and Play Among the Baining of Papua New Guinea*. Chicago: University of Chicago Press.

Farah, Martha J. 2002. Emerging ethical issues in neuroscience. *Nature Neuroscience* 5, no. 11: 1123–1129.

Fausto-Sterling, Anne. 1994. *Myths of Gender: Biological Theories about Women and Men*. New York: Basic Books.

Fausto-Sterling, Anne. 2000. *Sexing the Body: Gender, Politics and the Construction of Sexuality*. New York: Basic Books.

Fehr, Ernst, and Urs Fischbacher. 2004. Social norms and human cooperation. *Trends in Cognitive Sciences* 8, no. 4: 185–190.

Fellner, Markus. 2006. *Psycho movie: Zur Konstruktion psychischer Störung im Spielfilm*. Bielefeld: transcript.

Fellous, Jean-Marc, and Michael A. Arbib (Eds.). 2005. *Who Needs Emotions? The Brain Meets the Robot*. Oxford and New York: Oxford University Press.

Ferber, Marianne A., and Julie A. Nelson (Eds.). 1993. *Beyond Economic Man: Feminist Theory and Economics*. Chicago: University of Chicago Press.

Ferris, Craig F., Charles T. Snowdon, Jean A. King, et al. 2004. Activation of neural pathways associated with sexual arousal in non-human primates. *Journal of Magnetic Resonance Imaging* 19: 168–175.

Fessler, Daniel M. T. 2007. Starvation, serotonin, and symbolism: A psychobiocultural perspective on stigmata. *Mind & Society.* www.sscnet.ucla.eud/anthro/faculty/fessler/ (accessed August 9, 2007).

Fiedler, Klaus, Jeannette Schmid, and Teresa Stahl. 2002. What is the current truth about polygraph lie detection? *Basic and Applied Social Psychology* 24, no. 4: 313–324.

Fineman, Stephen. 2004. Getting the measure of emotion—And the cautionary tale of emotional intelligence. *Human Relations* 57: 719–740.

Fischer, Klaus, Michael Florian, and Thomas Malsch (Eds.). 2005. *Socionics: Scalability of Complex Social Systems.* Berlin: Springer.

Fischer, Kurt W., Phillip R. Shaver, and Peter Carnochan. 1990. How emotions develop and how they organize development. *Cognition and Emotion* 4: 81–127.

Fischer, Kurt W., Daniel H. Bullock, Elaine J. Rotenberg, and Pamela Raya. 1993. The dynamics of competence: How context contributes directly to skill. In *Development in Context: Acting and Thinking in Specific Environments*, ed. R. Wozniak and K. W. Fischer, 93–117. Hillsdale: Lawrence Erlbaum Associates.

Fiske, Brian. 2004. The sexual brain. *Nature Neuroscience* 7, no. 10: 1029.

Fiske, Donald W. 1949. Consistency of the factorial structures of personality ratings from different sources. *Journal of Abnormal Social Psychology* 44, no. 3: 329–344.

Fitzgerald, Michael. 2005. *The Genesis of Art: Asperger's Syndrome and the Arts.* Philadelphia: Jessica Kingsley.

Fletcher, Joyce K. 1999. *Disappearing Acts: Gender, Power, and Relational Practice at Work.* Cambridge: MIT Press.

Flora, Carlin. 2006. The girl with a boy's brain. *Psychology Today Magazine.* November/December. http://psychologytoday.com/articles/pto-20061103-000002.xml (accessed September 1, 2007).

Flückiger, Barbara. 2002. *Sound Design: Die virtuelle Klangwelt des Films.* Marburg: Schüren Verlag.

Föllinger, Sabine. 1996. *Differenz und Gleichheit: Das Geschlechterverhältnis in der Sicht griechischer Philosophen des 4.-11. Jahrhunderts vor Christus.* Stuttgart: Steiner.

Fondas, Nanette. 1997. Feminization unveiled: Management qualities in contemporary writings. *Academy of Management Review* 22, no. 1: 257–282.

Fortenbaugh, William W. 2002. *Aristotle on Emotion: A Contribution to Philosophical Psychology, Rhetoric, Poetics, Politics, and Ethics.* 2nd ed. London: Duckworth.

Foucault, Michel. 1979. Governmentality. *Ideology and Consciousness* 7: 5–21.

Foucault, Michel. 1980. *The History of Sexuality*. New York: Vintage.

Foucault, Michel. 1988. Technologies of the self. In *Technologies of the Self: A Seminar with Michel Foucault*, ed. Luther H. Martin, Huck Gutman, and Patrick H. Hutton, 16–49. Amherst: University of Massachusetts Press.

Fraisse, Geneviève. 1993. *Reason's Muse: Sexual Difference and the Birth of Democracy*, transl. Jane Marie Todd. Chicago: University of Chicago Press.

Fraisse, Geneviève. 2007. *Du Consentement*. Paris: Seuil.

Fraisse, Geneviève, and Michelle Perrot (Eds.). 1995. *A History of Women in the West* (5 vols., series ed. Georges Duby and Michelle Perrot), *vol. 4: Emerging Feminism from Revolution to World War*. Cambridge: Harvard University Press.

Freeman, Walter, and James Watts. 1942. *Psychosurgery: Intelligence, Emotion and Social Behavior Following Prefrontal Lobotomy for Mental Disorders*. Springfield and Baltimore: C. C. Thomas.

Freud, Sigmund. 1963. Lecture XXII: Some thoughts on development and regression aetiology. In *Introductory Lectures. The Standard Edition of the Complete Psychological Works of Sigmund Freud*, vol. 16, transl. James Strachey. London: The Hogarth Press.

Freud, Sigmund. [1883] 1975. *Letters of Sigmund Freud*. New York: Basic Books.

Freud, Sigmund. 1991. *Drei Abhandlungen zur Sexualtheorie*. Frankfurt am Main: Fischer Verlag (1965. *Three Essays on the Theory of Sexuality*, transl. and ed. James Strachey. New York: Avon Books, Division of the Hearst Corp.).

Freud, Sigmund. 1999. *Gesammelte Werke*. Frankfurt am Main: Fischer.

Friedland, Roger, and John Mohr. 2004. The cultural turn in American sociology. In *Matters of Culture*, ed. Roger Friedland and John Mohr, 1–68. Cambridge: Cambridge University Press.

Friedrich, Walter. 1981. Die Legende vom genetischen IQ. Marxistisch-Leninistische Philosophie und wissenschaftliches Weltbild. Zum 70. Geburtstag von Walter Hollitscher. *Wissenschaftliche Zeitschrift der Karl-Marx-Universität Leipzig, Gesellschafts- und Sprachwissenschaftliche Reihe* 30: 174–182.

Frith, Uta. 2003. *Autism: Explaining the Enigma*. 2nd ed. Malden: Blackwell.

Frith, Uta, and Christopher D. Frith. 2003. Development and neurophysiology of mentalizing. *Philosophical Transactions of the Royal Society of London: Series B* 358: 459–473.

Fromm, Erich. 1955. *The Sane Society*. New York: Henry Holt.

Fuchs, Thomas. 2006/2007. Neuromythologien. *Scheidewege* 36: 184–202.

Fukuyama, Francis. 1995. *Trust: The Social Virtues and the Creation of Prosperity*. New York: Free Press.

Fullbrook, Edward (Ed.). 2003. *The Crisis in Economics: The Post-autistic Economics Movement: The First 600 Days*. New York: Routledge.

Furedi, Frank. 2004. *Therapy Culture: Cultivating Vulnerability in an Uncertain Age*. London and New York: Routledge.

Gächter, Simon. 2005. Ist Rache wirklich süß? Die Bedeutung der Gefühle für die Wirtschaftswissenschaften. http://wznrw.de/Neuro2005/Dokumentationen/G%C4CHTER%20FORMATIERT.pdf (accessed January 25, 2007).

Gaffin, Dennis. 1995. The production of emotion and social control: Taunting, anger, and the Rukka in the Faeroe Islands. *Ethos* 23: 149–172.

Galbraith, James K. 2001. A contribution to the state of economics in France and the world. *Post-autistic Economics Newsletter* 4. http://www.paecon.net/PAEReview/wholeissues/issue4.htm (accessed March 3, 2007).

Gallese, Vittorio. 2002. The roots of empathy: The shared manifold hypothesis and the neural basis of intersubjectivity. *Psychopathology* 36: 171–180.

Gallese, Vittorio. 2005. Embodied simulation: From neurons to phenomenal experience. *Phenomenology and the Cognitive Sciences* 4: 23–48.

Gallese, Vittorio, Luciano Fadiga, Leonardo Fogassi, and Giacomo Rizzolatti. 1996. Action recognition in the premotor cortex. *Brain* 119, no. 2: 593–609.

Gallese, Vittorio, Christian Keysers, and Giacomo Rizzolatti. 2004. A unifying view of the basis of social cognition. *Trends in Cognitive Sciences 8*, no. 9: 396–403.

Galton, Francis. 1869. *Hereditary Genius*. London: MacMillan.

GAO. 1998. Report to the Subcommittee on Personnel, Committee on Armed Services, U.S. Senate. Military Recruiting: The Department of Defense Could Improve Its Recruiter Selection and Incentive Systems. *GAO-NSIAD-98-58*, January.

Gardener, Helen H. 1893. Sex in brain. [1887]. In idem: *Facts and Fictions of Life*. 97–125. Chicago: Kerr.

Gardner, Beatrice T., and R. Allen Gardner. 1969. Teaching language to a chimpanzee. *Science* 165, no. 894: 664–672.

Gardner, Beatrice T., and R. Allen Gardner. 1975. Early signs of language in child and chimpanzee. *Science* 187, no. 4178: 752–753.

Gardner, Howard. 1983. *Frames of Mind: The Theory of Multiple Intelligences*. New York: Basic Books.

Gardner, Howard. 1999. *Intelligence Reframed*. New York: Basic Books.

Garland, Brent (Ed.). 2004. *Neuroscience and the Law: Brain, Mind, and the Scales of Justice*. New York: Dana Press.

Gaut, Berys. 1999. Identification and emotion in narrative film. In *Passionate Views: Film, Cognition and Emotion*, ed. Carl Plantinga and Greg Smith, 200–217. Baltimore: Johns Hopkins University Press.

Gazzaniga, Michael S. (Ed.). 1995. *The Cognitive Neurosciences*. Cambridge: MIT Press.

Geary, David C. 1998. *Male, Female: The Evolution of Human Sex Differences*. Washington, DC: American Psychological Association.

Geher, Glenn (Ed.). 2005. *Measuring Emotional Intelligence: Common Ground and Controversy*. New York: Nova Science.

Geher, Glenn, and Geoffrey Miller (Eds.). 2007. *Mating Intelligence: Sex, Relationships, and the Mind's Reproductive System*. Mahwah: Lawrence Erlbaum Associates.

Geimer, Peter (Ed.). 2002. *Ordnungen der Sichtbarkeit*. Frankfurt am Main: Suhrkamp.

Gelb, Adhémar, and Kurt Goldstein (Eds.). 1920. *Psychologische Analysen hirnpathologischer Fälle*, vol. 1. Leipzig: Barth.

Geschwind, Norman, and Albert Galaburda. 1985. Cerebral lateralization, biological mechanisms, associations, and pathology: I. A hypothesis and a program for research. *Archive of Neurology* 42: 428–459.

Ghiselin, Michael T. 1974. *The Economy of Nature and the Evolution of Sex*. Berkeley: University of California Press.

Giardini, Angelo, and Michael Frese. 2006. Reducing the negative effects of emotion work in service occupations: Emotional competence as a psychological resource. *Journal of Occupational Health Psychology* 11, no. 1: 63–75.

Gibbs, Nancy. 1995. The E.Q. factor. *Time*, October 2.

Giddens, Anthony. 1979. *Central Problems in Social Theory: Action, Structure and Contradiction in Social Analysis*. Berkeley: University of California Press.

Giddens, Anthony. 1991. *Modernity and Self-Identity: Self and Society in the Late Modern Age*. Cambridge: Polity Press.

Gillberg, Christopher. 1992. The Emanuel Miller Memorial Lecture 1991. Autism and autistic-like conditions: Subclasses among disorders of empathy. *The Journal of Child Psychology and Psychiatry, and Allied Disciplines* 33, no. 5: 813–842.

Glimcher, Paul W. 2003. *Decisions, Uncertainty, and the Brain: The Science of Neuroeconomics*. Cambridge: MIT Press.

Glimcher, Paul W., Michael C. Dorris, and Hannah M. Bayer. 2005. Physiological utility theory and the neuroeconomics of choice. *NIH Public Access Author Manuscript*, http://www.pubmedcentral.nih.gov/articlerender.fcgi?artid=1502377 (accessed January 25, 2007).

Godfrey-Smith, Peter. 1998. *Complexity and the Function of Mind in Nature*. Cambridge: Cambridge University Press.

Goffman, Erving. 1963. *Stigma: Notes on the Management of Spoiled Identity*. Hamondsworth: Pelican.

Gohm, Carol L., Grant C. Corser, and David J. Dalsky. 2005. Emotional intelligence under stress: Useful, unnecessary, or irrelevant? *Personality and Individual Differences* 39, no. 6: 1017–1028.

Golden, Daniel. 2006. *The Price of Admission: How America's Ruling Class Buys Its Way into Elite Colleges—And Who Gets Left Outside the Gates*. New York: Crown Publishers.

Goleman, Daniel. 1995. *Emotional Intelligence: Why It Can Matter More than IQ*. New York: Bantam Books.

Goleman, Daniel. 1996. *Emotional Intelligence: Why It Can Matter More than IQ*. London: Bloomsbury.

Goleman, Daniel. 1997a. *Inteligentzia Rigshit,* transl. Amir Carmeli. Tel Aviv: Matar.

Goleman, Daniel (Ed.). 1997b. *Healing Emotions: Conversations with the Dalai Lama on Mindfulness, Emotions, and Health*. Boston: Shambala.

Goleman, Daniel. 1998. *Working with Emotional Intelligence*. New York: Bantam Books.

Goleman, Daniel. 2006. *Social Intelligence: The New Science of Human Relationships*. New York: Bantam Books (London: Hutchinson).

Goleman, Daniel, Richard Boyatzis, and Annie McKee. 2002. *Primal Leadership: Learning to Lead with Emotional Intelligence*. Boston: Harvard Business School Press.

Gombrich, E. H. 2000. *Art and Illusion: A Study in the Psychology of Pictorial Representation*. Princeton: Princeton University Press.

Gopnik, Alison, and Andrew Meltzoff. 1994. "Minds, bodies, and persons": Young children's understanding of the self and others reflected in imitation and theory of mind research. In *Self-Awareness in Animals and Humans: Developmental Perspectives*, ed. Sue Taylor Parker and Robert W. Mitchell, 166–186. Cambridge: Cambridge University Press.

Gordon, Robert M. 1995. Sympathy, simulation, and the impartial spectator. *Ethics* 105: 727–742.

Goswami, Usha. 2004. Neuroscience, education and special education. *British Journal of Special Education* 31, no. 4: 175–183.

Goswami, Usha. 2006. Neuroscience and education: From research to practice? *Nature Reviews Neuroscience* 7, no. 5: 406–413.

Gottman, John M., Lynn F. Katz, and Carole Hooven. 1997. *Meta-Emotion: How Families Communicate Emotionally*. Mahwah: Lawrence Erlbaum Associates.

Gough, Harisson G. 1957. *California Psychological Inventory*. Palo Alto, CA: Consulting Psychologists Press.

Gould, Stephen Jay. 1982. *The Panda's Thumb: More Reflections in Natural History*. New York: Norton.

Gould, Stephen Jay. 1996. *The Mismeasure of Man*. Rev. and expanded ed. New York: Norton.

Gräb-Schmidt, Elisabeth. 2002. *Technikethik und ihre Fundamente: Dargestellt in Auseinandersetzung mit den technikethischen Ansätzen von Günter Ropohl und Walter Christoph Zimmerli*. Berlin and New York: De Gruyter.

Grandin, Temple, and Catherine Johnson. 2005. *Animals in Translation: Using the Mysteries of Autism to Decode Animal Behavior*. New York: Scribner.

Gray, Jeffrey A. 1995. A model of limbic system and basal ganglia: Applications to anxiety and schizophrenia. In *The Cognitive Neurosciences*, ed. Michael S. Gazzaniga, 1165–1176. Cambridge: MIT Press.

Greely, Henry T. 2004. "Prediction, litigation, privacy, and property": Some possible legal and social implications of advances in neuroscience. In *Neuroscience and the Law: Brain, Mind, and the Scales of Justice*, ed. Brent Garland, 114–156. New York: Dana Press.

Greene, Sheila. 2004. Biological determinism: Persisting problems for the psychology of women. *Feminism and Psychology* 14: 431–435.

Griem, Julika. 2008. *Monkey Business: Affen als Figuren anthropologischer und ästhetischer Reflexion seit 1800*. Freiburg: Rombach (in press).

Griesemer, James R. 2005. The informational gene and the substantial body: On the generalization of evolutionary theory by abstraction. In *Idealization XII: Correcting the Model: Idealization and Abstraction in the Sciences*, ed. Martin R. Jones and Nancy Cartwright. *Pozna Studies in the Philosophy of the Sciences and the Humanities* 86: 59–115. Amsterdam and New York: Rodopi.

Grima, Benedicte. 1992. *The Performance of Emotion among Paxtun Women*. Austin: University of Texas Press.

Groß, Dominik, and Sabine Müller. 2006. Mit bunten Bildern zur Erkenntnis? Neuroimaging und Wissenspopularisierung am Beispiel des Magazins "Gehirn&Geist." In *Farbe—Erkenntnis—Wissenschaft: Zur epistemischen Relevanz von Farbe in der Medizin*, ed. Dominik Groß and Tobias H. Duncker, 77–92. Berlin and Münster: Lit.

Gruber, Malte-Christian. 2006. *Rechtsschutz für nichtmenschliches Leben: Der moralische Status des Lebendigen und seine Implementierung in Tierschutz-, Naturschutz- und Umweltrecht*. Baden-Baden: Nomos.

Grundy, Isobel. 1999. *Lady Mary Wortley Montagu*. Oxford: Oxford University Press.

Guilford, Joy P. 1967. *The Nature of Human Intelligence*. New York: McGraw-Hill.

Habermas, Jürgen. 2004. *Zwischen Naturalismus und Religion: Philosophische Aufsätze*. Frankfurt am Main: Suhrkamp.

Hackbert, Lucianne, and Julia R. Heiman. 2002. Acute dehydroepiandrosterone (DHEA) effects on sexual arousal in postmenopausal women. *Journal of Women's Health & Gender-Based Medicine* 11, no. 2: 155–162.

Hacking, Ian. 1983. *Representing and Intervening*. Cambridge: Cambridge University Press.

Hacking, Ian. 1998. *Rewriting the Soul: Multiple Personality and the Science of Memory*. 2nd and corr. ed. Princeton: Princeton University Press.

Hacking, Ian. 2005. *The Taming of Chance*. Cambridge: Harvard University Press.

Hacking, Ian. 2006. What is Tom saying to Maureen? In *The London Review of Books* (LRB) 28, no. 9: May 11th 2006. http://www.lrb.co.uk/v28/n09/hack01_.html (accessed October 30, 2006).

Haferkamp, Hans, and Neil J. Smelser (Eds.). 1992. *Social Change and Modernity*. Berkeley: University of California Press.

Hagemann, Rudolf. 1988. Der Beitrag der Zwillingsforschung zur Analyse der genetischen Grundlagen der Intelligenzleistung des Menschen. In *Vom Gen zum Verhalten: Der Mensch als biopsychosoziale Einheit*, ed. Erhard Geissler and Herbert Hörz, 33–52. Berlin (East): Akademie-Verlag.

Hagner, Michael. 1994. Lokalisation, Funktion, Cytoarchitektonik: Wege zur Modellierung des Gehirns. In *Objekte, Differenzen, Konjunkturen: Experimentalsysteme im historischen Kontext*, ed. Michael Hagner, Hans-Jörg Rheinberger, and Bettina Wahrig-Schmidt, 121–150. Berlin: Akademie-Verlag.

Hagner, Michael. 1997. *Homo cerebralis: Der Wandel vom Seelenorgan zum Gehirn*. Berlin: Berlin-Verlag.

Hagner, Michael. 2004. *Geniale Gehirne: Die Geschichte der Elitegehirnforschung*. Göttingen: Wallstein.

Haig, David. 2002. *Genomic Imprinting and Kinship*. New Brunswick: Rutgers University Press.

Haig, David. 2004. The inexorable rise of gender and the decline of sex: Social change in academic titles. *Archives of Sexual Behavior* 33, no. 2: 87–96.

Hamann, Stephan. 2005. Sex differences in the responses of the human amygdala. *The Neuroscientist* 11, no. 4: 288–293.

Hamilton, Antonia F. de C., and Anne Krendl. 2007. Overturning stereotypes of and with autism. *Current Biology* 17, no. 6: R641–642.

Happe, Francesca G. E. 1994. An advanced test of theory of mind: Understanding of story characters' thoughts and feelings by autistic, mentally handicapped, and normal children and adults. *Journal of Autism and Developmental Disorders* 24: 129–154.

Haraway, Donna J. 1985. Manifesto for cyborgs. *Socialist Review* 80: 65–108.

Haraway, Donna J. 1989. *Primate Visions: Gender, Race, and Nature in the World of Modern Science.* London and New York: Routledge.

Haraway, Donna J. 1997. *Modest_Wittnes@Second_Millenium. FemaleMan@_Meets_OncoMouseTM.* Feminism and Technoscience. New York and London: Routledge.

Harding, Sandra. 1991. *Whose Science? Whose Knowledge? Thinking from Women's Lives.* Ithaca: Cornell University Press.

Hariri, Ahmad R., Venkata S. Mattay, Allesandro Tessitore, Bhaskar Kolachana, Francesco Fera, David Goldman, Michael F. Egan, and Daniel R. Weinberger. 2002. Serotonin transporter genetic variation and the response of human amygdala. *Science* 297: 400–402.

Harris, Marvin. 2001. *The Rise of Anthropological Theory: A History of Theories of Culture.* Updated ed. Walnut Creek: AltaMira Press.

Harrison, Ted. 1996. *Stigmata: A Medieval Mystery in a Modern Age.* New York: Penguin.

Harrowitz, Nancy A., and Barbara Hyams (Eds.). 1995. *Jews and Gender: Responses to Otto Weininger.* Philadelphia: Temple University Press.

Hartmann, Michael. 2002. *Der Mythos von den Leistungseliten: Spitzenkarrieren und soziale Herkunft in Wirtschaft, Politik, Justiz und Wissenschaft.* Frankfurt am Main: Campus.

Hassan, Robert. 2003. The MIT Media Lab: Techno dream factory or alienation as a way of life? *Media, Culture & Society* 25: 87–106.

Hatcher, Caroline. 2003. Refashioning a passionate manager: Gender at work. *Gender, Work and Organization* 10, no. 4: 391–412.

Hatfield, Elaine, John Cacioppo, and Richard Rapson. 1994. *Emotional Contagion.* Cambridge: Cambridge University Press.

Hathaway, Starke, R., and J. Charnley McKinley. 1942. A multiphasic personality schedule (Minnesota): III. The measurement of symptomatic depression. *Journal of Psychology* 14: 73–84.

Hatzimoysis, Anthony (Ed.). 2003. *Philosophy and the Emotions.* Cambridge: Cambridge University Press.

Hauser, Jens. 2008. Observations on an art of growing interest. In *Tactical Biopolitics: Art, Activism, and Technoscience,* ed. Beatriz DaCosta and Kavita Philip, 83–103. Cambridge: MIT Press.

Hausman, Bernice. 1995. *Changing Sex: Transsexualism, Technology, and the Idea of Gender.* Durham: Duke University Press.

Haviland, John B. 1977. *Gossip, Reputation and Knowledge in Zinacantan.* Chicago: University of Chicago Press.

Haviland-Jones, Jeannette, Holly Hale Rosario, Patricia Wilson, and Terry R. McGuire. 2005. An environmental approach to positive emotions: Flowers. *Evolutionary Psychology* 3: 104–132.

Hayek, Friedrich August von. 1976. *The Sensory Order: An Inquiry into the Foundations of Theoretical Psychology*. Chicago: University of Chicago Press.

Heath, Robert G. 1972. Pleasure and brain activity in man: Deep and surface electroencephalograms during orgasm. *The Journal of Nervous and Mental Disease* 154, no. 1: 318.

Hegarty, Peter, and Felicia Pratto. 2001. Sexual orientation beliefs: Their relationship to anti-gay attitudes and biological determinist arguments. *Journal of Homosexuality* 41, no. 1: 121–135.

Hegel, Georg Wilhelm Friedrich. 1970. *Enzyklopädie der philosophischen Wissenschaften im Grundrisse*. 3rd ed. 1830. Frankfurt am Main: Suhrkamp.

Heidegger, Martin. 1929. *Was ist Metaphysik?* Bonn: Cohen.

Heidegger, Martin. 2005. *Die Grundprobleme der Phänomenologie*. Frankfurt am Main: Klostermann.

Heintz, Kathrin. 2006. Assessing the validity of the Multifactor Leadership Questionnaire: Discussing new approaches to leadership. http://deposit.ddb.de/cgi-bin/dokserv?idn=979242258 (accessed July 27, 2007).

Helmreich, Stefan. 2000. *Silicon Second Nature: Culturing Artificial Life in a Digital World*. Updated ed. with a new preface. Berkeley: University of California Press.

Helmreich, Stefan. 2007. An archaelogy of artificial life, underwater. In *Genesis Redux: Essays in the History and Philosophy of Artificial Life*, ed. Jessica Riskin, 321–333. Chicago: University of Chicago Press.

Herlitz, A., L. G. Nilsson, and L. Backman. 1997. Gender differences in episodic memory. *Memory and Cognition* 25, no. 6: 801–811.

Herrnstein, Richard J., and Charles A. Murray. 1994. *The Bell Curve: Intelligence and Class Structure in American Life*. New York: Free Press.

Hess, Ursula, Arvid Kappas, Gregory J. McHugo, John T. Lanzetta, and Robert E. Kleck. 1992. The facilitative effect of facial expression on the self-generation of emotion. *International Journal of Psychophysiology* 12: 251–265.

Hill, Elisabeth, and Uta Frith. 2003. Understanding autism: Insights from mind and brain. *Philosophical Transactions of the Royal Society of London: Series B* 358: 281–289.

Hill, Elisabeth, and David Sally. 2003. Dilemmas and bargains: Autism, theory-of-mind, cooperation and fairness. http://ssrn.com/abstract=407040 (accessed February 6, 2007).

Hill, Jason. 2000. *Becoming a Cosmopolitan: What It Means to be a Human Being in the New Millenium*. Lanham: Rowman and Littlefield.

Hines, Melissa. 2004. *Brain Gender*. Oxford: Oxford University Press.

Hirschfeld, Lawrence, Elizabeth Bartmess, Sarah White, and Uta Frith. 2007. Can autistic children predict behavior by social stereotypes? *Current Biology* 17, no. 12: 451–452.

Hochschild, Arlie R. 1979. Emotion work, feeling rules, and social structure. *American Journal of Sociology* 85: 551–575.

Hochschild, Arlie R. 1983. *The Managed Heart: Commercialization of Human Feeling*. Berkeley: University of California Press (1990. *Das gekaufte Herz: Zur Kommerzialisierung der Gefühle*, transl. Ernst von Kardorff. Frankfurt/New York: Campus).

Hodgson, Geoffry M. 1993. *Economics and Evolution: Bringing Life Back into Economics*. Ann Arbor: University of Michigan Press.

Hoffmann-Lange, Ursula. 1992. *Eliten, Macht und Konflikt in der Bundesrepublik*. Opladen: Leske + Budrich.

Hogan, Robert, and Louis W. Stokes. 2006. Business susceptibility to consulting fads: The case for emotional intelligence. In *The Emotional Intelligence Bandwagon: The Struggle Between Science and Marketing for the Soul of EI*, ed. Kevin R. Murphy, 263–280. Mahwah: Lawrence Erlbaum Associates.

Holland, Owen, and Rod Goodman. 2003. "Robots with internal models": A route to machine consciousness? In *Machine Consciousness*, ed. Owen Holland, 77–110. Exeter: Imprint Academic.

Hollon, Steven D., and Philip C. Kendall. 1980. Cognitive self-statements in Depression: Development of an automatic thoughts questionnaire. *Cognitive Therapy and Research* 4: 383–395.

Holstege, Gert, Janniko R. Georgiadis, Anne M. J. Paans, Linda C. Meiners, Ferdinand H.C.E. van der Graaf, and A.A.T. Simone Reinders. 2003. Brain activation during human male ejaculation. *The Journal of Neuroscience* 23, no. 27: 9185–9193.

Holstege, Gert, and Janniko R. Georgiadis. 2004. The emotional brain: Neural correlates of cat sexual behavior and human male ejaculation. *Progress in Brain Research* 143: 39–45.

Honegger, Claudia. 1991. *Die Ordnung der Geschlechter: Die Wissenschaften vom Menschen und das Weib 1750–1850*. Frankfurt am Main and New York: Campus.

Honneth, Axel. 1996. *The Struggle for Recognition: The Moral Grammar of Social Conflicts*. Cambridge: MIT Press.

Honneth, Axel. 2005. *Verdinglichung*. Frankfurt am Main: Suhrkamp.

Hosoda, Megumi, and Dianna L. Stone. 2000. Current gender stereotypes and their evaluative content. *Perceptual and Motor Skills* 90, no. 3: 1283–1294.

Huber, Wolfgang. 1996. *Gerechtigkeit und Recht: Grundlinien christlicher Rechtsethik*. Gütersloh: Kaiser, Gütersloher Verlagshaus.

Hubig, Christoph. 1978. *Dialektik und Wissenschaftstheorie*. Berlin and New York: DeGruyter.

Hubig, Christoph. 2006. *Die Kunst des Möglichen I*. Bielefeld: transcript.

Huettel, Scott A., C. Jill Stowe, Evan M. Gordon, Brent T. Warner, and Michael L. Platt. 2006. Neural signatures of economic preferences for risk and ambiguity. *Neuron* 49: 765–775.

Hughes, Jason. 2005. Bringing emotion to work: Emotional intelligence, employee resistance and the reinvention of character. *Work, Employment & Society* 19: 603–625.

Humphrey, Nicholas. 2002. *The Inner Eye: Social Intelligence in Evolution.* Oxford and New York: Oxford University Press.

Hunter, J. E., F. L. Schmidt, and M. K. Judiesch. 1990. Individual differences in output variability as a function of job complexity. *Journal of Applied Psychology* 75: 28–42.

Huschke, Emil. 1854. *Schädel, Hirn und Seele des Menschen und der Thiere nach Alter, Geschlecht und Rasse: Dargestellt nach neuen Methoden und Untersuchungen.* Jena: Mauke.

Hüsing, Bärbel, Lutz Jäncke, and Brigitte Tag (Eds.). 2006. *Impact Assessment of Neuroimaging.* Amsterdam: IOS Press.

Husserl, Edmund. [2nd ed. 1922] 2002. *Ideen zu einer reinen Phänomenologie und phänomenologischen Philosophie.* Tübingen: Max Niemeyer.

Illes, Judy, Matthew P. Kirschen, Kim Karetsky, Megan Kelly, Arnold Saha, Thomas A. Raffin, John E. Desmond, Gary H. Glover, and Scott W. Atlas. 2004. Discovery and disclosure of incidental findings in neuroimaging research. *Journal of Magnetic Resonance Imaging* 20, no. 5: 743–747.

Illouz, Eva. 2008. *Saving the Modern Soul: Therapy, Emotions, and the Culture of Self-Help.* Berkeley: University of California Press.

Imbusch, Peter, and Dieter Rucht. 2007. Wirtschaftseliten und ihre gesellschaftliche Verantwortung. *Aus Politik und Zeitgeschichte* 4–5: 3–10.

Institute of Medicine. 2001. *Exploring the Biological Contributions to Human Health: Does Sex Matter?* Ed. Theresa M. Wizemann and Mary-Lou Pardue. Washington DC: National Academy Press.

International Molecular Genetic Study of Autism Consortium. 1998. A full genome screen for autism with evidence for linkage to a region on chromosome 7q. *Journal for Human Molecular Genetics* 7: 571–578.

Irausquin, Rosemarie S., and Beatrice de Gelder. 1997. Serial recall of poor readers in two presentation modalities: Combined effects of phonological similarity and word length. *Journal of Experimental Child Psychology* 65: 342–369.

Jacobsen, Joyce P. 2007. *The Economics of Gender.* 3rd ed. Malden, Oxford, and Carlton: Blackwell.

Jacoby, Russell, and Nancy Glauberman. 1995. *The Bell Curve Debate: History, Documents, Opinions.* New York: Random House.

James, Nicky. 1989. Emotional labour: Skill and work in the social regulation of feelings. *The Sociological Review* 37, no. 1: 15–42.

James, William. 1884. What is an emotion? *Mind* 9: 188–205.

James, William. 1890. *The Principles of Psychology*. New York: H. Holt (1983. Cambridge: Harvard University Press).

Janich, Peter, and Michael Weingarten. 1999. *Wissenschaftstheorie der Biologie*. Heidelberg: UTB.

Jefferson, Geoffrey. 1949. The mind of mechanical man. The Lister Oration delivered at the Royal College of Surgeons of England. *British Medical Journal* 1: 1105–1121.

Jellonnek, Burkhard, and Rüdiger Lautmann (Eds.). 2002. *Nationalsozialistischer Terror gegen Homosexuelle: Verdrängt und ungesühnt*. Paderborn: Schöningh.

Jensen, Arthur R. 1998. *The g Factor: The Science of Mental Ability*. Westport: Praeger.

Jobe, Lisa E., and Susan Williams White. 2007. Loneliness, social relationships, and a broader autism phenotype in college students. *Personality and Individual Differences* 42, no. 8: 1479–1489.

John, Warren St. 1999. Agent Provocateur. *WIRED* issue 7.09. http://www.wired.com/wired/archive/7.09/brockman.html (accessed June 22, 2006).

Johnson, Mark. 1987. *The Body in the Mind: The Bodily Basis of Meaning, Imagination, and Reason*. Chicago: University of Chicago Press.

Jusserow, Adrie S. 1999. "De-homogenizing American individualism": Socializing hard and soft individualism in Manhattan and Queens. *Ethos* 27, no. 2: 210–234.

Kafetsios, Konstantinos. 2004. Attachment and emotional intelligence abilities across the life course. *Personality and Individual Differences* 37, no. 1: 129–145.

Kaiser, Jocelyn. 2005. Gender in the pharmacy: Does it matter? *Science* 308, no. 5728: 15–73.

Kanazawa, Satoshi, and Griet Vandermassen. 2005. Engineers have more sons, nurses have more daughters: An evolutionary psychological extension of Baron-Cohen's extreme male brain theory of autism. *Journal of Theoretical Biology* 233, no. 4: 589–599.

Kanner, Leo. 1943. Autistic disturbances of affective contact. *Nervous Child* 2: 217–250.

Kant, Immanuel. 1974. *Kritik der Urteilskraft*. In *Werkausgabe in 12 Bänden*, ed. Wolfgang Weischedel, vol. 10, Frankfurt am Main: Suhrkamp.

Karafyllis, Nicole C. 2001. *Biologisch, Natürlich, Nachhaltig: Philosophische Aspekte des Naturzugangs im 21. Jahrhundert*. Tübingen and Basel: A. Francke.

Karafyllis, Nicole C. (Ed.). 2003. *Biofakte—Versuch über den Menschen zwischen Artefakt und Lebewesen*. Paderborn: Mentis.

Karafyllis, Nicole C. 2004. Lebewesen als Programme. Die wissenschaftstheoretische Verflechtung von Life Sciences und Techno Sciences und ihre anthropologische Bedeutung. In *Disziplinen des Lebens: Zwischen Anthropologie, Literatur und Politik*, ed. Ulrich Bröckling, Benjamin Bühler, Marcus Hahn, Matthias Schöning, and Manfred Weinberg, 35–54. Tübingen and Basel: A. Francke.

Karafyllis, Nicole C. 2006a. *Die Phänomenologie des Wachstums*. Habilitationsschrift Philosophy. Stuttgart: University of Stuttgart (completed manuscript) (2008. Bielefeld: transcript, in press).

Karafyllis, Nicole C. 2006b. Notwendigkeit, Möglichkeiten und Grenzen einer Cultural Philosophy of Science. *Erwägen Wissen Ethik / Deliberation Knowledge Ethics* 17, no. 4: 613–633.

Karafyllis, Nicole C. 2007a. Growth of biofacts: The real thing or metaphor? In *Tensions and Convergences: Technological and Aesthetical (Trans)Formations of Society*, ed. Reinhard Heil, Andreas Kaminski, Marcus Stippack, Alexander Unger, and Marc Ziegler, 141–152. Bielefeld: transcript.

Karafyllis, Nicole C. 2007b. "Den Bösen sind sie los, die Bösen sind geblieben." Hegels Bedingungen der Freiheit und die Rolle der Philosophie als Geisteswissenschaft: Ein Lehrstück für aktuelle Bosheiten zur Hirnforschung als PopScience. In *Bilder und Begriffe des Bösen*, ed. Gisela Engel and Malte-Christian Gruber, 59–87. Berlin: trafo.

Karafyllis, Nicole C. 2008a. "Bruno ist tot!" Über die Raubtiernatur des eigenen und des anderen Lebens. In *Ist Technik die Zukunft der menschlichen Natur?*, ed. Armin Grunwald et al. Hannover: Wehrhahn (in press).

Karafyllis, Nicole C. 2008b. Die Medialität pflanzlicher Reproduktion im *Science Fiction*-Film. In *Sexualität als Experiment. Identität, Lust und Reproduktion zwischen Science und Fiction*, ed. Nicolas Pethes and Silke Schicktanz, 365–388. Frankfurt am Main: Campus (in press).

Karafyllis, Nicole C. 2008c. Endogenous Design of Biofacts: Tissues and Networks in Bio Art and Life Science. In *sk-interfaces. Exploding Borders—Creating Membranes in Art, Technology and Society*, ed. Jens Hauser, 43–58. Liverpool: University of Liverpool Press).

Karafyllis, Nicole C. 2008d. Biofacts and bodyshopping. In *Ethical Considerations on Today's Science and Technology: A German–Chinese Approach*, ed. Wenchao Li and Hans Poser. Münster: LIT (in press).

Karafyllis, Nicole C. 2008e. Hybride und Biofakte. Ontologische und anthropologische Probleme der aktuellen Hochtechnologien. In *Herausforderung Technik*, ed. Hans Poser, 195–216. New York, Frankfurt am Main: Peter Lang.

Karafyllis, Nicole C., and Jan C. Schmidt (Eds.). 2002. *Zugänge zur Rationalität der Zukunft*. Stuttgart and Weimar: Metzler.

Katz, Jack. 1999. *How Emotions Work*. Chicago: University of Chicago Press.

Kaufman, Alan S., and James C. Kaufman. 2001. Emotional intelligence as an aspect of general intelligence: What would David Wechsler say? *Emotion* 1, no. 3: 258–264.

Keller, Evelyn Fox. 1995. The origin, history, and politics of the subject called "gender and science"—A first person account. In *Handbook of Science and Technology Studies*, ed. Sheila Jasanoff, Gerald E. Markle, James C. Petersen, and Trevor Pinch, 80–94. Thousand Oaks: Sage.

Keller, Evelyn Fox. 2002. *Making Sense of Life: Explaining Biological Development with Models, Metaphors, and Machines*. Cambridge: Harvard University Press.

Keller, Evelyn Fox. 2005. Revisiting scale-free networks. *BioEssays* 27: 1060–1068.

Keller, Suzanne. 1963. *Beyond the Ruling Class: Strategic Elites in Modern Society*. New York: Random House.

Kenning, Peter, Hilke Plassmann, Michael Deppe, Harald Kugel, and Wolfram Schwindt. 2005. Wie eine starke Marke wirkt. *Harvard Business Manager 3*: 53–57.

Kennison, Shelia M., and Jessie C. Trofe. 2003. Comprehending pronouns: A role for word-specific gender stereotype in information. *Journal of Psycholinguistic Research* 32, no. 3: 355–378.

Kern, Kathi L. 1996. Gray matters: Brains, identities, and natural rights. In *The Social and Political Body*, ed. Theodore R. Schatzki and Wolfgang Natter, 103–121. New York: Guilford.

Kiesow, Rainer Maria, and Martin Korte (Eds.). 2005. *Emotionales Gesetzbuch: Dekalog der Gefühle*. Cologne: Böhlau.

Kiloh, L. G., R. S. Gye, R. G. Rushworth, D. S. Bell, and R. T. White. 1974. Stereotactic amygdaloidotomy for aggressive behaviour. *Journal of Neurology, Neurosurgery, and Psychiatry* 37, no. 4: 437–444.

Kimura, Doreen. 1999. *Sex and Cognition*. Cambridge: MIT Press.

Klinkenborg, Verlyn. 2005. What do animals think? Temple Grandin says animals think like autistic humans. She should know. *Discover* (January 5), http://discovermagazine.com/2005/may/what-do-animals-think (accessed June 12, 2007).

Knorr-Cetina, Karin. 1999. *Epistemic Cultures: How the Sciences Make Knowledge*. Cambridge: Harvard University Press (2002. *Wissenskulturen*. Frankfurt am Main: Suhrkamp).

Knorr-Cetina, Karin. 2005. Culture in global knowledge societies. In *The Blackwell Companion to the Sociology of Culture*, ed. Marc Jacobs and Nancy Weiss Hanrahan, 65–79. Oxford: Blackwell.

Kobayashi, Chiyoko, Gary H. Glover, and Elise Temple. 2007. Children's and adults' neural bases of verbal and nonverbal "theory of mind." *Neuropsychologia* 45: 1522–1532.

Kochinka, Alexander. 2004. *Emotionstheorien: Begriffliche Arbeit am Gefühl*. Bielefeld: transcript.

Köchy, Kristian. 2003. *Perspektiven des Organischen*. Paderborn: Schöningh.

Köchy, Kristian. 2005. Zur Funktion des Bildes in den Biowissenschaften. In *Bild—Zeichen: Perspektiven einer Wissenschaft vom Bild*, ed. Stefan Majetschak, 215–239. Munich: Wilhelm Fink.

Köchy, Kristian, and Gregor Schiemann (Eds.). 2006. *Natur und Labor*. Frankfurt am Main: Vittorio Klostermann.

Koertge, Noretta. 2003. Feminist values and the value of science. In *Scrutinizing Feminist Epistemology: An Examination of Gender in Science,* ed. Cassandra L. Pinnick, Noretta Koertge, and Robert F. Almeder, 222–233. New Brunswick: Rutgers University Press.

Komisaruk Barry R., Beverly Whipple, Sherry Grimes, Audrita Crawford, Wen-Ching Liu, Andrew Kalnin, and Kristine Mosier. 2004. Brain activation during vaginocervical self-stimulation and orgasm in women with complete spinal cord injury: fMRI evidence of mediation by the vagus nerves. *Brain Research* 1024: 77–88.

König, Josef. 1994. Bemerkungen zur Metapher. In *Kleine Schriften,* ed. Josef König, 156–176. Freiburg and Munich: Karl Alber.

Konner, Melvin. 2002. *The Tangled Wing: Biological Constraints and the Human Spirit*. Rev. ed. New York: Henry Holt.

Konnertz, Ursula, Hille Haker, and Dietmar Mieth (Eds.). 2006. *Ethik—Geschlecht—Wissenschaft*. Paderborn: Mentis.

Kosslyn, Stephen M. 1994. *Image and Brain: The Resolution of the Imagery Debate*. Cambridge: MIT Press.

Kourany, Janet A. (Ed.). 2002. *The Gender of Science*. Englewood Cliffs: Prentice Hall.

Kozel, F. Andrew, Kevin A. Johnson, Qiwen Mu, Emily L. Grenesko, Steven J. Laken, and Mark S. George. 2005. Detecting deception using functional magnetic resonance imaging. *Biological Psychiatry* 58, no. 8: 605–613.

Kreimer, Margarete. 2006. Stillstand bei Einkommensunterschied zwischen den Geschlechtern: Zur Notwendigkeit der Erweiterung des ökonomischen Diskriminierungsgesetzes. In *Genus Oeconomicum: Ökonomie—Macht—Geschlechterverhältnisse,* ed. Meike Lemke, Cornelia Ruhe, Marion Woelki, and Béatrice Ziegler, 159–172. Konstanz: UKV.

Krendl, Anne C., Neil Macrae, William M. Kelly, Johanthan A. Fugelsang, and Todd F. Heatherton. 2006. The good, the bad, and the ugly: An fMRI investigation of the functional anatomic correlates of stigma. *Social Neuroscience* 1, no. 1: 5–15.

Kripke, Saul A. 1982. *Wittgenstein on Rules and Private Language*. Cambridge: Harvard University Press.

Kroeger, Matthias, and Kathrin Tartler. 2002. Multifactor Leadership Questionnaire: From the American to the German Culture. In *Organizational Development and Leadership,* ed. Jörg Felfe, 125–140. Frankfurt am Main: Peter Lang.

Krohn, Wolfgang. 2007. Realexperimente—Die Modernisierung der "offenen Gesellschaft" durch experimentelle Forschung. *Erwägen Wissen Ethik / Deliberation Knowledge Ethics* 18, no. 3: 343–365.

Kulick, Don, and Christopher Stroud. 1993. Conceptions and uses of literacy in a Papua New Guinean village. In *Cross-Cultural Approaches to Literacy*, ed. Brian V. Street, 30–61. Cambridge: Cambridge University Press.

Kunda, Gideon, and John van Maanen. 1999. Changing scripts at work: Managers and professionals. *Annals of the American Academy of Political and Social Science* 561, 64–80.

Lakoff, George. 1987. *Women, Fire, and Dangerous Things: What Categories Reveal about the Mind.* Chicago: University of Chicago Press.

Lakoff, George, and Mark Johnson. 1999. *Philosophy in the Flesh: The Embodied Mind and Its Challenge to Western Thought.* New York: Basic Books.

Landy, Frank J. 2005. Some historical and scientific issues related to research on emotional intelligence. *Journal of Organizational Behavior* 26, no. 4: 411–424.

Landy, Frank J. 2006. The long, frustrating, fruitless search for social intelligence. In *The Emotional Intelligence Bandwagon: The Struggle between Science and Marketing for the Soul of EI*, ed. Kevin R. Murphy, 81–124. Mahwah: Lawrence Erlbaum Associates.

Lang, Peter J. 1995. The emotion probe: Studies of motivation and attention. *American Psychologist* 50: 372–385.

Langton, Rae. 2000. The musical, the magical, and the mathematical soul. In *History of the Mind–Body Problem*, ed. Tim Crane and Sarah Patterson, 13–33. London: Routledge.

Laqueur, Thomas. 1990. *Making Sex: Body and Gender from the Greeks to Freud.* Cambridge: Harvard University Press.

Laqueur, Thomas. 2003. *Solitary Sex: A Cultural History of Masturbation.* New York: Zone Books.

Latour, Bruno. 1993. *We Have Never Been Modern.* Cambridge: Harvard University Press.

Latour, Bruno. 2004. *Politics of Nature: How to Bring the Sciences into Democracy.* Cambridge: Harvard University Press.

Latour, Bruno, and Steve Woolgar. 1986. *Laboratory Life: The Construction of Scientific Facts.* 2nd ed. Princeton: Princeton University Press.

Lavie, Smadar. 1990. *The Poetics of Military Occupation: Mzeina Allegories of Bedouin Identity under Israeli and Egyptian Rule.* Berkeley: University of California Press.

Lawson, John, Simon Baron-Cohen, and Sally Wheelwright. 2004. Empathizing and systemizing in adults with and without Asperger syndrome. *Journal of Autism and Developmental Disorders* 34, no. 3: 301–310.

Le Breton, David. 1996. *L'anthropologie de la douleur.* Paris: Editions Metailié.

LeDoux, Joseph E. 1995. In search of an emotional system in the brain: Leaping from fear to emotion and consciousness. In *The Cognitive Neurosciences*, ed. Michael S. Gazzaniga, 1049–1062. Cambridge: MIT Press.

LeDoux, Joseph E. 1996. *The Emotional Brain: The Mysterious Underpinnings of Emotional Life*. New York: Simon & Schuster.

LeDoux, Joseph E. 2002. *Synaptic Self: How Our Brains Become Who We Are*. New York: Viking.

LeDoux, Joseph E., and William Hirst (Eds.). 1986. *Mind and Brain: Dialogues in Cognitive Neuroscience*. New York: Cambridge University Press.

Leicht-Scholten, Carmen (Ed.). 2007. *"Gender and Science": Perspektiven in den Natur- und Ingenieurwissenschaften*. Bielefeld: transcript.

Lemke, Thomas. 2000. Neoliberalismus, Staat und Selbsttechnologien. Ein kritischer Überblick über die governmentality studies. *Politische Vierteljahresschrift* 41, no. 1: 31–47.

Lemke, Thomas. 2001. "The birth of bio-politics"—Michel Foucault's lecture at the Collège de France on neo-liberal governmentality. *Economy & Society* 30, no. 2: 190–207.

Leuner, Barbara. 1966. Emotionale Intelligenz und Emanzipation. *Praxis der Kinderpsychologie und Kinderpsychiatry* 15: 196–203.

LeVay, Simon. 1991. A difference in hypothalamic structure between heterosexual and homosexual men. *Science* 235: 1034–1037.

Lewens, Tim. 2004. *Organisms and Artifacts*. Cambridge: MIT Press.

Lewenstein, Bruce V. (Ed.). 1992. *When Science Meets the Public*. Washington, DC: American Association for Advancement of Science.

Lewenstein, Bruce V. 1997. Communiquer la science au public: L'emergence d'un genre américain, 1820–1939. In *La science populaire dans la presse et l'edition: XIXe et XXe siècles*, ed. Bernadette Bensaude-Vincent and Anne Rassmussen, 143–153. Paris: CNRS-Editions.

Lewis, Michael, Jeannette M. Haviland-Jones, and L. F. Barrett (Eds.). 2008. *Handbook of Emotions*. 3rd ed. New York: Guilford (in press). (2nd ed. 2001).

Lieberman, Leonard. 2001. How "Caucasoids" got such big crania and why they shrank: From Morton to Rushton. *American Anthropologist* 42, no. 1: 69–95.

Lieberman, Matthew D., Ahmad Hariri, Johanna M. Jarcho, Naomi I. Eisenberger, and Susan Y. Bookheimer. 2005. An fMRI investigation of race-related amygdala activity in African-American and Caucasian-American individuals. *Nature Neuroscience* 8: 720–722.

Lilienfeld, Scott O., Steven Jay Lynn, and Jeffrey M. Lohr (Eds.). 2004. *Science and Pseudoscience in Clinical Psychology*. New York: Guilford.

Lo, Andrew W., and Dmitry V. Repin. 2002. The psychophysiology of real-time financial risk processing. *Journal of Cognitive Neuroscience* 14, no. 3: 323–339.

Longino, Helen. 1990. *Science as Social Knowledge: Values and Objectivity in Scientific Inquiry*. Princeton: Princeton University Press.

Loori, Ali A. 2005. Multiple intelligences: A comparative study between the preferences of males and females. *Social Behavior and Personality* 33, no. 1: 77–88.

Lopes, Paulo N., Marc A. Brackett, John B. Nezlek, Astrid Schütz, Ina Sellin, and Peter Salovey. 2004. Emotional intelligence and social interaction. *Personality and Social Psychology Bulletin* 30, no. 8: 1018–1034.

Lopes, Paulo N., Stephane Côté, and Peter Salovey. 2006. An ability model of emotional intelligence: Implications for assessment and training. In *Linking Emotional Intelligence and Performance at Work: Current Research Evidence with Individuals and Groups*, ed. Vannessa U. Druskat, 53–80. Mahwah: Lawrence Erlbaum Associates.

Lorenz, Konrad. 1980. Tiere sind Gefühlsmenschen, *Der Spiegel* 47, November 17: 251–262.

Löther, Andrea. 2006. Von der Studentin zur Professorin: Eine Analyse zum Frauen- und Männeranteil im wissenschaftlichen Qualifikationsprozeß. *Forschung und Lehre* 11: 634–635.

Lovelock, James. 1988. *The Ages of Gaia: A Biography of Our Living Earth*. New York: Norton.

Low, Bobbi S. 2000. *Why Sex Matters: A Darwinian Look at Human Behavior*. Princeton: Princeton University Press.

Luckner, Andreas. 2005. *Klugheit*. Berlin and New York: DeGruyter.

Luhmann, Niklas. 1995. *Social Systems*. Stanford: Stanford University Press.

Lutchmaya, Svetlana, Simon Baron-Cohen, P. Raggatt, Rebecca Knickemeyer, and J. T. Manning. 2004. 2nd to 4th digit ratios, fetal testosterone and estradiol. *Early Human Development* 77: 23–28.

Lutz, Catherine A. 1988. *Unnatural Emotion: Everyday Sentiments on a Micronesian Atoll and Their Challenge to Western Theory*. Chicago: University of Chicago Press.

Lutz, Catherine A., and Lila Abu-Lughod. 1990a. Introduction. In *Language and the Politics of Emotion*, ed. Catherine A. Lutz and Lila Abu-Lughod, 1–23. Cambridge: Cambridge University Press.

Lutz, Catherine A., and Lila Abu-Lughod (Eds.). 1990b. *Language and the Politics of Emotion*. Cambridge: Cambridge University Press.

Lynch, Owen M. (Ed.). 1990. *Divine Passions: The Social Construction of Emotions in India*. Berkeley: University of California Press.

Lynn, Richard. 2006. *Race Differences in Intelligence: An Evolutionary Analysis*. Atlanta: Washington Summit Books.

Lynn, Richard, Paul Irwing, and Thomas Cammock. 2001. Sex differences in general knowledge. *Intelligence* 30, no. 1: 27–39.

Lynn, Richard, and Paul Irwing. 2004. Sex differences on the Progressive Matrices: A meta-analysis. *Intelligence* 32, no. 5: 481–498.

Macha, Hildegard. 2004. Rekrutierung von weiblichen Eliten. *Aus Politik und Zeitgeschichte* 10: 25–33.

Maio, Gregory R., and Victoria M. Esses. 2001. The need for affect: Individual differences in the motivation to approach or avoid emotions. *Journal of Personality* 69: 583–615.

Mäki, Uskali. 2002. Economic ontology: What? Why? How? In *The Economic World View: Studies in the Ontology of Economics*, ed. Uskali Mäki, 3–14. Cambridge: Cambridge University Press.

Manifest der Hirnforscher. 2004. Elf führende Neurowissenschaftler über Gegenwart und Zukunft der Hirnforschung. *Gehirn & Geist* 6: 30–37.

Mansfield, Harvey C. 2006. *Manliness*. New Haven: Yale University Press.

Maravilla, Kenneth R., and Claire C. Yang. 2007. Sex and the brain: The role of fMRI for assessment of sexual function and response. *International Journal of Impotence Research* 19: 25–29.

Marcoulatos, Iordanis. 2003. The secret life of things: Rethinking social ontology. *Journal for the Theory of Social Behaviour* 33, no. 3: 245–278.

Margerison, Charles J. 1987. *Conversation Control Skills for Managers*. London: Mercury Books.

Marshall, Alfred. 1890. *Principles of Economics: An Introductory Volume*. London: Macmillan.

Martin, Emily. 1994. *Flexible Bodies: Tracking Immunity in American Culture from the Days of Polio to the Age of AIDS*. Boston: Beacon Books.

Massaro, Dominic W., and Michael M. Cohen. 2000. Tests of auditory–visual integration efficiency within the framework of the fuzzy logical model of perception. *Journal of the Acoustic Society of America* 108: 784–789.

Mathes, Bettina. 2006. *Under Cover: Das Geschlecht in den Medien*. Bielefeld: transcript.

Matthews, Gerald, Moshe Zeidner, and Richard D. Roberts. 2002. *Emotional Intelligence: Science and Myth*. Cambridge: MIT Press.

Matthews, Gerald, Moshe Zeidner, and Richard D. Roberts (Eds.). 2007. *Science of Emotional Intelligence: Knowns and Unknowns*. New York: Oxford University Press.

Mayer, John D., and Yvonne N. Gaschke. 1988. The experience and meta-experience of mood. *Journal of Personality and Social Psychology* 55: 105–111.

Mayer, John D., and Peter Salovey. 1993. The intelligence of emotional intelligence. *Intelligence* 17, no. 4: 433–442.

Mayer John D., and Glenn Geher. 1996. Emotional intelligence and the identification of emotion. *Intelligence* 22, no. 2: 89–113.

Mayer, John D., David R. Caruso, and Peter Salovey. 1999. Emotional intelligence meets traditional standards for an intelligence. *Intelligence* 27, no. 4: 267–298.

Mayer, John D., David R. Caruso, and Peter Salovey. 2000. Selecting a measure of emotional intelligence: The case for ability scales. In *The Handbook of Emotional Intelligence*, ed. Reuven Bar-On and James D. A. Parker, 320–342. San Fransisco: Jossey-Bass.

Mayer, John D., Peter Salovey, and David R. Caruso. 2000. Models of emotional intelligence. In *Handbook of Intelligence*. , ed. R. J. Sternberg, 396–420. New York: Cambridge Press.

Mayer, John D., Peter Salovey, and David R. Caruso. 2002a. *Mayer–Salovey–Caruso Emotional Intelligence Test (MSCEIT) Item Booklet*. Toronto: MHS Publishers.

Mayer, John D., Peter Salovey, and David R. Caruso. 2002b. *Mayer–Salovey–Caruso Emotional Intelligence Test (MSCEIT) User's Manual*. Toronto: MHS Publishers.

Mayer, John D., Peter Salovey, David R. Caruso, and Gil Sitarenios. 2003. Measuring emotional intelligence with the MSCEIT V2.0. *Emotion* 3, no. 1: 97–105.

Mayer, John D., Richard D. Roberts, and Seigal Barsade. 2008. Human abilities: Emotional intelligence. *Annual Review of Psychology* 59: 507–536.

Maynard-Smith, John. 1982. *Evolution Theory and the Theory of Games*. Cambridge: Cambridge University Press.

Maza, Sarah C. 1993. *Private Lives and Public Affairs: The Causes Célèbres of Prerevolutionary France*. Berkeley: University of California Press.

McCabe, Kevin. 2003. Neuroeconomics. In *Encyclopedia of Cognitive Science*, ed. Lynn Nadel, 294–298. New York: Nature Publishing Group. Macmillian Publishing.

McGhee, Paul E., and Terry Frueh. 1980. Television viewing and the learning of sex-role stereotypes. *Sex Roles* 6: 179–188.

McLaren, Angus. 1990. *A History of Contraception from Antiquity to the Present Day*. Oxford: Blackwell.

McLaren, Angus. 1999. *Twentieth-Century Sexuality*. Oxford: Blackwell.

McMahon, Anthony. 1999. *Taking Care of Men: Sexual Politics in the Public Mind*. Cambridge: Cambridge University Press.

Mehler, Barry. 1997. Raymond B. Cattell and the New Eugenics. *Genetica* 99: 153–163.

Meier, Marietta. 2007. Psychochirurgie: Eingriffe am Gehirn als Massnahme gegen "asoziales" Verhalten 1945–1970. In *Zwang zur Ordnung: Psychiatrie im Kanton Zürich, 1870–1970*, ed. Marietta Meier, Brigitta Bernet, Roswitha Dubach, and Urs Germann, 235–270. Zurich: Chronos.

Meinel, Christoph, and Monika Renneberg (Eds.). 1996. *Geschlechterverhältnisse in Medizin, Naturwissenschaft und Technik*. Bassum, Stuttgart: GNT-Verlag.

Meltzoff, Andrew N. 1990. Towards a developmental cognitive science: The implications of cross-modal matching and imitation for the development of representation and memory in infancy. *Annals of the New York Academy of Sciences* 608: 1–31.

Meltzoff, Andrew N. 1996. "The human infant as imitative generalist": A 20-year progress report on infant imitation with implications for comparative psychology. In *Social Learning in Animals: The Roots of Culture,* ed. Cecilia M. Heyes and Bennett G. Galef, 347–370. San Diego: Academic Press.

Meltzoff, Andrew N., and Jean Decety. 2003. What imitation tells us about social cognition: A rapprochement between developmental psychology and cognitive neuroscience. *Philosophical Transactions of the Royal Society of London: Series B: Biological Sciences,* 358: 491–500.

Menke, Bettine, and Barbara Vinkenly. 2004. *Stigmata: Poetiken der Körperinschrift.* Munich: Wilhelm Fink.

Merleau-Ponty, Maurice. 1962. *Phenomenology of Perception,* transl. Colin Smith. New York: Routledge. (1966. *Phänomenologie der Wahrnehmung,* transl. Rudolf Boehm. Berlin: DeGruyter).

Merleau-Ponty, Maurice. 1996. *Le primat de la perception et ses consequences philosophiques.* Lagrasse: Edition Verdier. (2003. *Das Primat der Wahrnehmung,* transl. Jürgen Schröder. Frankfurt am Main: Suhrkamp).

Metzinger, Thomas. 2004. *Being No One: The Self-Model Theory of Subjectivity.* Cambridge: MIT Press.

Meyer, John, John Boli, Thomas George, and Francisco Ramirez. 1997. World society and the nation–state. *American Journal of Sociology* 103, no. 1: 144–181.

Meyer, Jürgen Bona. 1870. *Philosophische Zeitfragen: Populäre Aufsätze.* Bonn: A. Marcus.

Meyerowitz, Joanne. 2002. *How Sex Changed: A History of Transsexuality.* Cambridge: Harvard University Press.

Miller, Barbara Diane (Ed.). 1993. *Sex and Gender Hierarchies.* Cambridge and New York: Cambridge University Press.

Miller, Peter, and Nikolas Rose. 1990. Governing economic life. *Economy and Society* 19, no. 1: 1–31.

Miller, Peter, and Nikolas Rose. 1995. Production, identity, and democracy. *Theory and Society* 24, no. 3: 427–467.

Millikan, Ruth. 1984. *Language, Thought, and Other Biological Categories.* Cambridge: MIT Press.

Mills, Charles Wright. 1956. *The Power Elite.* New York: Oxford University Press.

Minagar, Alireza, Eduardo Gonzalez-Toledo, James Pinkston, and Stephen L. Jaffe. 2006. Neuro-imaging in multiple sclerosis. *International Review of Neurobiology, Neuroimaging Part B* 67: 165–201.

Minkowski, Eugène. 1927. *La schizophrénie: Psychopathologie des schizoïdes et des schizophrènes.* Paris: Payot.

Minkowski, Eugène. 1933. *Etudes phenomenologiques et psychopathologiques*. Paris: College de l'Evolution Psychiatrique.

Minsky, Marvin. 2006. *The Emotion Machine: Commonsense Thinking, Artificial Intelligence, and the Future of the Human Mind*. New York: Simon & Schuster.

Mises, Ludwig von. 1981. *The Theory of Money and Credit*. Indianapolis: Liberty Fund, transl. H.E. Batson. http://www.econlib.org/library/mises/msT0.html (accessed July 28, 2007).

Mittal, Sandeep, and Peter M. Black. 2006. Intraoperative magnetic resonance imaging in neurosurgery: The Brigham concept. *Acta Neurochirurgica: Supplement* 98: 77–86.

Moir, Anne, and David Jessel. 1992. *Brain Sex: The Real Difference between Men and Women*. New York: Dell.

Moll, Jorge, Frank Krueger, Roland Zahn, Matteo Pardini, Ricardo de Oliveira-Souza, and Jordan Grafman. 2006. Human fronto-mesolimbic networks guide decisions about charitable donations. *Proceedings of the National Academy of Sciences* 103, no. 42: 15623–15628 (http://www.pnas.org/cgi/doi/10.1073/pnas.0604475103).

Moller-Okin, Susan. 1989. *Justice, Gender and the Family*. New York: Basic Books.

Montagu, Lady Mary Wortley. 1997. *Selected Letters,* ed. Isobel Grundy. London: Penguin Books.

Morbeck, Mary E., Allison Galloway, and Adrienne L. Zihlman. 1997. *The Evolving Female: A Life History Perspective*. Princeton: Princeton University Press.

Morris, John. S., M. deBonis, and R. J. Dolan. 2002. Human amygdala responses to fearful eyes. *NeuroImage* 17: 214–222.

Moss, Fred A., and Thelma Hunt. 1930. *Social Intelligence Test*. George Washington University series. Washington, DC: Center for Psychological Service, George Washington University.

Mosse, George L. 1996. *The Image of Man: The Creation of Modern Masculinity*. New York: Oxford University Press.

Muir, Hazel. 2003. Einstein and Newton showed sings of autism. *New Scientist* (April 30). http://www.newscientist.com/article/dn3676.html (accessed September 4, 2007).

Münkler, Herfried. 2006. Vom gesellschaftlichen Nutzen und Schaden der Eliten. In *Deutschlands Eliten im Wandel,* ed. Herfried Münkler, Grit Straßenberger, and Matthias Bohlender, 25–45. Frankfurt am Main: Campus.

Münsterberg, Hugo. 1913. *Psychology and Industrial Efficiency*. Boston: Mifflin.

Münte, Thomas F., Eckart Altenmüller, and Lutz Jäncke. 2002. The musician's brain as a model for neuroplasticity. *Nature Reviews Neuroscience* 3, no. 6: 473–478.

Murphy, Kevin R. (Ed.). 2006. *A Critique of Emotional Intelligence: What Are the Problems and How Can They Be Fixed?* London: Lawrence Erlbaum Associates.

Mutter, Joachim, Johannes Naumann, Rainer Schneider, Harald Walach, and Boyd Hadley. 2005. Mercury and autism: Accelerating evidence. *Neuroendocrinology Letters* 16, no. 5: 431–436.

Myers, Fred R. 1986. *Pintupi Country, Pintupi Self: Sentiment, Place, and Politics among Western Desert Aborigines.* Berkeley: University of California Press.

Nadeau, Robert. 1996. *S/He Brain: Science, Sexual Politics, and the Myths of Feminism.* Westport: Praeger.

Nagel, Thomas. 1970. *The Possibility of Altruism.* London: Oxford University Press.

Nazeer, Kamran. 2003. *Send in the Idiots: Or How We Grew to Understand the World.* London: Bloomsbury.

Negroponte, Nicolas. 2000. From being digital to digital beings. *IBM Systems Journal* 39, no. 3–4: 417–418.

Nelson, Julie. 2001. Why the PAE movement needs feminism. *Post-autistic Economics Newsletter* 9. http://www.paecon.net/PAEtexts/Nelson1.htm (accessed February 3, 2007).

Newberg, Andrew, Abass Alavi, Michael Baime, Michael Pourdehnad, Jill Santanna, and Eugene d'Aquili. 2001. The measurement of regional cerebral blood flow during the complex cognitive task of meditation: A preliminary SPECT study. *Psychiatry Research: Neuroimaging Section* 106: 113–122.

Newberg, Andrew B., and Bruce Y. Lee. 2005. The neuroscientific study of religious and spiritual phenomena: Or why God doesn't use biostatistics. *Zygon* 40, no. 2: 469–489.

Newsome, Shaun, Arla L. Day, and Victor M. Catano. 2000. Assessing the predictive validity of emotional intelligence. *Personality and Individual Differences* 29, no. 6: 1005–1016.

Nieden, Susanne zur. 2005a. Erbbiologische Forschungen zur Homosexualität an der Deutschen Forschungsanstalt für Psychiatrie während der Jahre des Nationalsozialismus. *Ergebnisse des Forschungsprogramms "Geschichte der Kaiser-Wilhelm-Gesellschaft im Nationalsozialismus"* 25.

Nieden, Susanne zur (Ed.). 2005b. *Homosexualität und Staatsräson: Homophobie und Politik in Deutschland, 1900–1945.* Frankfurt am Main: Campus.

Nimchinsky, Esther A., Emmanuel Gillison, John M. Allman, Daniel P. Pearl, Joseph M. Erwing, and Patrick R. Hof. 1999. A neuronal morphologic type unique to humans and great apes. *Proceedings of the National Academy of Sciences* 96, no. 9: 5268–5273.

Noyes, John K. 1997. *The Mastery of Submission: Invention of Masochism.* Ithaca: Cornell University Press.

Nussbaum, Martha C. 1999a. The feminist critique of liberalism. In *Sex and Social Justice*, ed. Martha C. Nussbaum, 55–80. Oxford: Oxford University Press.

Nussbaum, Martha C. 1999b. Objectification. In *Sex and Social Justice*, ed. Martha C. Nussbaum, 213–239. Oxford: Oxford University Press.

Nussbaum, Martha C. 2001 (Reprint 2003). *Upheavals of Thought: The Intelligence of Emotions.* Cambridge: Cambridge University Press.

Nye, Robert A. 1998. *Masculinity and Male Codes of Honor in Modern France.* Berkeley: University of California Press.

Nye, Robert A. (Ed.). 1999. *Sexuality.* Oxford: Oxford University Press.

Oliver, Mary Beth. 1993. Exploring the paradox of the enjoyment of sad films. *Human Communication Research* 19: 315–342.

Oosterhuis, Harry. 2000. *Stepchildren of Nature: Kraft-Ebbing, Psychiatry and the Making of Sexual Identity.* Chicago: University of Chicago Press.

Orland, Barbara (Ed.). 2005. *Artifizielle Körper- Lebendige Technik.* Zurich: Chronos.

Ortner, Sherry B. 1972. Is female to male as nature is to culture? *Feminist Studies* 2: 5–31.

Ortner, Sherry B. 1999. "Thick resistance": Death and the cultural construction of agency in Himalayan mountaineering. In *The Fate of "Culture": Geertz and Beyond*, ed. Sherry Ortner, 136–164. Berkeley: University of California Press.

Ortony, Andrew (Ed.). 1993. *Metaphor and Thought*, 2nd ed. Cambridge: Cambridge University Press.

Ortony, Andrew, and Terence J. Turner. 1990. What's basic about basic emotions? *Psychological Review* 97: 315–331.

Otis, Laura. 1999. *Membranes: Metaphors of Invasion in Nineteenth-Century Literature, Science, and Politics.* Baltimore: Johns Hopkins University Press.

Oudshoorn, Nelly. 1994. *Beyond the Natural Body: An Archaeology of Sex Hormones.* New York: Routledge.

Paglia, Camille. 1990. *Sexual Personae: Art and Decadence from Nefertiti to Emily Dickinson.* New Haven: Yale University Press.

Panksepp, Jaak. 1998. *Affective Neuroscience: The Foundations of Human and Animal Emotions.* Oxford and New York: Oxford University Press.

Panksepp, Jaak. 2003. Feeling the pain of social loss. *Science* 302: 237–239.

Papez, James W. 1927. The brain of Helen Gardener (Alice Chenoweth Day). *American Journal of Physical Anthropology* 11: 29–88.

Park, Kwangsung, Heoung-Keun Kang, Jeong-Jin Seo, Hyung Joong Kim, Soo-Bang Ryu, and Gwang-Woo Jeong. 2001. Blood-oxygenation-level-dependent functional magnetic resonance imaging for evaluating cerebral regions of female sexual arousal response. *Urology* 57: 1189–1194.

Parker, Patricia S., and dt ogilvie. 2003. Gender, culture, and leadership: Towards a culturally distinct model of African-American women executives' leadership strategies. In *Reader in Gender,*

Work and Organization, ed. Robin J. Ely, Erica Gabrielle Foldy, and Maureen Scully, 181–203. Oxford: Blackwell.

Parkinson, Brian, and A. S. R. Manstead. 1992. Appraisal as a cause of emotion. *Review of Personality and Social Psychology* 13: 122–149.

Parnas, Josef, Piérre Bovet, and Dan Zahavi. 2002. Schizophrenic autism: Clinical phenomenology and pathogenic implications. *World Psychiatry* 1, no. 3: 131–136.

Parsons, Talcott. 1977. *Social Systems and the Evolution of Action Theory*. New York: Free Press.

Paul, Annie Murphy. 2004. *Cult of Personality: How Personality Test Are Leading Us to Miseducate Our Children, Mismanage Our Companies, and Misunderstand Ourselves*. New York: Free Press.

Paul, Elizabeth S., Emma J. Harding, and Michael Mendl. 2005. Measuring emotional processes in animals: The utility of a cognitive approach. *Neuroscience and Biobehavioral Reviews* 29: 469–491.

Paulhus, Delroy L., Daria C. Lysy, and Michelle S. M. Yik. 1998. Self-report measures on intelligence: Are they useful as proxy IQ tests? *Journal of Personality* 66, no. 4: 525–554.

Payne, Wayne, L. 1985. *A Study of Emotion: Developing Emotional Intelligence; Self-Integration; Relating to Fear, Pain and Desire (Theory, Structure of Reality, Problem-Solving, Contraction/Expansion, Tuning in/Coming out/Letting Go)*. PhD dissertation, Cincinnati: The Union For Experimenting Colleges And Universities (now The Union Institute).

Payne, Wayne L. 1986. A study of emotion: Developing emotional intelligence; self-integration; relating to fear, pain and desire. *Dissertation Abstracts International 47 (1-A)*, 203.

Pearson, Helen. 2006. Lure of lie detectors spooks ethicists. *Nature* 441, no. 7096: 918–919.

Pentland, Alex P. 2000. Perceptual intelligence. *Communications of the ACM* 43, no. 3: 35–40.

Persaud, Raj. 2004. Faking it: The emotional labour of medicine. *BMJ Career Focus* 329: 87.

Persky, Joseph J. 1995. Retrospectives: The ethology of *Homo economicus*. *Journal of Economic Perspectives* 9, no. 2: 221–231.

Pervin, Lawrence A. 1980. *Personality: Theory, Assessment, and Research*. New York: Wiley.

Petrides, K. V., and Adrian Furnham. 2001. Trait emotional intelligence: Psychometric investigation with reference to established trait taxonomies. *European Journal of Personality* 15, no. 6: 425–448.

Pfeifer, Rolf, and Josh Bongard. 2006. *How the Body Shapes the Way We Think: A New View of Intelligence*. Cambridge: MIT Press.

Phelps, Elizabeth, and Laura A. Thomas. 2003. Race, behavior, and the brain: The role of neuroimaging in understanding complex social behaviors. *Political Psychology* 24, no. 4: 747–758.

Philippi, Anne, Elke Roschmann, Frédéric Tores, Pierre Lindenbaum, Abdel Benajjou, L. Germain-Leclerc, C. Marcaillou, Karine Fontaine, M. Vanpeene, S. Roy, S. Maillard, V. Decaulne, J. P. Saraiva, Peter Brooks, Francis Rousseau, and Jörg Hager. 2005. Haplotypes in the gene encoding protein kinase c-beta (PRKCB1) on chromosome 16 are associated with autism. *Molecular Psychiatry* 10: 950–960.

Philippot, Pierre, Gaëtane Chapelle, and Sylvie Blairy. 2002. Respiratory feedback in the generation of emotion. *Cognition and Emotion* 16: 605–627.

Picard, Rosalind W. 1998. *Affective Computing.* Cambridge: MIT Press.

Picard, Rosalind W. 2000. Toward computers that recognize and respond to user emotion. *IBM Systems Journal* 39, no. 3–4: 705–719.

Picard, Rosalind W., and Charles Q. Du. 2002. Monitoring stress and heart health with a phone and wearable computing. *Offspring* 1, no. 1: 14–22.

Picard, Rosalind W., and Jonathan Klein. 2002. Computers that recognize and respond to user emotion: Theoretical and practical implications. *Interacting With Computers* 14: 141–169.

Pickering, Andrew. 1995. *The Mangle of Practice: Time, Agency, and Science.* Chicago: University of Chicago Press.

Pinch, Adela. 1996. *Strange Fits of Passion: Epistemologies of Emotion, Hume to Austen.* Stanford: Stanford University Press.

Pincus, Tamar, and Stephen Morley. 2001. Cognitive-processing bias in chronic pain: A review and integration. *Psychological Bulletin* 127: 599–617.

Piven, Joseph. 2001. The broad autism phenotype: A complementary strategy for moleculargenetic studies of autism. *American Journal of Medical Genetics* 105: 34–35.

Plantinga, Carl. 1999. The scene of empathy and the human face on film. In *Passionate Views: Film, Cognition and Emotion,* ed. Carl Plantinga and Greg Smith, 239–257. Baltimore: Johns Hopkins University Press.

Plantinga, Carl. 2007. Synästhetische Affekte: Szenarios von Schuld und Scham in Hitchcocks Filmen. In *Audiovisuelle Emotionen: Emotionsdarstellung und Emotionsvermittlung durch audiovisuelle Medienangebote,* ed. Anne Bartsch, Jens Eder, and Kathrin Fahlenbrach, 350–362 Cologne: Herbert von Halem-Verlag.

Plantinga, Carl, and Greg M. Smith (Eds.). 1999. *Passionate Views: Film, Cognition and Emotion.* Baltimore: Johns Hopkins University Press.

Plato. 1961. *The Collected Dialogues of Plato,* ed. Edith Hamilton and Huntington Cairns. *Theaetetus,* 845–919. *Sophist,* 957–1017. Transl. F. M. Cornford, vol. 71 of Bollingen Series. Princeton: Princeton University Press.

Plessner, Helmuth. 1968. *Die Frage nach der Conditio humana.* Frankfurt am Main: Suhrkamp.

Portes, Alejandro. 1998. Social capital: Its origins and applications in modern sociology. *Annual Review of Sociology* 24: 1–24.

Powell, Gary N., Anthony D. Butterfield, and Jane D. Parent. 2002. Gender and managerial stereotypes: Have the times changed? *Journal of Management* 28: 177–193.

Premack, David. 1971. Language in a chimpanzee. *Science* 171: 808–822.

Premack, David, and Guy Woodruff. 1978. Does the chimpanzee have a theory of mind? *Behavioral and Brain Sciences* 4: 515–526.

Priddat, Birger P. 2007. The *affective turn* in economics: Neuroeconomics. In *Neuroökonomie: Neue Theorien zu Konsum, Marketing und emotionalem Verhalten in der Ökonomie*, ed. Birger P. Priddat, 213–224. Marburg: Metropolis.

Prinz, Jesse J. 2006. *Gut Reactions: A Perceptual Theory of Emotion*. Oxford: Oxford University Press.

Pruetz, Jill D., and Paco Bertolani. 2007. Savanna chimpanzees, *Pan troglodytes verus*, hunt with tools. *Current Biology* 17: 412–417.

Putnam, Hilary. 1994. *Words and Life*, ed. James Conant. Cambridge: Harvard University Press.

Putnam, Hilary. 1997. "Fuctionalism": Cognitive science or science fiction? In *The Future of the Cognitive Revolution*, ed. David Martel Johnson and Christina E. Erneling, 32–44. Oxford: Oxford University Press.

Quine, Willard van Orman. 1951. Two dogmas of empiricism. *The Philosophical Review* 60: 20–43.

Quine, Willard van Orman. 1969. *Ontological Relativity and Other Essays*. New York: Columbia University Press.

Racine, Eric, Ofek Bar-Ilan, and Judy Illes. 2005. fMRI in the public eye. *Nature Reviews Neuroscience* 6, no. 2: 159–164.

Radcliff-Browne, Alfred. [1935] 1952. On the concept of function in social science. In *Structures and Functions in Primitive Society: Essays and Addresses*, ed. Alfred Radcliff-Browne, 178–187. London: Cohen and West.

Radner, Daisie, and Michael Radner. 1989. *Animal Consciousness*. Buffalo: Prometheus.

Rammel, Christian. 2002. Sir Isaac Newton, Dr. Pangloss und die unbegrenzte Welt—Neoklassische Ökonomie und Nachhaltige Entwicklung. *Kurswechsel* 4. http://www.iff.ac.at/socec/backdoor/ws03-vose-trans/rammel.pdf (accessed July 24, 2007).

Ravetz, Jerome R. 1990. *The Merger of Knowledge with Power: Essays in Critical Science*. New York and London: Mansell.

Reddy, Kavita S. 2005. Cytogenetic abnormalities and fragile-X syndrome in autism spectrum disorder. *BMC Medical Genetics* 6 (January 18, 2005).

Reddy, William M. 1999. Emotional liberty: History and politics in the anthropology of emotions. *Cultural Anthropology* 14: 256–288.

Reddy, William M. 2001. *The Navigation of Feeling: A Framework for the History of Emotions*. Cambridge: Cambridge University Press.

Reichle, Ingeborg, Steffen Siegel, and Achim Spelten (Eds.). 2007. *Verwandte Bilder: Die Fragen der Bildwissenschaften*. Berlin: Kadmos.

Reiss, Allan L., and Lisa Freund. 1990. Fragile-X syndrome. *Biological Psychiatry* 27: 223–240.

Rhode, Deborah. 2003a. The difference "difference" makes. In *Reader in Gender, Work and Organization*, ed. Robin J. Ely, Erica Gabrielle Foldy, and Maureen Scully, 159–180. Oxford: Blackwell.

Rhode, Deborah (Ed.). 2003b. *The Difference "Difference" Makes: Women and Leadership*. Palo Alto: Stanford University Press.

Richardson, Diane. 2000. *Re-thinking Sexuality*. London: Sage.

Richeson, Jennifer A., Abigail A. Baird, Heather L. Gordon, Todd F. Heatherton, Carrie L. Wyland, Sophie Trawalter, and J. Nicole Shelton. 2003. An fMRI investigation of the impact of interracial contact on executive function. *Nature Neuroscience* 6, no. 12: 1323–1328.

Rick, Scott, and George F. Loewenstein. 2007. The role of emotion in economic behavior. *Social Science Research Network*, http://ssrn.com/abstract=954862 (accessed July 20, 2007).

Ricœur, Paul. 1992. *Oneself as Another,* transl. K. Blamey. Chicago and London: University of Chicago Press.

Rimé, Bernard. 2005. *Le partage social des emotions*. Paris: Presses Universitaires de France.

Rinn, William. 1991. Neuropsychology of facial expression. In *Fundamentals of Nonverbal Behavior*, ed. Robert Feldman and Bernd Rimé, 3–30. Cambridge: Cambridge University Press.

Rist, John M. 1977. *Stoic Philosophy*. Cambridge: Cambridge University Press.

Ritvo, E. R., L. B. Jorde, et al. 1989. The UCLA–University of Utah epidemiology survey of autism recurrence risk estimates and genetic counseling. *The American Journal of Psychiatry* 146: 1032–1038.

Rizzolatti, Giacomo, and Laila Craighero. 2004. The mirror-neuron system. *Annual Review of Neurosience* 27: 169–192.

Roberts, Richard D., Moshe Zeidner, and Gerald Matthews. 2001. Does emotional intelligence meet traditional standards for an intelligence? Some new data and conclusions. *Emotion* 1, no. 3: 196–231.

Roberts, Richard D., Ralf Schulze, Moshe Zeidner, and Gerald Matthews. 2005. Understanding, measuring, and applying emotional intelligence: What have learned? What have missed? In

Emotional Intelligence: An International Handbook, ed. Ralf Schulze and Richard D. Roberts, 311–341. Cambridge: Hogrefe & Huber.

Roberts, Richard D., Ralf Schulze, and Carolyn MacCann (in press). The measurement of emotional intelligence: A decade of progress? In *Handbook of Personality Theory and Assessment*, 2 vols., eds. Gregory J. Boyle, Gerald Matthews, and Donald Saklofske. London: Sage.

Robinson, Michael D. 1998. Running from William James' bear: A review of preattentive mechanisms and their contributions to emotional experience. *Cognition and Emotion* 12: 667–696.

Rodd, Melissa. 2006. Essentialism and mathematical agency: A critique of Simon Baron-Cohen's book "The Essential Difference." *IOWME Newsletter* 20, no. 2 (July). London: International Organisation of Women Mathematics Education.

Roelcke, Voker. 2004. Introduction: Historical perspectives on human subjects research during the 20th century, and some implications for present day issues in bioethics. In *Twentieth Century Ethics of Human Subject Research: Historical Perspectives on Values, Practices and Regulations*, ed. Volker Roelcke and Giovanni Maio, 11–18. Stuttgart: Steiner.

Rolls, Edmund T. 1995. A theory of emotion and consciousness, and its application to understanding the neural basis of emotion. In *The Cognitive Neurosciences*, ed. Michael S. Gazzaniga, 1091–1106. Cambridge: MIT Press.

Romanucci-Ross, Lola, and Laurence Tancredi. 2004. Criminal behaviour and brain imaging techno-science. In *When Law and Medicine Meet: A Cultural View*, ed. Lola Romanucci-Ross and Laurence Tancredi, 61–73, vol. 24, *International Library of Ethics, Law and the New Medicine*. Dordrecht, Boston, London: Kluwer Academic Publishers.

Ropohl, Günter. 1999. *Allgemeine Technologie*. Munich and Vienna: Carl Hanser.

Rorty, Richard. 1995. Is truth a goal of enquiry? Davidson vs. Wright. *Philosophical Quarterly* 45: 281–300.

Rosaldo, Michelle Z. 1980. *Knowledge and Passion: Ilongot Notions of Self and Social Life*. Cambridge: Cambridge University Press.

Rose, Nikolas. 1997. *Inventing Our Selves: Psychology, Power and Personhood*. Cambridge: Cambridge University Press.

Rosenblueth Arturo, Norbert Wiener, and Julian Biegelow. 1943. Behavior, purpose, teleology. *Philosophy of Science* 10: 18–24.

Rosenthal, Elisabeth. 2006. When bad people are punished, men smile (but women don't). *The New York Times* (January 19, 2006).

Rosenthal, Robert, and Bella M. DePaulo. 1979. Sex differences in eavesdropping on nonverbal cues. *Journal of Personality and Social Psychology* 37, 273–285.

Ross, Colin A., and Alvin Pam. 1995. *Pseudoscience in Biological Psychiatry: Blaming the Body*. New York: Wiley.

Ross, Don. 2005. *Economic Theory and Cognitive Science: Microexplanation*. Cambridge: MIT Press.

Ross, Michael, and Diane Holmberg. 1992. Are wives' memories for events in relationships more vivid than their husbands' memories? *Journal of Social and Personal Relationships* 9, no. 4: 585–604.

Rotundo, E. Anthony. 1994. *American Manhood: Transformation in Masculinity from the Revolution to the Modern Era*. New York: Basic Books.

Rouse, Joseph. 1996. Feminism and the social construction of scientific knowledge. In *Feminism, Science, and the Philosophy of Science*, ed. Lynn Hankinson Nelson and Jack Nelson, 195–215. Dordrecht: Kluwer.

Rüdinger, Nikolaus. 1882. Ein Beitrag zur Anatomie der Affenspalte und der internen Interparietalfurche beim Menschen nach Race, Geschlecht und Individualität. In *Beiträge zur Anatomie und Embryologie als Festgabe Jacob Henle zum 4. April 1882 dargebracht von seinen Schülern*. 186–198. Bonn: Cohen.

Rushton, J. Philippe. 2000. *Race, Evolution, and Behavior: A Life History Perspective*. 3rd ed. Port Huron: Charles Darwin Research Institute.

Rushton, J. Philippe. 2003. Race, brain size, and IQ: The case for consilience. *Behavioral and Brain Sciences* 26: 648–649.

Russell, James A. 2003. Core affect and the psychological construction of emotion. *Psychological Review* 110: 145–172.

Russell, James A., Jo-Anne Bachorowski, and José-Miguel Fernández-Dols. 2003. Facial and vocal expressions of emotions. *Annual Review of Psychology* 54: 329–349.

Russett, Cynthia Eagle. 1989. *Sexual Science: The Victorian Construction of Womanhood*. Cambridge: Harvard University Press.

Rustin, Michael. 1991. *The Good Society and the Inner World: Psychoanalysis, Politics and Culture*. London and New York: Verso.

Rutter, Michael. 1978. Diagnosis and definition. In *Autism: A Reappraisal of Concepts and Treatment*, ed. Michael Rutter and Eric Schopler, 1–26. New York: Plenum Press.

Ryback, David. 1998. *Putting Emotional Intelligence to Work: Successful Leadership Is More than IQ*. Woburn: Butterworth-Heinemann.

Sackett, G. P. 1966. Monkeys reared in isolation with pictures as visual input: Evidence for an innate releasing mechanism. *Science* 154: 1468–1473.

Sacks, Oliver. 1995. *An Anthropologist on Mars: Seven Paradoxical Tales*. New York: Knopf.

Saint-Simon, Louis de Rouvroy, Duc de. 1947–1961. *Mémoires*. 7 vols. Paris: Gallimard.

Salovey, Peter, and John D. Mayer. 1990. Emotional intelligence. *Imagination, Cognition, and Personality* 9, no. 3: 185–211.

Salovey, Peter, John D. Mayer, Susan L. Goldman, Carolyn Turvey, and Tibor P. Palfai. 1995. Emotional attention, clarity, and repair: Exploring emotional intelligence using the Trait Meta-Mood Scale. In *Emotion, Disclosure, and Health*, ed. James W. Pennebaker, 125–154. Washington, DC: American Psychological Association.

Salovey, Peter, and John D. Mayer. 1997. What is emotional intelligence? In *Emotional Development and Emotional Intelligence*, ed. Peter Salovey and David J. Sluyter, 3–31. New York: Basic Books.

Sanfey, Alan G., George Loewenstein, Samuel M. McClure, and Jonathan D. Cohen. 2006. Neuroeconomics: Cross-currents in research on decision-making. *Trends in Cognitive Sciences* 10, no. 3: 108–116.

Sano, K., and Y. Mayanagi. 1988. Posteromedial hypothalamotomy in the treatment of violent, aggressive behaviour. *Acta Neurochirurgica (Wien) Suppl.* 44: 145–151.

Sapolsky, Robert M. 1997. *The Trouble with Testosterone: And Other Essays on the Biology of the Human Predicament.* New York: Scribner.

Satzinger, Helga. 1996. Das Gehirn, die Frau und ein Unterschied in den Neurowissenschaften des 20. Jahrhunderts: Cécile Vogt (1875–1962). In *Geschlechterverhältnisse in Medizin, Naturwissenschaft und Technik*, ed. Christoph Meinel and Monika Renneberg, 75–82. Bassum/Stuttgart: Verlag für Geschichte der Naturwissenschaften und der Technik.

Savage-Rumbaugh, E. Sue, Jeannine Murphy, Rose A. Sevcik, Karen E. Brakke, Shelly L. Williams, and Duane M. Rumbaugh. 1993. *Language Comprehension in Ape and Child*, vol. 58 of *Monographs of the Society for Research in Child Development.* Chicago: University of Chicago Press.

Sayer, Andrew. 2005. *The Moral Significance of Class.* Cambridge: Cambridge University Press.

Schein, Louisa. 1999. Performing modernity. *Cultural Anthropology* 14: 361–395.

Schiebinger, Londa. 1993. *Nature's Body: Gender in the Making of Modern Science.* Boston: Beacon Press.

Schiebinger, Londa. 1999. *Has Feminism Changed Science?* Cambridge: Harvard University Press.

Schiemann, Gregor. 2007. *The Loss of Certainty.* New York, Berlin: Springer.

Schmitz, Hermann. 2007. *Der Leib, der Raum und die Gefühle.* Bielefeld and Locarno: Edition Sirius.

Schmitz, Sigrid. 2003. Vom kleinen Unterschied. *Das Magazin* 2, http://www.wz.nrw.de/magazin/inhalt.asp?ausgabe=2003/2&magname=Bildgebende^Verfahren^der^Hirnforschung (accessed July 21, 2007).

Schmitz, Sigrid. 2006a. Frauen- und Männergehirne: Mythos oder Wirklichkeit? In *Geschlechterforschung und Naturwissenschaften: Einführung in ein komplexes Wechselspiel*, ed. Smilla Ebeling and Sigrid Schmitz, 211–234. Wiesbaden: VS-Verlag.

Schmitz, Sigrid. 2006b. Jägerinnen und Sammler: Evolutionsgeschichten zur Menschwerdung. In *Geschlechterforschung und Naturwissenschaften: Einführung in ein komplexes Wechselspiel*, ed. Smilla Ebeling and Sigrid Schmitz, 191–210. Wiesbaden: VS-Verlag.

Schooler, Jonathan, Stellan Ohlsson, and Kevin Brooks. 1993. Thoughts beyond words: When language overshadows insight. *Journal of Experimental Psychology* 122, no. 2: 166–183.

Schooler, Jonathan W., and Stephen M. Fiore. 1997. "Consciousness and the limits of language": You can't always say what you think or think what you say. In *Scientific Approaches to Consciousness*, ed. Jonathan D. Cohen and Jonathan W. Schooler, 241–257. Mahwah: Lawrence Erlbaum Associates.

Schopler, Eric, and Gary B. Mesibov (Eds.). 1992. *High-Functioning Individuals with Autism*. New York: Plenem Press.

Schore, Allan. 1994. *Affect Regulation and the Origin of the Self: The Neurobiology of Emotional Development*. Hillsdale: Lawrence Erlbaum Associates.

Schreibman, Laura. 2005. *The Science and Fiction of Autism*. Cambridge: Harvard University Press.

Schulze, Harri. 1986. *Methodische und methodologische Probleme bei der Erfassung der menschlichen Intelligenz in klassischen Zwillingsstudien*. Dissertation, Karl-Marx-University Leipzig.

Schulze, Ralf, Oliver Wilhelm, and Patrick Kyllonen. 2007. Approaches to the assessment of emotional intelligence. In *Science of Emotional Intelligence: Knowns and Unknowns*, ed. Gerald Matthews, Moshe Zeidner, and Richard D. Roberts, 199–229. New York: Oxford University Press.

Schutte, Nicola S., John M. Malouff, Lena E. Hall, Donald J. Haggerty, Joan T. Cooper, Charles J. Golden, and Liane Dornheim 1998. Development and validation of a measure of emotional intelligence. *Personality and Individual Differences* 25, no. 2: 167–177.

Schütz, Alfred, and Thomas Luckmann. 2003. *Strukturen der Lebenswelt*. Konstanz: UVK.

Schwartz, Marie Jenkins. 2006. *Birthing a Slave: Motherhood and Medicine in the Antebellum South*. Cambridge: Harvard University Press.

Scott, Joan W. 2005. *Parité! Sexual Equality and the Crisis of French Universalism*. Chicago: University of Chicago Press.

Searle, John. 1992. *The Rediscovery of Mind*. Cambridge: MIT Press.

Searle, John. 2004. *Freiheit und Neurobiologie*. Frankfurt am Main: Suhrkamp (2007. *Freedom and Neurobiology: Reflections on Free Will, Language, and Political Power*, transl. Jürgen Schröder. *Columbia Themes in Philosophy*. New York: Columbia University Press).

Searle, John R. 2005. *Mind: A Brief Introduction*. Oxford: Oxford University Press.

Seidlitz, Larry, and Ed Diener. 1998. Sex differences in the recall of affective experiences. *Journal of Personality and Social Psychology* 74, no. 1: 262–271.

Seitz, Rüdiger J., Janpeter Nickel, and Nina P. Azari. 2006. Functional modularity of the medial prefrontal cortex: Involvement in human empathy. *Neuropsychology* 20: 743–751.

Sellner, Judith A., and James G. Sellner. 1991. *Loving for Life: Your Self-Help Guide to a Successful, Intimate Relationship*. North Vancouver: Self-Counsel Press.

Senn, Josianne Bodart. 2004. Le neuromanagement débarque en Suisse. *PME Magazine* 9: 80–83.

Sennett, Richard. 1998. *Corrosion of Character: The Personal Consequences of Work in the New Capitalism*. New York: Norton.

Sennett, Richard. 2006. *The Culture of the New Capitalism*. New Haven and London: Yale University Press.

Sewell, William H., Jr. 1992. A theory of structure: Duality, agency, and transformation. *American Journal of Sociology* 98: 1–29.

Sewell, William H., Jr. 1999. "Geertz, cultural systems, and history": From synchrony to transformation. In *The Fate of "Culture": Geertz and Beyond*, ed. Sherry Ortner, 35–55. Berkeley: University of California Press.

Seyfarth, Robert M. 1987. Vocal communication and its relation to language. In *Primate Societies*, ed. Barbara B. Smuts, Dorothy L. Cheney, Robert M. Seyfarth, Richard W. Wrangham, and Thomas T. Struhsaker, 440–451. Chicago and London: University of Chicago Press.

Shapin, Steven, and Simon Schaffer. 1985. *Leviathan and the Air-Pump: Hobbes, Boyle, and the Experimental Life*. Princeton: Princeton University Press.

Sinclair, Robert C., Curt Hoffman, and Melvin M. Mark. 1994. Construct accessibility and the misattribution of arousal: Schachter and Singer revisited. *Psychological Science: A Journal of the American Psychological Society* 5: 15–19.

Singer, Peter (Ed.). 2005. *In Defense of Animals: The Second Wave*. 4th rev. ed. London: Blackwell.

Singer, Tania, Ben Seymour, John O'Doherty, Holger Kaube, Raymond J. Dolan, and Chris D. Frith. 2004a. Empathy for pain involves the affective but not sensory components of pain. *Science* 303, no. 5661: 1157–1162.

Singer, Tania, Stefan J. Kiebel, Joel S. Winston, Raymond J. Dolan, and Chris D. Frith 2004b. Brain responses to the acquired moral status of faces. *Neuron* 41, no. 4: 653–662.

Singer, Tania, and Ernst Fehr. 2005. The neuroeconomics of mind reading and empathy. *The American Economic Review* 95, no. 2: 340–345.

Singer, Tania, Ben Seymour, John P. O'Dougherty, Klaas E. Stephan, Raymond J. Dolan, and Chris D. Frith. 2006. Empathic neural responses are modulated by the perceived fairness of others. *Nature* 439: 466–469.

Skuse, David H. 2007. Rethinking the nature of genetic vulnerability to autistic spectrum disorders. *Trends in Genetics* 23, no. 8: 387–395.

Smalley, Susan L., Vlad Kustanovich, Sonia L. Minassian, et al. 2002. Genetic linkage of attention-deficit/hyperactivity disorder on chromosome 16p13, in a region implicated in autism. *The American Journal of Human Genetics* 71: 959–963.

Smelser, Neil J. 1998. The rational and the ambivalent in the social sciences. *American Sociological Review* 63, no. 1: 1–16.

Smith, Adam. [1759] 1790. *Theory of Moral Sentiments*. 6th ed. http://www.ibilio.org/ml/libri/S/SmithA_MoralSentiments_p.pdf (accessed August 8, 2006).

Smith, Adam. [1790] 1982. *The Theory of Moral Sentiments*, ed. David D. Raphael and Alexander L. Macfie. Indianapolis: Liberty Classics.

Smith, Greg M. 1999. Local emotions, global moods, and film structure. In *Passionate Views: Film, Cognition and Emotion*, ed. Carl Plantinga and Greg Smith, 103–127. Baltimore: Johns Hopkins University Press.

Smith, Greg M. 2003. *Film Structure and the Emotion System*. Cambridge: Cambridge University Press.

Smith, Jeff 1999. Movie music as moving music: Emotion, cognition, and the film score. In *Passionate Views: Film, Cognition and Emotion*, ed. Carl Plantinga and Greg Smith, 146–168. Baltimore: Johns Hopkins University Press.

Smith, Murray. 1999. Gangsters, cannibals, aesthetes, or apparently perverts allegiances. In *Passionate Views: Film, Cognition and Emotion*, ed. Carl Plantinga and Greg Smith, 217–239. Baltimore: Johns Hopkins University Press.

Smith, Vernon L. 2002. *Constructivist and Ecological Rationality in Economics*. Nobel Prize Lecture. http://nobelprize.org/nobel_prizes/economics/laureates/2002/smith-lecture.pdf (accessed May 29, 2007).

Soares, Angelo. 2003. Tears at work: Gender, interaction, and emotional labor. *Just Labor* 2: 36–44.

Sokolon, Marlene K. 2006. *Political Emotions: Aristotle and the Symphony of Reason and Emotion*. DeKalb: Northern Illinois University Press.

Sommer, Iris E. C., André Aleman, Anke Bouma, and Renée S. Kahn. 2004. Do women really have more bilateral language representation than men? A meta-analysis of functional image studies. *Brain* 127: 1845–1852.

Spearman, Charles. 1904. General intelligence, objectively determined and measured. *American Journal of Psychology* 15, no. 2: 201–293.

Spearman, Charles. 1927. *The Abilities of Man, Their Nature and Measurement*. New York: Macmillan.

Spencer, Lyle M., Jr., and Singe M. Spencer. 1993. *Competence at Work: Models for Superior Performance*. New York: Wiley.

Spencer, Lyle M., Jr., David C. McClelland, and Signe M. Spencer. 1992. *Competency Assessment Methods: History and State of the Art*. Boston: Hay/McBer Research and Innovation Group.

Stanton, William Ragan. 1982. *The Leopard's Spots: Scientific Attitudes toward Race in America, 1815–1859*. Reprint of 1960. Chicago: University of Chicago Press.

Star, Susan L., and James R. Griesemer. 1989. Institutional ecology, "translations," and boundary objects: Amateurs and professionals in Berkeley's Museum of Vertebrate Zoology, 1907–1939. *Social Studies of Science* 19: 387–420 (Reprint 1999. In *The Science Studies Reader*, ed. Mario Biagioli, 505–524. New York: Routledge).

Stearns, Carol Z., and Peter N. Stearns. 1990. Introducing the history of emotion. *Psychohistory Review* 18: 263–291.

Stearns, Peter N. 1994. *American Cool: Constructing a Twentieth-Century Emotional Style*. New York: New York University Press.

Stearns, Peter N., and Jan Lewis (Eds.). 1998. *An Emotional History of the United States*. New York: New York University Press.

Stein, Steven J., and Howard E. Book. 2000. *The EQ Edge: Emotional Intelligence and Your Success*. Toronto: Stoddart.

Steiner, Claude. 1997. *Achieving Emotional Literacy: A Personal Program to Improve your Emotional Intelligence*. New York: Avon Books.

Steinmetzer, Jan, and Sabine Müller. 2007. Zwischen Kundenorientierung und Manipulation: Medizinethische Reflexion zum Neuromarketing. In *Sind die Gedanken frei? Die Neurowissenschaften in Geschichte und Gegenwart*, ed. Dominik Groß and Sabine Müller, 134–142. Berlin: Medizinisch Wissenschaftliche Verlagsgesellschaft.

Stepan, Nancy. 1982. *The Idea of Race in Science: Great Britain, 1800–1960*. London: Macmillan.

Stephan, Inge. 2000. Geniekult und Männerbund: Zur Ausgrenzung des "Weiblichen" in der Sturm- und Drang-Bewegung. *Text und Kritik* 146: 46–54.

Stephan, Inge. 2001. Das Haar der Frau: Motiv des Begehrens, Verschlingens und der Rettung. In *Körperteile: Eine kulturelle Anatomie*, ed. Claudia Benthien and Christoph Wulf, 27–48. Reinbeck/Hamburg: Rowohlt.

Stepper, Sabine, and Fritz Strack. 1993. Proprioceptive determinants of emotional and nonemotional feelings. *Journal of Personality and Social Psychology* 64: 211–220.

Stern, Daniel. 1985. *The Interpersonal World of the Infant: A View from Psychoanalysis and Developmental Psychology*. New York: Basic Books.

Stern, Elsbeth, Roland Grabner, Ralph Schumacher, Christa Neuper, and Henrik Saalbach. 2005. *Lehr-Lern-Forschung und Neurowissenschaften—Erwartungen, Befunde, Forschungsperspektiven*, ed. Bundesministerium für Bildung und Forschung, *Bildungsreform, Band 13*. Bonn, Berlin: Bundesministerium für Bildung und Forschung.

Sternberg, Robert J. 1985. *Beyond IQ: A Triarchic Theory of Intelligence*. Cambridge: Cambridge University Press.

Sternberg, Robert J., Barbara E. Conway, Jerry L. Ketron, and Morty Bernstein. 1981. People's conceptions of intelligence. *Journal of Personality and Social Psychology* 41, no. 1: 37–55.

Stocker, Michael, and Elizabeth Hegeman. 1996. *Valuing Emotions*. Cambridge: Cambridge University Press.

Stocking, George. 1968. *Race, Culture, and Evolution: Essays in the History of Anthropology*. New York: Free Press.

Stocking, S. Holly. 1998. On drawing attention to ignorance. *Science Communication* 20: 165–178.

Stoff, Heiko. 2004. *Ewige Jugend: Konzepte der Verjüngung vom späten neunzehnten Jahrhundert bis ins Dritte Reich*. Cologne: Böhlau.

Stokes, Mark A., and Archana Kaur. 2005. High-functioning autism and sexuality. *Autism* 9: 266–289.

Stolz, Jennifer A., and Derek Besner. 1997. Visual word recognition: Effort after meaning but not (necessarily) meaning after effort. *Journal of Experimental Psychology: Human Perception and Performance* 23: 1314–1322.

Stümke, Hans-Georg. 1989. *Homosexuelle in Deutschland: Eine politische Geschichte*. Munich: Beck.

Sullivan, Mark D. 2001. Finding pain between minds and bodies. *Clinical Journal of Pain* 17: 146–156.

Tague, Ingrid H. 2001. Love, honor, and obedience: Fashionable women and the discourse of marriage in the early eighteenth century. *Journal of British Studies* 40: 76–106.

Tan, Ed S. (Ed.). 1996. *Emotion and the Structure of Narrative Film: Film as an Emotion Machine*, transl. Barbara Fasting. Mahwah: Lawrence Erlbaum Associates.

Tan, Ed S. 2005. Three views of facial expression and its understanding in the cinema. In *Moving Image Theory: Ecological Considerations*, ed. Joseph D. Anderson and Barbara Fisher Anderson, 107–128. Carbondale: Southern Illinois University Press.

Tancredi, Laurence R. 2004. Neuroscience developments and the law. In *Neuroscience and the Law: Brain, Mind, and the Scales of Justice*, ed. Brent Garland, 71–113. New York: Dana Press.

Tanner, Nancy. 1981. *On Becoming Human*. Cambridge: Cambridge University Press.

Tay, Liz. 2007. Finger length could point out technophobia. *Australian PC World*, published May 29, 2007 (http://www.pcworld.idg.com.au/index.php/id;1646444287).

Terada, Rei. 2001. *Feeling in Theory: Emotion after the "Death of the Subject."* Cambridge: Harvard University Press.

Teubner, Gunther. 1988. New industrial policy and the "essence" of the legal person. *The American Journal of Comparative Law* 36: 130–155.

Teubner, Gunther. 2006. Rights of non-humans? Electronic agents and animals as new actors in politics and law. *Journal of Law and Society* 33: 497–521.

Thirion, Bertrand, Philippe Pinel, Sebastien Meriaux, Alexis Roche, Stanislas Dehaene, and Jean Baptiste Poline. 2007. Analysis of a large fMRI cohort: Statistical and methodological issues for group analyses. *NeuroImage* 35, no. 1: 105–120.

Thorndike, Edward L. 1920. Intelligence and its uses. *Harper's Magazine* 140: 227–235.

Tietzel, Manfred. 1981. Die Rationalitätsannahme in den Wirtschaftswissenschaften oder Der homo oeconomicus und seine Verwandten. *Jahrbuch für Sozialwissenschaften* 32: 115–138.

Tiger, Lionel, and Heather T. Fowler (Eds.). 2007. *Female Hierarchies*. New Brunswick: Transaction.

Tomasello, Michael. 1990. Cultural transmission in the tool use and communicatory signaling of chimpanzees? In *"Language" and Intelligence in Monkeys and Apes: Comparative Developmental Perspectives*, ed. Sue T. Parker and Kathleen R. Gibson, 274–311. New York: Cambridge University Press.

Trinidad, Dennis R., and C. Anderson Johnson. 2002. The association between emotional intelligence and early adolescent tobacco and alcohol use. *Personality and Individual Differences* 32, no. 1: 95–105.

Trinidad, Dennis R., Jennifer B. Unger, Chih-Ping Chou, and C. Anderson Johnson. 2004. The protective association of emotional intelligence with psychosocial smoking risk factors for adolescents. *Personality and Individual Differences* 36, no. 4: 945–954.

Tuana, Nancy. 1989. The weaker seed: The secret bias of reproductive theory. In *Feminism and Science*, ed. Nancy Tuana, 147–191. Bloomington: Indiana University Press.

Tucker, William H. 1994. *The Science and Politics of Racial Research*. Urbana: University of Illinois Press.

Tucker, William H. 2002. *The Funding of Scientific Racism: Wickliffe Draper and the Pioneer Fund*. Urbana: University of Illinois Press.

Turing, Alan. 1950. Computing machinery and intelligence. *Mind* 50: 433–460.

Turnbull, Colin. 1965. *Wayward Servants: The Two Worlds of the African Pygmies*. New York: Natural History Press.

Turner, John R. G., and B. Glass. 1976. Genetics, intelligence, and society. *The Quarterly Review of Biology* 51: 85–88.

Ulshöfer, Gotlind. 2001. *Ökonomie und Theologie: Beiträge zu einer prozeßtheologischen Wirtschafts-ethik.* Gütersloh: Kaiser, Gütersloher Verlagshaus.

Ulshöfer, Gotlind. 2003. Biotechnischer Fortschritt als Herausforderung für den *homo oeconomicus.* Wirtschaftsethische Überlegungen. In *Biofakte: Versuch über den Menschen zwischen Artefakt und Lebewesen,* ed. Nicole C. Karafyllis, 121–130. Paderborn: Mentis.

United Nations Educational, Scientific, and Cultural Organization's (UNESCO's) Gender Mainstreaming Implementation Framework (GMIF) for 2002–2007. Brussels: UNESCO. http://unesdoc .unesco.org/images/0013/001318/131854e.pdf (accessed May 26, 2007).

Van Bourgondien, Mary E., Nancy D. Reichle, and Ann Palmer. 1997. Sexual behavior in adults with autism. *Journal of Autism and Developmental Disabilities* 27, no. 2: 113–125.

Van Essen, David C., H. A. Drury, J. Dickson, John Harwell, Donna Hanlon, and Charles H. Anderson. 2001. An integrated software suite for surface-based analyses of cerebral cortex. *Journal of American Medical Informatics Association* 8, no. 5: 199–216.

Veyne, Paul. 2005. Passion, perfection et âme matérielle dans l'utopie stoïcienne et chez saint Augustine. *L'Empire greco-romain,* 683–712. Paris: Seuil.

Vidal, Catherine (Ed.). 2006. *Féminin Masculin: Mythes et Idéologies.* Paris: Belin.

Vidal, Catherine, and Dorothée Benoit-Browaeys. 2005. *Cerveau, sexe et pouvoir.* Paris: Belin.

Vignemont, Frederique de, and Tania Singer. 2006. The empathic brain: How, when and why? *Trends in Cognitive Sciences* 10, no. 10: 435–441.

Villemagne, Victor L., Christopher C. Rowe, S. Macfarlane, K. E. Novakovic, and Colin L. Masters. 2005. Imaginem oblivionis: The prospects of neuroimaging for early detection of Alzheimer's disease. *Journal of Clinical Neuroscience* 12, no. 3: 221–230.

Vogt, Oskar. 1912. Bedeutung, Ziele und Wege der Hirnforschung. *Nord und Süd* 36: 309–314.

Voracek, Martin, and Stefan G. Dressler. 2006. Lack of correlation between digit ratio (2D:4D) and Baron-Cohen's "Reading the Mind in the Eyes" test, empathy, systemizing, and autism spectrum quotients in general population sample. *Personality and Individual Differences* 41, no. 8: 1481–1491.

Voskuhl, Adelheid. 2005. "Bewegung" und "Rührung": Musik spielende Androiden und ihre kulturelle Bedeutung im späten 18. Jahrhundert. In *Artifizielle Körper—lebendige Technik,* ed. Barbara Orland, 87–103. Zurich: Chronos.

Vroomen, Jean, and Beatrice de Gelder. 1995. Metrical segmentation and lexical inhibition in spoken word recognition. *Journal of Experimental Psychology: Human Perception and Performance* 21: 98–108.

Vroomen, Jean, Monique van Zon, and Beatrice de Gelder. 1996. Cues to speech segmentation: Evidence from juncture misperceptions and word spotting. *Memory and Cognition* 24: 744–755.

Wager, Tor D., and Kevin N. Ochsner. 2005. Sex differences in the emotional brain. *Neuroreport* 16, no. 2: 85–87.

Wahrig, Bettina. 2006. Wissenschaftsgeschichte und die Kategorie "Geschlecht." In *Ethik—Geschlecht—Wissenschaft*, ed. Ursula Konnertz, Hille Haker, and Dietmar Mieth, 123–243. Paderborn: Mentis.

Waiter, Gordon, Justin H. G. Williams, Alison D. Murray, Anne Gilchrist, David L. Perrett, and Andrew Whiten. 2004. A voxel-based investigation of brain structure in male adolescents with autistic spectrum disorders. *NeuroImage* 22, no. 2: 619–625.

Wajcman, Judy. 2004. *TechnoFeminism.* Cambridge: Polity Press.

Wallace, B. Alan (Ed.). 2003. *Buddhism and Science: Breaking New Ground.* New York: Columbia University Press.

Walsh, W. Bruce, and Nancy E. Betz. 1985. *Tests and Assessment.* Englewood Cliffs: Prentice Hall.

Walter, Henrik, Birgit Abler, Angela Ciaramidaro, and Susanne Erk. 2005. Motivating forces of human actions: Neuroimaging reward and social interaction. *Brain Research Bulletin* 67: 368–381.

Walzer, Michael. 1983. *Spheres of Justice: A Defense of Pluralism and Equality.* Oxford: Martin Robertson.

Waniak, Eva. 2005. Meaning in gender theory: Clarifying a basic problem from a linguistic-philosophical perspective. *Hypatia* 20, no. 2: 48–68.

Wardhaugh, Benjamin. 2008. Formal causes and mechanical causes: The analogy of the musical instrument in late seventeenth-century natural philosophy. In *Philosophies of Technology: Francis Bacon and His Contemporaries*, ed. Claus Zittel, Gisela Engel, Romano Nanni, and Nicole C. Karafyllis. Boston and Leiden: Brill (in press).

Wassmann, Claudia. 2002. *Die Macht der Emotionen: Wie Gefühle unser Denken und Handeln beeinflussen.* Darmstadt: WBG.

Wassmann, Claudia. 2007. The brain as icon—Reflections on the representation of brain imaging on American television, 1984–2002. In *Tensions and Convergences: Technological and Aesthetical (Trans)Formations of Society*, ed. Reinhard Heil, Andreas Kaminski, Marcus Stippack, Alexander Unger, and Marc Ziegler, 153–162. Bielefeld: transcript.

Weber, Jutta. 2003. *Umkämpfte Bedeutungen: Naturkonzepte im Zeitalter der Technoscience.* Frankfurt am Main: Campus.

Weber, Max. 1956. *Wirtschaft und Gesellschaft.* 4th ed. Tübingen: Mohr.

Wegner, Daniel M. 1997. Why the mind wanders. In *Scientific Approaches to Consciousness*, ed. Jonathan D. Cohen and Jonathan W. Schooler, 295–315. Mahwah: Lawrence Erlbaum Associates.

Wegner, Daniel M., and Daniel B. Gold. 1995. Fanning old flames: Emotional and cognitive effects of suppressing thoughts of a past relationship. *Journal of Personality and Social Psychology* 68: 782–792.

Wehling, Peter. 2006. *Im Schatten des Wissens? Perspektiven der Soziologie des Nichtwissens.* Konstanz: UVK.

Weiler, Bernd. 2006. *Die Ordnung des Fortschritts: Zum Aufstieg und Fall der Fortschrittsidee in der "jungen" Anthropologie.* Bielefeld: transcript.

Weinberg, Richard. 1904–1905. Gehirnform und Geistesentwicklung. *Politisch-anthropologische Revue* 3: 686–698.

Weininger, Otto. 1980. *Geschlecht und Charakter: Eine prinzipielle Untersuchung.* Reprint of 1st ed. Vienna 1903. Munich: Matthes & Seitz.

Weininger, Otto. 2004. *Sex and Character—With Interlinear Translation*, transl. R. Willis. http://www.lulu.com (accessed June 23, 2007).

Weiss, Elisabeth M., Eberhard A. Deisenhammer, Hartmann Hinterhuber, and Josef Marksteiner. 2005. Geschlechtsunterschiede kognitiver Leistungen—Populärwissenschaftliche Stereotypien oder evidenzbasierte Studienergebnisse? *Fortschritte der Neurologie & Psychiatrie* 73, no. 10: 587–595.

Wenzlaff, Richard M., and Danielle E. Bates. 1998. Unmasking a cognitive vulnerability to depression: How lapses in mental control reveal depressive thinking. *Journal of Personality and Social Psychology* 75: 1559–1571.

Wexler, Bruce E. 2006. *Brain and Culture: Neurobiology, Ideology, and Social Change.* Cambridge: MIT Press.

Whiten, Andrew, and Richard W. Byrne (Eds.). 1997. *Machiavellian Intelligence II:* Extensions and Evaluations. Cambridge: Cambridge University Press.

Wiener, Margaret J. 1995. *Visible and Invisible Realms: Power, Magic, and Colonial Conquest in Bali.* Chicago: University of Chicago Press.

Wiener, Norbert. [1948] 1961. *Cybernetics, or: Control and Communication in the Animal and the Machine.* 2nd rev. ed. Cambridge: MIT Press (1963. *Kybernetik. Regelung und Nachrichtenübertragung im Lebewesen und in der Maschine.* 2nd rev. ed. Düsseldorf and Vienna: Econ Verlag).

Wierzbicka, Anna. 1999. *Emotions across Languages and Cultures: Diversity and Universals.* Cambridge: Cambridge University Press.

Wijngaard, Marianne, van den. 1997. *Reinventing the Sexes: The Biomedical Construction of Femininity and Masculinity.* Bloomington: Indiana University Press.

Wikan, Unni. 1989. Managing the heart to brighten face and soul: Emotions in Balinese morality and health care. *American Ethnologist* 16: 294–312.

Wikan, Unni. 1990. *Managing Turbulent Hearts: A Balinese Formula for Living*. Chicago: University of Chicago Press.

Wild, Barbara, Michael Erb, and Mathias Bartels. 2001. Are emotions contagious? Evoked emotions while viewing emotionally expressive faces: Quality, quantity, time course and gender differences. *Psychiatry Research* 102: 109–124.

Willis, Paul E. 1980. *Learning to Labour: How Working Class Kids Get Working Class Jobs*. Farnborough: Saxon House.

Wing, Lorna. 1981. Sex ratio in early childhood autism and related conditions. *Psychiatry Research* 5: 129–137.

Wilson, Edward O. 1978. *On Human Nature*. Cambridge: Harvard University Press.

Wilson, Timothy, and Jonathan W. Schooler. 1991. Thinking too much: Introspection can reduce the quality of preferences and decisions. *Journal of Personality and Social Psychology* 60, no. 2: 181–192.

Wittmann, Axel D., Jens Frahm, and Wolfgang Hänicke. 1999. Magnetresonanz-Tomografie des Gehirns von Carl Friedrich Gauß. *Mitteilungen der Gauß-Gesellschaft* 36: 9–19.

Wolpe, Paul Root. 2004. Ethics and social policy in research on the neuroscience of human sexuality. *Nature Neuroscience* 7, no. 10: 1031–1033.

Woodmansee, Martha. 1984. The genius and the copyright: Economic and legal conditions of the emergence of "the Author." *Eighteenth-Century Studies* 17, no. 4: 425–448.

Wulff, Hans J. 2002. Das empathische Feld. In *Film und Psychologie—Nach der kognitiven Phase?* ed. Jan Sellmer, and Hans J. Wulff, 109–123. Marburg: Schüren Verlag.

Yang, Yaling, Adrian Raine, Todd Lencz, Susan Bihrle, Lori LaCasse, and Patrick Colletti. 2005. Volume reduction in prefrontal gray matter in unsuccessful criminal psychopaths. *Biological Psychiatry* 57, no. 10: 1103–1108.

Yarom, Nitza. 1992. *Body, Blood, and Sexuality: A Psychoanalytic Study of St. Francis' Stigmata and Their Historical Context*. New York: Peter Lang.

Young, Iris Marion. 1990. *Justice and the Politics of Difference*. Princeton: Princeton University Press.

Young, Robert M. 1973. The historiographic and ideological contexts of the nineteenth-century debate on man's place in nature. In *Changing Perspectives in the History of Science: Essays in Honour of Joseph Needham*, ed. Mikuláš Teich, Joseph Needham, and Robert M. Young, 344–438. London: Heinemann.

Young, Robert M. 1990. *Mind, Brain and Adaptation in the Nineteenth Century: Localization and Its Biological Context from Gall to Ferrier*. Cambridge and London: Oxford University Press (Reprint of 1970).

Zahn-Harnack, Agnes. 1928. *Die Frauenbewegung. Geschichte, Probleme, Ziele*. Berlin: Deutsche Buch-Gemeinschaft.

Zak, Paul J. 2004. Neuroeconomics. *Philosophical Transactions of the Royal Society of London: Series B* 359: 1737–1748.

Zak, Paul J. 2007. The neuroeconomics of trust. http://www.neuroeconomicstudies.org/pdf/Zak %20Trust%20chapter%20FINAL.pdf (accessed June 25, 2007); printed version: 2007. *Renaissance in Behavioral Economics*, ed. Roger Frantz, 17–33. New York: Routledge.

Zak, Paul J., Karla Borja, William T. Matzner, and Robert Kurzban. 2005. The neuroeconomics of distrust: Sex differences in behavior and physiology. *American Economic Review, Papers, and Proceedings* 95, no. 2: 360–363.

Zapf, Dieter, Claudia Seifert, Heidrun Mertini, Christoph Voigt, Melanie Holz, E. Vondran, Amela Isic, and Barbara Schmutte. 2000. Emotionsarbeit in Organisationen und psychische Gesundheit. In *Psychologie der Arbeitssicherheit: Beiträge zur Förderung von Sicherheit und Gesundheit in Arbeitssystemen*, ed. Hans-Peter Musahl and Thomas Eisenhauer, 99–106. Heidelberg: Asanger.

Zapf, Dieter, and Melanie Holz. 2006. On the positive and negative effects of emotion work. *European Journal of Work and Organizational Psychology* 15: 1–28.

Zeidner, Moshe, Gerald Matthews, Richard D. Roberts, and Carolyn MacCann. 2003. Development of emotional intelligence: Towards a multi-level investment model. *Human Development* 46, no. 2–3: 69–96.

Zeller, Anne C. 1987. Communication by sight and smell. In *Primate Societies*, ed. Barbara B. Smuts, Dorothy L. Cheney, Robert M. Seyfarth, Richard W. Wrangham, and Thomas T. Struhsaker, 433–439. Chicago and London: University of Chicago Press.

Zerilli, Linda M. G. 1998. Doing without knowing: Feminism's politics of the ordinary. *Political Theory* 26: 435–458.

Ziegenfuss, Jennifer. 2005. Neuromarketing: Evolution of advertising or unethical use of medical technology? *The Brownstone Journal* 12 www.bu.edu/brownstone/issues/12/ziegenfuss.html (accessed August 7, 2007).

Zillmann, Dolf. 1991. Empathy: Affect from bearing witness to the emotions of others. In *Responding to the Screen: Reception and Reaction Processes*, ed. Jennings Bryant and Dolf Zillmann, 135–167. Hillsdale NJ: Lawrence Erlbaum Associates.

Zilsel, Edgar. 1918. *Die Geniereligion: Ein Versuch über das moderne Persönlichkeitsideal mit einer historischen Begründung*. Vienna and Leipzig: Wilhelm Braumüller.

Zilsel, Edgar. 1926. *Die Entstehung des Geniebegriffs: Ein Beitrag zur Ideengeschichte der Antike und des Spätkapitalismus*. Tübingen: Mohr.

Zimmermann, Ralf. 2006. *Neuromarketing und Markenwirkung: Was das Marketing von der modernen Hirnforschung lernen kann*. Saarbrücken: VDM.

Zittel, Claus, Gisela Engel, Romano Nanni, and Nicole C. Karafyllis (Eds.). 2008. *Philosophies of Technology: Francis Bacon and His Contemporaries*. Boston and Leiden: Brill.

Zweigenhaft, Richard L., and G. William Domhoff. 2006. *Diversity in the Power Elite: How It Happened, Why It Matters*. Lanham: Rowman and Littlefield.

About the Authors

Chapter 1

Nicole C. Karafyllis is a philosopher and biologist and Assistant Professor at the Institute of Society and Policy Analysis at Johann Wolfgang Goethe–University Frankfurt/ M. (since 1998), where she teaches Science & Technology Studies and Philosophy. Since finishing her Habilitation (postdoctoral thesis) in Philosophy on *The Phenomenology of Growth: Philosophy of Productive Life between the Concepts of Nature and Technology* (Stuttgart 2006), she also teaches at the Institute of Philosophy at the University of Stuttgart (Germany). In 2008, she was Visiting Professor for Applied Philosophy of Science at the University of Vienna (Austria). Karafyllis studied both biology and philosophy in Erlangen-Nuremberg (Germany), Stirling (UK), Cairo (Egypt), Tübingen, and Frankfurt/M. (Germany). She obtained her doctorate (Dr. rer. nat.) at the Interfacultary Center for Ethics in the Sciences and Humanities at the University of Tübingen (1999); her dissertation on methods of vision-based technology assessment was awarded the Franzke Prize for Technology and Responsibility at the Technical University Berlin 2001. Since 2004 she has been a Permanent Fellow at the Center for Early Modern Studies in Frankfurt/M. Her main areas of research are philosophy of life science and technology, cultural anthropology and societal change, phenomenology and perceptions of nature, biofacts and bioethics, gender studies, history of science and technology, especially Early Modern Era and nineteenth century. Selected publications: 2001. *Biologisch, Natürlich, Nachhaltig. Philosophische Aspekte des Naturzugangs im 21. Jahrhundert*. Tübingen: A. Francke; 2003. *Biofakte—Versuch über den Menschen zwischen Artefakt und Lebewesen* (ed.). Paderborn: Mentis; 2004. *Technikphilosophie im Aufbruch. Festschrift für Günter Ropohl* (ed. with T. Haar). Berlin: edition sigma; 2008 (forthcoming). *Die Phänomenologie des Wachstums*. Bielefeld: transcript; 2008 (forthcoming). *Philosophies of Technology: Francis Bacon and his Contemporaries* (ed. with C. Zittel, R. Nanni and G. Engel). Boston and Leiden: Brill.

Gotlind B. Ulshöfer is a program director for economics, business ethics and gender issues at the Protestant Academy of Arnoldshain, Germany. She teaches economics and business ethics at the Faculty for Economics and Business Administration, and has been lecturer at the Faculty of Social Sciences of the Johann Wolfgang Goethe–University Frankfurt/M. She also taught ethics at the University of Hannover. Ulshöfer holds a doctorate in theological ethics from the University of Heidelberg and was a doctoral fellow at the Interfacultary Center for Ethics in the Sciences and Humanities at the University of Tübingen, where she wrote a dissertation on the relation of theology, economics and economic ethics. She studied economics and Protestant theology at the universities of Tübingen (diploma in economics 1998, diploma in Protestant theology 1994), Heidelberg (Germany), and at the Hebrew University in Jerusalem (Israel). In 1993 she graduated with a Master of Theology from Princeton Theological Seminary (USA). She is also an ordained minister (1st Church exam 1994; 2nd Church exam 2001). She was a visiting scholar at the Beyers-Naudé-Centre at the University of Stellenbosch (South Africa) 2005, and at the Center for Process Studies at Claremont School of Theology (USA) 1996. She is working on a habilitation (postdoctoral thesis) project on "Social Responsibility," which deals with a systematic-theological analysis of social responsibility in a globalized economy. Her areas of research span economics and business ethics, social ethics, gender studies, diaconic theology and finances, public theology, business and society. Selected publications: 2001. *Ökonomie und Theologie. Beiträge zu einer prozeßtheologischen Wirtschaftsethik.* Gütersloh: Gütersloher Verlagshaus; 2004. *Vom Sein zum Sollen und zurück. Zum Verhältnis von Faktizität und Normativität,* ed. with B. Emunds, G. Horntrich, G. Kruip. Frankfurt/M.: Haag and Herchen; 2004. Corporate Social Responsibility in the Context of the European Union—Is an Ethics of Responsibility adequate? In *Pluralism in Europe? Pluralismus in Europa?, Annual Report/ Jahresbericht,* ed. Societas Ethica , 222–235. Paper presented at the 41st annual conference, August 25–29, in Ljubljana, Slovenia; 2005. *Unternehmensleitbild Generationengerechtigkeit—Theorie und Praxis,* ed. with J. Tremmel. Frankfurt/M.: IKO—Verlag für interkulturelle Kommunikation; 2005. *Religion und Theologie im öffentlichen Diskurs. Hermeneutische und ethische Perspektiven* (ed.). Frankfurt/M.: Haag and Herchen; 2007. *Generationengerechtigkeit als Aufgabe von Wirtschaft, Politik und Gesellschaft,* ed. with M. S. Aßländer and A. Suchanek. Munich and Mering: Rainer Hampp.

Chapter 2

Michael Hagner is Professor of Science Studies at the ETH Zurich (Switzerland). Hagner studied medicine and philosophy at the Free University Berlin. After he took his final medical degree (1986), he worked as a neurophysiologist, before turning to history of science in 1989. He was a Visiting Fellow at the Wellcome Institute for the History of Medicine in London and taught at the Medical University in Lübeck and at the Georg August-University Göttingen. In 1995, he moved to the Max Planck Institute for the History of Science, where he worked until 2003. Hagner was invited as a visiting professor at the universities of Salzburg, Tel Aviv, Frankfurt/M., and Cologne. He was a Fellow at the Collegium Helveticum (ETH Zurich) and at the Zentrum für Literatur- und Kulturforschung (Berlin). His current research projects include the history of cybernetics and the role of images in the sciences and humanities. Selected publications: 1995; 2nd ed. 2005. *Der* falsche *Körper. Beiträge zu einer Geschichte der Monstrositäten.* Göttingen: Wallenstein; 1997; pb 2000. *Homo cerebralis. Der Wandel vom Seelenorgan zum Gehirn.* Berlin: Berlin-Verlag; 2004; 2nd ed. 2005. *Geniale Gehirne. Zur Geschichte der Elitegehirnforschung.* Göttingen: Wallstein (French translation in preparation); 2005. *Einstein on the Beach. Der Physiker als Phänomen* (ed.). Frankfurt/M.: S. Fischer; 2006, 2nd ed. 2007. *Der Geist bei der Arbeit. Historische Untersuchungen zur Hirnforschung.* Göttingen: Wallstein; 2008. *Die Transformation des Humanen. Beiträge zur Kulturgeschichte der Kybernetik*, ed. with E. Hörl. Frankfurt/M.: Suhrkamp.

Chapter 3

Robert A. Nye   is Professor of History Emeritus at Oregon State University (USA), and teaches European Intellectual History and History of Sexuality. Nye took History degrees from San Jose State (1964) and the University of Wisconsin (1965, 1969) and taught at the University of Oklahoma for 25 years, becoming a George Lynn Cross Research Professor in 1992. In 1994 he came to Oregon State University where he became the Thomas Hart and Mary Jones Horning Professor of the Humanities and Professor of History. Nye has also taught at Harvard University. He was a Fellow of Churchill College, Cambridge, and has won Fellowships from the National Endowment for the Humanities, the Harry Frank Guggenheim Foundation, and the Rutgers Center for Historical Analysis. He was a Fellow in history at the Australian National University in Canberra in summer 1999. Nye was elected to a three-year term on the editorial board of the American Historical Review, 2003–2006. His research interests are in the history of the social sciences, medicine and society, and sexuality, particularly in France and Great Britain. He is also presently working on a comparative history of the professions as instances of masculine culture, with a special emphasis on medicine. A longer-term project is a complete history of French sexuality since World War

I. Selected publications: 1993. *Masculinity and Male Codes of Honor in Modern France*. New York, Berkeley: University of California Press (pb); 1999. *Sexuality* (ed.). Oxford: Oxford University Press.

Chapter 4

William M. Reddy is W. T. Laprade Professor of History and Professor of Cultural Anthropology at Duke University, NC (USA). He studied history at the University of Chicago (PhD 1974). His awards and honors include Guggenheim Fellowships and Fulbright Fellowships (1987–1988), Directeur d'études associé, Ecole des Hautes Etudes en Sciences Sociales, Paris (1987); Professeur invité, Ecole des Hautes Etudes en Sciences Sociales, Paris (1997). Current areas of research are comparative history of romantic love, emotions and family life in France (1750–1850), history and cultural variability of emotions. Methodological interests include theories of culture, cognitive psychology, and interpretive method. Selected publications: 1997. *The Invisible Code: Honor and Sentiment in Postrevolutionary France 1814–1848*. Berkeley: University of California Press; 2001. *The Navigation of Feeling: A Framework for the History of Emotions*. Cambridge and New York: Cambridge University Press.

Chapter 5

Bärbel Hüsing is coordinator of the business unit Biotechnology and Life Sciences at the Competence Center Emerging Technologies at the Fraunhofer Institute for Systems and Innovation Research (Fraunhofer ISI) in Karlsruhe (Germany). She studied biology at the University of Hannover (Germany), worked as a junior researcher at the Research Centre Jülich GmbH, Jülich (Germany), receiving her doctoral degree at Heinrich-Heine-University Düsseldorf (Germany) in 1991. Since 1991 she has been a Senior Researcher and Project Manager at Fraunhofer ISI, from 1996 to 2007 she was deputy head and head of the departments Innovations in Biotechnology and Emerging Technologies, respectively. Her research areas are scientific innovation analyses, strategic and policy advice regarding emerging technologies, scientific-technical developments and prospective studies in biotechnology, nanotechnology, and neurotechnology, the contribution of emerging technologies to the ability to cope with societal challenges, frame conditions and influencing factors for innovation processes in these technologies, impact and technology assessment in emerging technologies, new technologies in the pharmaceutical industry, medicine and the health care system. The chapter in this book emerged from the project "Impact Assessment of Neuroimaging," commissioned and funded by the Swiss Centre for Technology Assessment TA-SWISS and the

Swiss Academy of Medical Sciences (SAMS), and jointly carried out with L. Jäncke and B. Tag. Selected publications: 2005. Human tissue-engineered products: Potential socio-economic impacts of a new European regulatory framework for authorisation, supervision and vigilance. In *Technical Report EUR 21838 EN*. Brussels: EC (with Bock, A.-K., E. Rodriguez-Cerezo, B. Bührlen, and M. Nusser); 2006. Fallstudien im Forschungsgebiet Life Sciences. In *Gender-Aspekte in der Forschung*, ed. S. Bührer and M. Schraudner. Stuttgart: Fraunhofer IRB Verlag; 2006. *Impact Assessment of Neuroimaging*. Amsterdam: IOS Press (with Jäncke, L., and B. Tag).

Chapter 6

Myriam N. Bechtoldt is Assistant Professor of Work and Organizational Psychology at the University of Amsterdam, Amsterdam (The Netherlands). She studied psychology at the Universities of Frankfurt/M. and Marburg (Germany). In 2004 she completed her training as a family and couples therapist accredited by the German Society of Systemic and Family Therapy (DGSF). She wrote her doctoral thesis on "The relevance of social competence to coping with interpersonal stressors at work" and received her doctorate from Johann Wolfgang Goethe University (Frankfurt/M.) in 2003. Currently she is a member of a European network of scientists funded by the EU that is studying the effects of cultural diversity (http://www.susdiv.org). Specifically, her task is to investigate the effects of personality-related diversity among staff members on organizational creativity and innovation. Other research areas of interest include social competence and emotion regulation. Selected publications: 2003. What is typical for call centre jobs? Job characteristics and service interactions in different call centres. *European Journal of Work and Organizational Psychology* 12, 311–340 (with Zapf, D., A. Isic, and P. Blau); 2004. Die Bedeutung Sozialer Kompetenz für die Bewältigung interpersoneller Stress-Situationen am Arbeitsplatz. Dissertation. http://publikationen. ub.uni-frank-furt.de/volltexte/–2004/—-382/; 2004. Kommunikation in Organisationen. In *Öffentlichkeitsarbeit für Non-Profit*, ed. Gemeinschaftswerk der Evangelischen Publizistik, 247–267. Wiesbaden: Gabler.

Chapter 7

Carolyn MacCann is a postdoctoral researcher at the Center for New Constructs, Educational Testing Service (ETS), Princeton, New Jersey (USA). **Ralf Schulze** is Assistant Professor at the Bergische Universität Wuppertal (Germany). His areas of specialization span the fields of psychometrics, research methods, individual differences, intelligence, and social psychology. **Gerald Matthews** is Professor of Psychology at McMicken College of Arts and Sciences at the University of Cincinnati (USA). **Moshe Zeidner** is past Dean of Research at the University of Haifa (Israel) and Director of the Center for Interdisciplinary Research on Emotions at Haifa University. **Richard D. Roberts** is a Senior Research Scientist at the Center for New Constructs, Educational Testing Service (ETS), Princeton, New Jersey (USA). Selected Publications: 2002. Matthews, G., R. D. Roberts, and M. Zeidner. *Emotional Intelligence: Science and Myth*. Cambridge, MA: MIT Press; 2004. MacCann, C., G. Matthews, R. D. Roberts, and M. Zeidner. The Assessment of Emotional Intelligence: On Frameworks, Fissures, and the Future. In *Measuring Emotional Intelligence. Common Ground and Controversy*, ed. Glenn Geher, 21–52. New York: Nova Science Publication; 2005. Schulze, R., and R. D. Roberts (eds.). *Emotional Intelligence: An International Handbook*. Cambridge: Hogrefe and Huber; 2006. Matthews, G., A. K. Emo, R. D. Roberts, and M. Zeidner. What is this thing called emotional intelligence? In *A Critique of Emotional Intelligence*, ed. K. R. Murphy, 3–36. Mahwah: Lawrence Erlbaum; (in press). Roberts, R.D., R. Schulze, and C. MacCann. The measurement of emotional intelligence: A decade of progress? In *Handbook of Personality Theory and Assessment*, ed. G. Boyle, G. Matthews and D. Saklofske. London: Sage.

Chapter 8

Eva Illouz is Professor for Sociology at the Hebrew University of Jerusalem (Israel). She received her PhD from the University of Pennsylvania (USA) in 1991. Her research interests include the role of culture in social action, the history and sociology of emotions, cultural critique applied to art and popular culture, the role of technology in social and cultural change, and the impact of capitalism on the cultural sphere. Selected publications: 1997. *Consuming the Romantic Utopia. Love and the Cultural Contradictions of Capitalism*. Berkeley: University of California Press (transl. into Hebrew and German); 2002. *The Culture of Capitalism*. Jerusalem: Israel University Broadcast (in Hebrew); 2003. *Oprah Winfrey and the Glamour of Misery: An Essay on Popular Culture*. New York: Columbia University Press; 2006. *Gefühle in Zeiten des Kapitalismus. Adorno-Vorlesungen 2004*. Frankfurt/M.: Suhrkamp; 2008. *Saving the Modern Soul. Therapy, Emotions, and the Culture of Self-Help*. Berkeley: University of California Press.

Chapter 9

Carmen Baumeler is a post-doc in Sociology at the University of Lucerne, Switzerland. She studied sociology, economics, and German literature at the University of

Zurich, Switzerland. After working as a personnel manager in private business for a short time, she returned to research at the ETH Zurich, working on an interdisciplinary project on computer science from 2001 to 2004. There she earned her doctorate with a dissertation on Wearable Computing. In addition she worked on a Swiss study on technology assessment (TA-Swiss) of Pervasive Computing. She teaches sociology at the University of Lucerne. Her main interests are in the fields of Sociology of Science and Technology, Organization Sociology, and Methodology in Social Sciences. Selected publications: 2003. Biotechnologie und Globalisierung: Eine Technikfolgenabschätzung. *Preprints zur Kulturgeschichte der Technik* 18; 2005. *Von kleidsamen Computern und unternehmerischen Universitäten. Eine ethnographische Organisationsstudie.* Münster: LIT; 2006. Die Etablierung der Geschlechterhierarchie im Computerlabor. Interaktionen im wissenschaftlichen Alltag. *Feministische Studien* 2, no. 11: 256–269.

Chapter 11

Kathrin Fahlenbrach   is Assistant Professor in Media Studies at Martin Luther University of Halle (Germany), and co-author **Anne Bartsch** is Research Associate at the Department of Media and Communication Studies at Martin Luther University of Halle (Germany). Fahlenbrach studied German and French Literature in Siegen and Berlin and was awarded a MA for a thesis on postmodernism in German literary critique. From 1996 to 1998 she worked on the research project "The literary system of the GDR" at the *Institute of Media and Communication Studies* at Halle. She received graduate funding from the Government of Sachsen-Anhalt for the years 1998–2000. She obtained her doctorate in media studies in 2000 with a dissertation on visual communication and collective identities in protest movements. In 2008 she finished her postdoctoral thesis (Habilitation) on "Audiovisual Metaphors. Embodied and Emotional Aethetics in Film and Television" ("Audiovisuelle Metaphern. Zur Körper- und Affektästhetik in Film und Fernsehen," Halle 2008). Selected publications: 2005. Aesthetics and Audiovisual Metaphors in Media Perception. In *Comparative literature and culture* 7, no. 4. Lafayette, Ind.: Purdue Univ. Press; 2005. The Emotional Design of Music Videos. Approaches to Audiovisual Metaphors. *Journal of Moving Image Studies* 3, no. 1. Anne Bartsch studied French and German Literature and Media Studies, and received her doctorate in Media and Communication Studies from the University of Halle in 2004 with a dissertation on "Emotional communication—an integrative model." Her current research project deals with gratification that is obtained from the emotions experienced during media use. Research interests: emotional communication, meta-emotion, and emotional gratification during media use. Selected publications: 2006. Emotional gratifications during media use—an integrative approach. *Communications* 31: 261–278 (with Mangold, R., R. Viehoff, and P. Vorderer); 2006. Meta-emotions. *Grazer Philosophische Studien* 73: 136–161 (with Jäger, C.); 2007: *Audiovisuelle Emotionen. Emotiondarstellung und Emotionsvermittlung durch audiovisuelle Medien,* ed. with J. Eder and K. Fahlenbrach. Halem: Cologne.

Chapter 13

Malte-Christian Gruber is a postdoctoral researcher at the Faculty of Law at the Johann Wolfgang Goethe University Frankfurt/M. (Germany). He studied law, philosophy, psychology, and classical philology in Frankfurt/M. and Mainz (successfully completed 1st state exam in 1998, 2nd exam in 2000). He received his doctorate in law (Dr. jur., Institute for Criminology and Philosophy of Law, Frankfurt) in 2005, with a dissertation entitled: "Rechtsschutz für nichtmenschliches Leben" ("Rights of Non-humans"). In 2006 he started working on his postdoctoral thesis (Habilitation) at the Institute of Economic Law in Frankfurt/M. (topic: "Self-Determination and Juridical Reconstruction of Collective Actors on the Basis of Supra-individual Self-Models"). Research interests: private law, philosophy of law, neurophilosophy, legal theory, sociology of law, and bioethics. Selected publications: 2003. Vom Kontinuum der Herkunft ins Kontinuum der Zukunft. Zur Relevanz von Argumenten der Potentialität bei der Bestimmung des rechtlichen Status von Biofakten. In *Biofakte. Versuch über den Menschen zwischen Artefakt und Lebewesen,* ed. N. C. Karafyllis, 131–154. Paderborn: Mentis; 2006. *Rechtsschutz für nichtmenschliches Leben. Der moralische Status des Lebendigen und seine Implementierung in Tierschutz-, Naturschutz- und Umweltrecht.* Baden-Baden: Nomos; 2007. *Bilder und Begriffe des Bösen,* ed. with G. Engel. Berlin: Trafo; 2007. Neuronale Normativität? Neurowissenschaften und Recht jenseits der Debatten um Willensfreiheit und Determinismus. In *Normativität und Rechtskritik,* ed. J. Bung, B. Valerius and S. Ziemann. Stuttgart: Steiner.

Name Index

Acker, Joan, 161–162, 189, 197
Adam, Alison, 325–326
Addison, Joseph, 82–83
Aguer, Hector, 71
Allen, Woody, 166
Angier, Natalie, 20, 298, 306
Aristotle, 32–33, 36, 40, 48n24, 168, 242
Asperger, Hans, 259, 293
Austin, John Langshaw, 87, 95

Bar-On, Reuven, 123, 140, 177n7
Baron-Cohen, Simon, xii, 1–4, 8, 17–21, 28, 40, 46n2, 208, 237–289, 292, 295, 299–305, 313n1, 314n7
Barres, Ben, 272
Bartsch, Anne, viii, xi, 34, 133, 137, 221–237
Bass, Bernhard, 208–209
Bateson, Gregory, 49n33
Baumeler, Carmen, viii, xi, 31, 45, 179–190, 195, 215, 226
Bechtoldt, Myriam N., vii, x, 34, 117–130, 139, 141, 176n3, 182
Becker, Gary S., 194
Bendelow, Gillian, 34
Benedikt, Moritz, 61
Bernays, Martha (later: Martha Freud), 151
Binet, Alfred, 21–22, 40, 42, 133
Bischoff, Theodor Ludwig Wilhelm, 59–61
Bleuler, Eugen, 259
Blumenberg, Hans, 311

Bollnow, Otto Friedrich, 47n20
Boltanski, Luc, 163, 177n11, 181, 191, 193
Bornstein, Kate, 79–80
Bourdieu, Pierre, 19–20, 87, 152, 161–163, 168–169, 209, 257, 270, 294
Briggs, Katherine C., 154
Brizendine, Louann, 1, 8, 20, 29, 46n2, 48n29, 77, 240, 244, 250, 260–262, 298–299, 301
Brockman, John, 44, 303–308, 314n13
Brosnan, Mark, 282–283
Büchner, Ludwig, 60
Burns, James G., 208
Butler, Judith, 13, 86

Caesar, Gaius Julius, 286
Camerer, Colin, 112, 192, 194, 199–200, 207, 213, 217n13
Caplan, Arthur, 285
Carroll, Lewis, 285
Carus, Carl Gustav, 56–57, color plate 6
Caruso, David, x, 156
Cassirer, Ernst, 248, 324–325
Cato, Marcus Portius (the Elder), 82
Cattell, Raymond Bernard, 41, 264
Chaplin, Charlie, 39
Chiapello, Ève, 163, 177n11, 181, 191, 193
Chion, Michel, 231
Chopin, Frédéric, 285
Cloninger, C. Robert, 291
Collins, Randall, 162

Coulter, Jeff, 86

Crary, Jonathan, 99n16

Cronbach, Lee, 119

Cruise, Tom, 277

Dahrendorf, Ralf, 17

Dalai Lama (14th) (Tenzin Gyatso), 43

Damasio, Antonio R., xii–xiii, 29, 32–33, 137, 222–223, 289, 296, 317–328

Darwin, Charles, 28, 34, 40, 60, 76, 205, 217n19, 255, 303, 323

Das, Veena, 86

Daum, Andreas, 295

Dawkins, Richard, 307

Dee, Georgette, 311

Dennett, Daniel C., 99n12, 303, 307–309

Descartes, René, 242

Devor, Holly, 78

Dewey, John, 133

Dickenson, Donna, 9

Djerassi, Carl, 306

Dreger, Alice, 76

Durkheim, Émile, 13, 162

Eastwood, Clint, 274

Edgeworth, Francis Ysidro, 193

Einstein, Albert, x, 255, 299

Ekman, Paul, 6, 34, 38–39, 46n2, 48n33, 272

Elias, Norbert, 85, 99n11

England, Paula, 194

Fahlenbrach, Kathrin, viii, xi, 34, 133, 137, 221–237

Fausto-Sterling, Anne, 29, 72–73, 77

Ferber, Marianne A., 194

Fletcher, Joyce K., 209

Foster, Jodie, 237–238, 277

Foucault, Michel, xi, 74, 179, 183–184, 189, 287, 292, 300

Freud, Sigmund, 32, 151–153, 163, 167, 258, 305–306, 314n5

Furedi, Frank, 171

Galbraith, James K., 193

Galen of Pergamon, 140

Gall, Franz Joseph, 55–56, 58, 68n3

Gallese, Vittorio, 36, 223, 231, 248, 273–274

Galton, Francis, 48n28

Gardener, Helen H., 61, 65

Gardner, Howard, 34, 119, 133–135, 155, 176n4, 264

Gates, Bill, 285

Gaut, Berys, 232–233

Gelder, Beatrice de, 88

Giddens, Anthony, 87, 169, 258

Ginsburg, Ruth Bader, 70

Glimcher, Paul, 213–214

Goffman, Erving, 25

Goleman, Daniel, xiv, 1, 5–11, 16, 20–21, 28, 33, 39, 43, 45n1, 46n2, 46n5, 117, 121–124, 128, 134–137, 147, 155, 164, 179, 182–185, 189, 196, 207–208, 239, 275, 262–265, 271, 274–277, 281, 286, 291, 297, 300–309, 314n10, 318, 321

Gordon, Robert M., 99n16

Grandin, Temple, 254, 270–273, 288, 299

Gruber, Malte-Christian, viii, xii, 8, 85, 317–328

Habermas, Jürgen, 308

Hacking, Ian, x, 22–23, 42, 99n12, 240, 243, 247–249, 255, 257, 263, 287, 290–298

Hagner, Michael, vii, x, xiv, 4, 7, 21, 41, 53–68, 72, 104, 210, 255, 299, 306

Haig, David, 69, 77

Hammond, William, 65

Hanks, Tom, 238

Haraway, Donna, 9, 30

Hartmann, Michael, 19

Hawking, Steven, 286

Hayek, Friedrich August von, 217n19

Hegel, Georg Wilhelm Friedrich, 32, 48n23, 272

Heidegger, Martin, 47n20, 246, 309–310

Helmreich, Stefan, 305, 307, 311n2

Herrnstein, Richard J., 121–123, 264

Hill, Jason, 314n17
Hines, Melissa, 8, 29, 243, 295
Hippocrates of Kos, 140
Hochschild, Arlie Russell, 38, 95, 100n29,
   177n10, 196, 226, 256, 302
Hoffman, Dustin, 237, 277
Homer, 242
Honneth, Axel, xii, 176, 217n16, 259
Hüsing, Bärbel, vii, x, 30, 78, 103–116, 191,
   319
Humboldt, Alexander von, 295
Hunt, Helen 237, 277
Huschke, Emil, 58–60
Husserl, Edmund, 31

Illes, Judy, 103, 109, 113–114
Illouz, Eva, viii, xi, xiv, 7, 19, 122, 137,
   151–177, 181, 189, 238, 296

James, Nicky, 38
James, William, 32–33, 133
Johnson, Mark, 5, 47n18, 232, 252

Kahneman, Daniel, 194, 216n5
Kanner, Leo, 259, 288, 293
Kant, Immanuel, 60, 272, 276
Karafyllis, Nicole C., vii–viii, xii, 1–49, 87,
   193, 208, 215, 223, 237–315, 321
Keller, Evelyn Fox, 7, 11–12, 279
Keller, Suzanne, 16–17
Kimura, Doreen, 2, 38, 46n2, 241, 283, 288
Knorr-Cetina, Karin, 5, 153, 240
Koertge, Noretta, 40–44, 48n33
Kosslyn, Stephen, 88–89, 324
Kourany, Janet A., 9
Krafft-Ebing, Richard von, 75
Krendl, Anne C., 22–27, 256, 278, color
   plates 4–5
Kunda, Gideon, 180

Lakoff, George, 5, 47n18, 232, 252
Langley, John Newport, 242
Laqueur, Thomas, 74–75

Lenin, Wladimir Iljitsch, 66
Leuner, Barbara, 134
Lewenstein, Bruce V., 295
Liebig, Justus von, 61, color plate 9
Longino, Helen, 44
Lovelock, James, 304

Maanen, John van, 180
MacCann, Carolyn, vii, xi, 18, 131–148, 208,
   262
McLaren, Angus, 73, 79
McMahon, Anthony, 256
Margulis, Lynn, 306
Marshall, Alfred, 217n19
Marx, Karl, 167, 217n16, 305–306
Matthews, Gerald, vii, xi, 18, 124, 131–148,
   183, 208, 262
Mayer, John ("Jack") D., x, xiii, 34, 117–118,
   123, 125, 134, 140, 142, 146, 156–160,
   176n3, 236n2
Mead, Margaret, 48n33, 77
Meltzoff, Andrew, 247, 323
Menezes, Marta de, 13
Merleau-Ponty, Maurice, 32, 47n21
Metzinger, Thomas, 320, 324
Meyer, John, 164–165
Meyer, Jürgen Bona, 60
Mills, Charles Wright, 16, 210
Minsky, Marvin, 7, 297
Mises, Ludwig von, 216n11
Money, John, 77
Montagu, Edward Mortley, 83–85, 97
Mother Teresa, 301
Münsterberg, Hugo, 176
Murray, Charles, 121–123, 264
Myers, Isabel, 154

Negroponte, Nicolas, 185, 283
Nelson, Julie A., 194
Newberg, Andrew, 43, 308
Newton, Isaac, 255
Nichols, Shona, 300
Nicholson, Jack, 237–238, 277, 291

Nussbaum, Martha, 33, 47n11, 48n24, 202, 217n16, 323
Nye, Robert A., vii, x, 36, 48n27, 69–80, 244, 255, 276, 283

Paglia, Camille, 285
Parsons, Talcott, 77
Payne, Wayne Leon, 117, 134
Pentland, Alex P., 186
Picard, Rosalind W., xiv, 185–188
Pierrepont, Lady Mary, 82–83, 85, 97
Pinker, Steven, 303
Plantinga, Carl, 221–222, 229, 232–233
Plato, 324
Pope Benedict XVI, 71
Pope John Paul II, 70
Portes, Alejandro, 163
Putnam, Hilary, 86, 99n14

Quine, Willard van Orman, 90, 99n25, 246

Reddy, William M., vii, x, 9, 34, 74, 81–100, 126, 163, 228, 232, 276, 321
Ricœur, Paul, xii, 6, 245, 324
Roberts, Richard, vii, xi, xiii, 18, 124, 131–148, 183, 208, 262
Roth, Gerhard, 299
Rüdinger, Nikolaus, 61–64, color plates 7–9
Rushton, J. Philippe, 41
Rustin, Michael, 168–169

Sacks, Oliver, 270, 288
Salovey, Peter, x, 34, 117–118, 125, 134, 140, 142, 156, 176n3, 222, 236n2
Sapolsky, Robert M., 29
Sayer, Andrew, 168
Scalia, Antonin, 70
Schaffer, Simon, 86, 88
Schiebinger, Londa, 9, 56, 72, 243, 253
Schiller, Friedrich, x, 57, color plate 6
Schmitz, Hermann, 32
Schmitz, Sigrid, 2, 41, 201, 269
Schooler, Jonathan, 90, 159–160

Schulze, Ralf, vii, xi, 18, 131–148, 208, 262
Sennett, Richard, 180, 195–196
Shaftesbury, Earl of, 81–82
Shapin, Steven, 86, 88
Simon, Théodore, 21
Singer, Peter, 273
Singer, Tania, xiv, 3–4, 14–16, 37–39, 48n30, 48n31, 193, 202–207, 260, 273, 319, color plates 1–3
Smith, Adam, 212–213, 217n19
Smith, Greg M., 228
Smith, Vernon, 194, 198
Spearman, Charles, 118–119, 122, 132
Špidla, Vladimir, 18
Sternberg, Robert J., 120–122, 137
Stocking, S. Holly, 294
Summers, Lawrence Henry ("Larry"), 53–54, 72, 272, 306–307

Talleyrand, Charles-Maurice de, 57, color plate 6
Theophrast, 286
Thorndike, Edward Bob, 118–119, 133
Turing, Alan, 241, 255

Ulshöfer, Gotlind, vii-viii, xi, 1–49, 112, 180, 191–217, 251, 289, 311

Varela, Francisco, 304, 308
Virgin Mary, 301
Vogt, Cécile, 66–67, 68n5
Vogt, Oskar, 66
Vroomen, Jean, 88

Wajcman, Judy, 19, 268
Walzer, Michael, 168
Wassmann, Claudia, 5, 29, 247, 296, 299
Wayne, John, 39
Weaver, Sigourney, 237, 275
Weber, Max, 167, 208
Wechsler, David, 133
Wehling, Peter, 257, 294, 296
Weil, Simone, 255

Weinberg, Richard, 65
Weininger, Otto, 4, 36, 48n27
Wexler, Bruce E., 8–9
Wiener, Norbert, 27, 30
Willis, Bruce, 268
Willis, Paul, 174
Wilson, Edward O., 214
Wilson, Timothy, 159–160
Winfrey, Oprah, 156, 176n5
Wittgenstein, Ludwig, 85–87, 91, 99n12,
    99n14
Woodmansee, Martha, 286

Zahn-Harnack, Agnes, 66, 68n5
Zak, Paul J., 198–202, 212–213
Zeidner, Moshe, vii, xi, 18, 124, 131–148,
    183, 208, 262
Zerilli, Linda, 86
Zillmann, Dolf, 232–233
Zilsel, Edgar, 286

Subject Index

Ability, x, 4, 6, 11, 53, 59, 65, 109, 113, 115, 118, 122–124, 127–129, 132–133, 139, 143, 155–156, 161, 163, 170, 174–175, 182, 185–186, 196–197, 215, 221, 246, 261, 263–264, 266, 270, 278, 287, 298, 301–302, 310, 318, 322–323. *See also* Emotional ability
communication, 38, 118, 222
cognitive, 107, 122, 161
hearing, 91, 245, 275, 293
mathematical, 106, 187, 245
mechanical, 22, 106, 161
perceptual, 118–119, 133, 143, 235n1
problem-solving, 120
reproductive, 73, 251
spatial, 104, 106, 145, 232, 271, 283
verbal, 120, 156, 287
Abnormality, 24, 103, 114, 137, 199, 238–240, 243–245, 249, 251–252, 259, 266, 277–278, 282–285, 291–296, 298, 301, 313n1, 327
Academic, 1, 2, 8–9, 22, 28, 34, 53–54, 59, 65, 69, 119, 131–132, 146, 148, 157, 226, 235, 254–255, 272, 278, 283, 294, 305, 307, 314n17
Acceptability, 17, 23, 183, 210–211, 257, 291, 297–298, 327
Acceptance, 22, 58, 65, 96, 120, 197, 216n10, 237, 250, 258, 275, 277–278, 294, 298, 319
Achievement, 17–20, 93, 121, 135, 182, 196–197, 209, 264, 285, 296, 327

Acting, 55, 68, 82, 122, 182, 184–185, 228–229, 318, 326
proactive, 70, 185–186
Action, ix, 35–36, 46n7, 70, 75, 81, 86, 90–92, 105, 113–114, 118, 125n4, 137, 141, 151, 153–154, 158, 160, 169, 171, 174, 184, 197, 210, 212, 217n14, 222, 227, 231–234, 317–318, 326–327. *See also* Affirmative action
appropriate, 113–114
performative, 300
recognition, 272
Actor, actorhood, 159, 161, 164, 168, 201, 250, 267, 318
professional, 37, 39, 228–229, 231, 237
rational, 158, 180
social, 158, 258, 271, 298, 326
Actuality, 38, 58, 88, 100n27, 169, 246
Adaptability, 76, 123–124, 135, 182
Adaptation, 27, 35, 73, 85, 122, 156, 175, 189, 198, 222–223, 290
Administration, 184, 313n3
business, 185
Adolescence, 79, 109, 146, 269
Adrenalin, 29
Adultery, 74
Aesthetics, aesthetic, xi, 10, 24, 221, 227–235, 271
Affect, affective, xii, 87, 91–92, 98n9, 286, 228–233, 241
affective computing, 175, 185–189
"affective mirror," 186

Affirmative action, 70, 197

African, 58, 61, 314n3, color plate 8

African-American, 41, 121, 172, 175, 264

Age, 11, 17, 78, 113, 129, 136, 152, 180, 186, 189, 253, 264, 276, 284, 287, 296, 313n3, 317–318, 323. *See also* Anti-Aging

Agency, 30, 98n8, 252, 310

Agent, 124, 186–187, 240, 252, 306, 313n3

Aggression, 6, 10, 29, 75, 94, 125, 129, 187, 210, 227, 264, 285, 289, 291, 299, 312

Agreeableness, 127, 136, 142–143, 290

Alien, 237, 286. *See also* Othering

Alife (artificial life), 304–305, 307, 313n2

Altruism, 37, 194, 199, 212, 290, 300–303, 309

Alzheimer's disease, 105, 110–111

Ambiguity, 11, 199, 216n12
  emotional, 159
  genital, 8

Amniocentesis, 283

Amniotic fluid, 243, 283

Amygdala, 2, 22, 27, 35, 41, 84, 108, 222–223, 261, 273, 289, 292, 318

Amygdaloidotomy, 291

Androgen, 283

Androgynous, 74, 171, 266

Angelman syndrome, 280–281

Anger, 10, 29, 33, 39, 90, 93–94, 125, 155, 174–175, 176n4, 177–187, 225

Angst, 311

Animal, xii, 8, 27, 239–244, 268, 270, 273, 275, 289, 292, 296–297, 321–325

Anterior cingulate cortex (ACC), 3, 14, 31, 35, 48n30

Anterior insula (AI), 48n30

Anthropology, 4, 29, 40, 84, 157, 288
  biological, 41, 59, 60, 61, 269
  cultural, xii, 86, 297, 328
  philosophical, 2, 42, 55, 211, 215, 239, 318

Anti-aging, 29, 260–261

Antiquity, 33, 36, 48n27, 256

Anxiety, 10, 29, 39, 97–98, 122, 124, 139, 146n2, 154, 167, 176n4, 182–183, 255, 283, 310–311
  anxiety disorder, 255

Ape, 35, 46n4, 268–269, 271, 322. *See also* Monkey

Application, 70, 84, 104–106, 108–110, 112–113, 115–116, 138, 145, 148, 179, 186–187, 235, 282, 284, 290, 300, 319
  context of, 39, 43, 104

Aptitude, 22, 54, 132, 134–135, 182

Archetype, 154

Aristocrat, aristocratic, 152

Army, U.S. Air Force, military, 16, 43, 65, 109, 160, 161n1, 166, 177n7, 185, 211

Arousal, arousability, 84, 90, 109, 225–226, 260–261
  a. state, 91–92

Art historian, 99n16

Artifact, 12, 19–20, 160, 241, 307, 319

Artificial, 9, 13, 36, 113, 229, 252
  agent, 319
  environment, 19

Artificial intelligence (AI), 5, 7, 19, 86, 241, 259, 268, 289, 304, 307, 319

Asia, Asian, 39, 41, 94–95, 280, 308

Asperger's syndrome (AS), 249, 253–254, 266, 270, 281, 285–286, 293, 298–300, 313n1. *See also* HFA

Assertiveness, 37, 124, 161

Assessing emotions scale (AES), 140

Asset, 151

Assimilation, 4, 125, 142, 144, 242

Asymmetry, 283

Attention, 12, 87–96, 108, 110–111, 225, 231, 292, 313n3

Attention-deficit hyperactivity disorder (ADHD), 108, 110–111, 248, 280, 292, 313n3

Attitude, 2, 22, 59, 70, 95, 121, 123, 154

Audiovisual, 221, 227-228, 230, 232, 234
  contract, 229
  setting, 229, 232

Augmented reality, 186
Authenticity, 33, 170, 177n16
Authority, 54, 59, 72, 208, 271–272, 291, 295, 306
Autism, autist, viii, xi–xii, xv–xvi, 28, 108, 186, 193–194, 200, 208, 216n2, 217n15, 237–312, 313n3, 314n7, 321. *See also* HFA
Autism rights movement, 238, 253–254, 278, 292, 296
Automatic evaluation, 27, 42
Autonomy, 13, 33, 47, 55, 180–181, 217n16, 243, 247, 258, 324
Avoidance, 27, 96, 226, 291
Awareness, 22, 115, 135–136, 246. *See also* Self-awareness
  emotional, 131, 134, 158
  mental, 159

Backlash, 247
Bargaining, 171
Beauty, beautiful, 24, 57, 92, 259, 278, 285, 299, 301, 311, 325
  beauty queen, 16
Behavior, xii, 6, 8, 27, 29–30, 33, 36, 38–39, 41, 55–56, 73–77, 93–95, 103, 106–109, 113, 116, 124, 127, 154–156, 171, 175, 193–198, 201–209, 213, 221–225, 230–235, 240–249, 251–259, 263, 269, 273–304, 310, 317, 319–322, 327–328. *See also* Conduct; Demeanor
  cultural, 20, 26, 45, 83, 132, 138, 161, 206, 238
  economic, 30, 154, 179, 192, 194, 197–202, 214, 251
  real-life, 11, 115, 120, 133, 217n15, 275
  sexual, 107, 302, 323
Behavioral economics, 194
Being (*esse*), 73, 309–310, 320
Belief, 41, 60, 73, 82, 91–92, 126, 139, 144, 193, 286, 328
Bell curve, 121, 263–266, 294
Benefit, 127, 144, 161, 183, 186, 197, 302
Benevolence, 33

Bestiality, 75
Beyondism, 42
Bias
  intentional, 27
  gender, 194, 215, 261, 326
  sexual, 8, 204
  unintentional, 27, 276
Bioethics, 46n4, 285. *See also* Ethics
Biofact, 35, 241
Biography, autobiography, 31, 37, 46n4, 83, 94, 145, 174, 289, 303, 325, 327–328
  cerebral, 55
Bioinformatics, 251, 279
Biology, biologist, xii, 3–7, 28, 30, 38, 72, 75, 79–80, 204, 212–216, 217n19, 241, 247, 251, 279, 282–293, 300–302, 309, 313–314
Biopolitics. *See* Politics
Biopsychology, 240, 243, 291
Birth, congenital, 11, 93, 129, 151–152, 238, 260, 363
Blackness (as cultural category), 12, 24, 41, 61, 175, 294
Blood, 8, 34, 84, 186–187, 201, 243–244, 289, 344, 369
  blood flow, 201
Bloodline, 40, 302
Body, 5, 12–13, 19–20, 26, 31–35, 42–44, 46n9, 47n17, 59, 61, 72–78, 89, 122, 132, 162–163, 184–186, 192, 198, 201, 211, 213, 221–232, 239–247, 256, 260–261, 268, 271–272, 278, 282–284, 291–298, 301, 305, 318–320, 324–327
Bonds 74, 136, 162, 167, 171, 175
Bourgeois, 55–56, 59–60, 167, 177n11
Boy, 118, 238, 259, 267, 269, 285, 347
Boyfriend, 299. *See also* Lover
Brain image, 1, 61, 296, 308. *See also* Neuroimage
Brain imaging, 1, 5, 195, 308, 319. *See also* Neuroimaging
Breast, 283
  cancer (in men), 284

Buddhism, Buddhist, 308
Business, 5, 10, 16–18, 110, 127, 165, 180, 195, 204, 215, 275, 301, 308, color plate 8

Calibration (of instruments), 23, 42
Calmness, 132, 292
Capability, 26, 182
Capacity, 7, 8, 12, 17, 19–21, 73, 75, 79, 109, 155, 159–160, 190, 239–241, 246, 252, 256, 298
  brain, 8, 11, 22, 47n10, 122, 256, 259, 266, 271–273, 278, 286, 288, 297, 305–310
  body, 5, 31, 73, 242, 275
  cognitive, 109–110, 160
  emotional, 3, 12, 95, 151, 154, 244, 249, 251, 271–276, 284, 322–323
  intellectual, 249, 291, 294, 298
  language, 241
  reproductive, procreative, 73, 78–79, 284
  sexual, 261
  social, 10, 133, 160–164, 175–176, 317
Capital, 19–20, 168, 176
  cultural, 19, 154, 161–163, 170
  economic, 19, 161
  emotional, 151, 153, 161–164
  social, 161, 163, 181
  symbolic, 19, 162, 170
Capitalism, xi, 43, 152, 162–163, 167, 171, 191, 193, 211, 298
  connectionist, 163–165, 175, 177n11
  flexible, 179–180, 183–186, 189, 195–201, 209, 214–125
Capital punishment, 100n30
Car, 17, 88, 205, 265, 275, 277
Care, caring, 10, 39, 152, 171, 189, 210, 238, 246, 248, 253, 256–257, 260, 276, 278
  child care, 39, 79, 303
  occupation of, 17, 196
Career, 17, 53, 60, 109, 163, 283, 306
Castration, 291
Category, categorization, 1, 3, 6, 11, 13, 21, 23, 26, 29–33, 35, 40, 43, 69, 71–73, 80, 154, 169, 176, 200, 237, 240–241, 247–255,

266–268, 274, 279, 282–286, 290, 292–293, 300–302, 309, 313n1, 314n7
Caucasian, 39, 41, 56, 58, 121, 264
Causality, 8, 42, 72, 129–130, 202, 241, 259, 263, 289, 313
Cell, cellular, 1, 35, 67, 77, 242, 247, 252, 305, 320
Central nervous system (CNS), 105, 325
Central processing unit (CPU), 19
Cerebellum, 3, 48n30, 56
Cerebralization, 54
Challenge, 4, 11, 36, 40, 67, 79–80, 90, 107, 113, 186, 191–192, 195, 213, 237, 246, 251, 282, 309, 318
  emotional, 132, 137, 196
Character, 2, 6, 21, 32, 36, 79, 86, 91, 96, 122, 134–135, 147, 166, 183, 192–193, 229, 230–234, 236n3, 268, 277, 327
Chauvinism, 327
Cheating, 38, 323. See also Faking; Lying; Pretending
Chief executive officer (CEO), 13, 186
Child(ren), ix, 8, 21, 33, 39, 74, 77, 122, 137, 172, 224–226, 245, 248, 252, 268, 276–285, 303, 313n3
Christian, 25, 81, 308
Chromosome, 72, 79, 106, 243, 264, 280
Church, 70
  Catholic, 70, 80n1, 309
Cinema, xi, 228–231, 238, 244–245, 257, 259, 267, 275, 277, 296
Cingulate gyrus, 26, 222
Class, 8, 11, 40–42, 48, 160, 167–168, 197, 258, 264
  middle, 10, 65, 75, 151–153, 167, 171, 174, 189, 283, 306, 314n10
  professional, 160
  propertied, 151
  social, 136, 152–153, 189
  under, lower, 46n6, 152, 327
  upper, 156, 160, 163, 210, 278
  working, 151–152, 172, 174, 189, 278
Class dynamics, 163–165

Classification, 8, 61, 154, 157, 160–161, 165

Client, 187

Clinic, clinical, 105, 108, 114, 131, 166, 195, 281, 292

application, 105–106

context, 28, 105, 204, 279, 287

clinician, 69, 110–111

Clitoris, 298

Coach, coaching, 6, 46, 225–228, 234

Code, x, 72, 86–91, 126, 177, 229, 231, 268

color, 13

cultural, 158, 272–276

Cognition, 4, 5, 6, 24, 31–32, 55, 84, 90, 104, 106–108, 111–112, 125, 144, 221, 235, 247, 256, 269, 274, 288, 292, 297, 310, 317

Cognitive science, ix, 5–7, 24, 29, 45, 47n18, 86, 194, 239–240, 247–248, 252, 268, 274, 279, 288, 292, 303- 304, 309, 315n17. *See also* Social cognitive science

neuroscience, 114–115, 240, 289

psychology, 90, 106–107, 121, 159, 241, 289

Cognitive unconscious, 5

Collective(s), 86, 91, 94, 258, 325–328

conscious, 61

interest, 189

sin, 74

system, 258, 262

emotional, 1, 274, 326–327

Combat, 29, 300

Commensuration, 161

Commodification, 162, 177n10

Commodity, 187

Communication, 135, 221, 322

Community, 33, 44, 68n1, 91–92, 212

"Coming out," 248

Company, 28, 80n3, 110–111, 128, 136, 177n12, 186, 188, 207, 304. *See also* Enterprise

Comparable worth, 197

Competence

cognitive, 156

cultural, 160–161

emotional, 127, 136, 153, 156–157, 160–162, 167, 170–171, 175, 182, 184, 322

personal, 135

professional, 154

social, 120, 135, 154, 157, 160, 168, 176n4, 322

Competition, 37, 41, 73, 180, 190, 215, 264, 300

Complicit, 37

Computational component, 185

Computed tomography (CT), 104–105

Computer, 12, 185–188, 201, 242, 252, 265, 267–269, 271–273, 290, 307, 326

age, 268, 286

"anxiety," 283

programmer, 137

science, 20, 179, 185–186, 247, 279, 288, 304

Computing, 31. *See also* Affect, affective computing

pervasive, 31

wearable, xi, 185

Condom, 78

Conduct, 81–82, 151, 155, 183. *See also* Behavior; Demeanor

Congregation for the Doctrine of the Faith (CDF), 70

Conscientiousness, 135, 142, 290

Consciousness, 27, 30–33, 46n4, 61, 94, 157, 304, 318, 322–328

Consensus, 81, 86, 141, 171, 212

Conservative, 59–60, 70, 271, 282, 288, 302

Constraint, 229

methodological, 31, 250, 272

emotional, 152, 158

Construction, construct, 24, 31, 44, 47n22, 192, 231–234, 243, 271

biological, 73–76, 282, 310

cultural, 84–85, 167, 326

(neuro)scientific, 11, 72, 104–105, 107, 120, 185, 201, 244, 260, 266, 319

psychological, 34, 36, 137–138, 142, 160–161, 182, 208, 224, 227, 259, 290, 293

Construction, construct (cont.)
  social, 19, 20, 70–71, 79–80, 168, 210, 275,
    296–297, 314n17, 326–328
Consultant, consulting firm, 111, 161,
    164–165
Consumer, consumerism, 30, 44, 185, 197
  Consumer Alert, 192, 195
Contempt, 33, 83, 233, 321
Control, 6, 10, 12, 19, 23–27, 30–31, 41, 66,
    82, 88–89, 99n24, 100n28, 109–110, 113,
    122, 133, 137, 144, 146, 156, 159–163, 171,
    179–180, 183, 186, 188, 194, 206, 208, 233,
    239, 243–245, 251–252, 261, 264, 267,
    274–275, 278, 290, 298, 309, 318, 325
Control concept, 92–94
Convolution, 66
Coping, 127, 129, 131, 146, 157–159, 163,
    171, 177n16, 196, 198, 226, 270, 290
  stress, 39, 109, 136
Corporation, corporate, 6, 13, 28, 154, 156,
    161–162, 171, 195, 252, 269, 299
  self (hood), 28, 168, 177n16
Correlation coefficient (r), 15, 124, 130n2,
    139–140, 142, 146–147
Cortex, 35, 55, 58, 67, 222–223. See also
  Anterior cingulate cortex (ACC); Prefrontal
  cortex; Orbit
Cost, 110
Courtship, 83–84, 97
CPI (California psychological inventory),
    124
Craftsmanship, 196
Cranioscopy, 57–59
Criminal, criminality, 68, 109, 327
Cultivation, 33, 74, 170–171, 175, 181, 297
Culture, x, 5–9, 11–13, 17, 24, 29, 33–34,
    36–44, 48n33, 51, 54–55, 60, 70–73, 81,
    84–87, 92, 94, 99n15, 113, 116, 126, 133,
    136, 148–165, 177n16, 181, 205–206,
    221–228, 232–235, 238, 242–248, 255,
    257–274, 284–288, 290, 293–296, 303,
    307–309, 314n17, 321, 325–327. See also
  Subculture

  studies, 4, 20, 221, 286
  popular, 39, 137, 155–156, 238, 245, 248,
    267, 296
  testing, 27, 42–43, 196
  "third," 305–306
Currency (emotional), 155, 163, 174
Curriculum, 71, 119, 133, 164, 305
Customer, 110, 128, 136
Cybernetics, 27
Cyberspace, 304
Cystic fibrosis, 278, 285
Cytoarchitectonics, 66

Danger, 29, 32, 44, 172, 255, 306, 321
Darwinism, 5, 28, 60, 260, 308
  social, 40, 215, 269, 310
Data, 1, 12, 16, 22, 42, 69, 104–105, 111,
    113–115, 121, 124, 136, 177n13–17,
    187–188, 192, 201, 204, 210, 252, 263 292,
    313n3
  biometric, 186, 188
  empirical, 10, 27, 36, 44, 120, 138, 265, 274,
    304
Death, 238, 275. See also Mortality
Decision, decision-making, 12, 16, 23, 30,
    34, 40, 44, 46n2, 108, 144, 156, 159, 182,
    191–195, 197–202, 207, 211–215, 216n5,
    223, 251, 294, 297, 311, 318, 326
Deductionism, 8, 43
Deep brain stimulation, 47n10, 291
Deliberation, 206
Demeanor, 152, 155, 160, 162. See also
  Behavior; Conduct
Democracy, 7, 16–17, 66, 157, 180, 184, 209,
    212, 215
Demography, 263
Depolitization, 256–257
Depression, 6, 108, 122, 128, 139, 166, 242,
    289–292
Deprivation, 6, 137, 151–152, 224
Design, 20
  experimental, 3, 12, 22, 27, 31, 41
  intelligent, 307

Desire, 3–4, 15, 29, 37–38, 43, 72, 75–79, 123, 145, 156, 203–207, 260–262, 286, 302

Determinism, 5, 8, 53, 55, 72, 75, 241, 256

Development, 7–8, 17, 23, 29, 36, 69, 200, 233, 243, 293

biological, 36, 56–58, 60, 77, 106, 115, 241–242, 247, 249, 281, 283

child, 122, 224–226, 238

disorder, 35 282

economic, 43, 74

emotional, 129, 134, 137, 152–153, 156, 169, 225, 229, 277, 319

personal, 17, 134, 152, 169, 179, 183, 196, 224, 254, 278, 325

prenatal, 77, 243, 245–249, 254, 262, 282, 287

scientific, 7, 18, 23, 27, 39, 45, 56, 67, 86–87, 91, 98n9, 99n16, 103–106, 112, 117–119, 123, 126, 131–133, 144, 147, 152, 179, 185, 188, 195, 197, 209, 214, 216n5, 217n19, 287, 289, 317, 319

sexual, 76

Deviance, 79, 92, 95–96, 103, 238, 240, 278, 291, 296, 317

Device, 104–105, 112, 186–189, 228, 234, 283, 320

Diagrammatic, 263

Difference

gender, 8, 12, 15, 17–19, 69, 75, 79, 128–129, 136, 144, 194, 197, 255, 323, 328

individual, 2–3, 129, 138, 160, 172, 174, 176, 206, 326

race, 41, 48n28, 121

sex, 8, 11–12, 18, 20–21, 29, 40–41, 44, 65–66, 69–72, 75, 106–108, 113, 129, 189, 197, 202, 204, 213, 241, 243, 255, 265, 269, 278–279, 282–283, 299, 306, 328

Digit ratio, 282–284

Dimorphism, 73, 76

Disability, 11, 243, 249, 265, 266, 270, 285, 302

Disclosure (of emotions), 300, 303

self, 177n16

Discourse, 1–9, 29, 46n2, 61, 65, 67, 75, 84–87, 91–92, 97, 168, 178, 186, 235, 253, 268–270, 285, 297, 299, 303, 308–309, 327

Discrimination, 42, 53, 70, 88, 115–116, 121, 134, 197, 216n8, 262, 272

Disease, 105, 110–111, 187

Disgust, 22–29, 125, 226, 233, 250, 278, 288

Disorder, 35, 108, 110–113, 137, 238–239, 242–249, 251–255, 280, 282, 284–285, 288–293, 302, 309, 313n1, 313n3

Display rules, 38, 272

Disposition, 21, 55–56

Distrust, 174–175. See also Trust

Division of labor, 4, 55, 66, 256, 261

DNA (deoxyribonucleic aid), 137, 242, 280

Documentary (TV), 299

Domestic, 74–75, 171, 326

self, 177n16

Domination, 70–71, 168, 184

Dopamine, 291

Down's syndrome, 280–281

Drama, 47n21, 82, 94, 312. See also Melodrama

Drive, 32, 56, 58, 135, 243–244, 252, 262, 267, 320. See also Trieb

achievement, 182

sex, 55, 75, 261

Drug, 6, 106, 134, 146

Dyslexia, 110, 143, 282

Early Modern Age, 9, 34, 87

Eccentric, 277, 287

Economics, xii, 4, 16, 30, 37, 43, 54, 112, 191–217

model, 37, 212

rationality, 44, 74, 180, 184, 192, 196

system, 184, 191, 212

feminist, 194–195, 214, 216n1

new home, 194

post-autistic (PAE), viii, xi, xvi, 191, 193, 214

Economic success, 121, 151, 153, 161, 168, 285, 294, 303–304

Economic theory, 30, 191–193, 199–200, 207, 214

Economic transformation 181–183

Economist, neuroeconomist, 30, 191–193, 199, 212, 216n3, 216n11, 217n19, 251, 304

Economy, 16, 18, 28, 42, 164, 191, 195, 212, 215, 253, 257, 264, 325

Economy of emotions, 152, 175

Education, 17–18, 33, 46n2, 47n14, 119, 135, 144, 169, 172, 179, 181, 196, 212, 217n18, 226, 245, 264, 302, 305

EEG (electroencephalography), 111, 187

Egg (cell), 76

Egocentrism, 258. See also Self-occupancy

Elite, elitist, ix, 5, 7, 9, 13, 16–21, 28, 38, 43, 45, 46n6, 47n12,n14, 53, 65–67, 68n2, 74, 103, 121, 132, 196, 207, 210, 237, 254, 257–258, 260, 262, 264, 270, 272, 285, 293, 301, 304, 307, 326–327, 328

Elitegehirn (elite brain), 7, 65

Emancipation, emancipatory, 39–40, 43, 45, 65, 204

Embodiment, 19, 33–34, 162, 232, 252, 258–259, 309–310

Emotional ability, 109, 127–128, 132, 136, 144, 185, 196

Emotional energy, 162–163

Emotional field, 160

Emotionality, 3, 9, 11, 28, 35, 147, 189, 242–245, 298, 315n17, 318, 326–327

Emotional labor, xi, 17, 38–39, 196, 265, 258, 302

Emotional literacy, 274. See also Illiteracy

Emotional makeup, 154, 160, 162, 165, 174, 177n10

Emotional quotient (EQ), 17, 34, 38–39, 117, 134–135, 140, 156, 265, 275–277, 287, 301, 303. See also Type, EQ-type

EQ-i (emotional quotient inventory), 124, 161

Emotional style, x, 85, 96, 100n30, 160, 163, 167, 175

Emotion script, 224, 228, 232, 234

Empathy, xii, 3, 6, 8, 31, 36–39, 94–95, 129, 135–136, 146, 171, 176n4, 189, 194, 199–203, 206–207, 210, 212, 221, 223, 227–228, 230–234, 236n4, 237, 245, 251, 256, 261, 263, 265–278, 284, 288–289, 301–303

Empathizer, empathizing (cognitive style), 2–3, 223, 262, 265–267, 271, 274, 300–303, 310. See also Type, E-type

Empiricism, 43, 246, 305

Employee, 13, 127–128, 136, 154, 171, 180–181, 189, 196, 207–209

flexible, viii, xi, 163, 179–188, 190, 195, 197, 302

Employment, employability, 16, 181, 226. See also Job; Unemployment

Emptiness, 309

Emulation, 33, 53

Endocrinology, 250. See also Hormone; Neuroendocrinology

Enterprise, 180. See also Company

Entrepreneur, 181–184, 190, 311

Environment, 8–9, 11, 68, 73, 77, 107, 116, 122–123, 136–137, 156–157, 180–185, 196, 201, 221, 224, 237, 240, 248, 254, 263, 272–273, 278, 304–310, 321, 324, 326

Epidemic, epidemiologic, 79, 245, 247, 280, 291

Epigenetic, 280

Epistemology, 25, 44, 260

Equality, 19–20, 37, 53, 60, 66, 174, 298

Equal opportunity, 18–19, 181, 197

Equity, 19, 37, 70, 265, 297–298

Essence (essentia), x, 2, 8, 24, 30, 47n20, 138, 164, 240, 243, 246, 271, 284, 296, 309–310, 322

Estradiol, 283

Estrogen, 29, 76, 252, 282

Ethics, 10, 328. See also Bioethics

Ethiopian, 56

Ethnicity, 8, 11, 109, 113, 169, 181, 210. See also Race

Ethos, 44, 152–153, 168, 171, 174

Europe, 71, 74, 80n3, 81–82, 95, 97, 197, 285, 293, 295, 304, 306, 313n3
  European Commission (EC), 16, 197
  European Union (EU), 16–18, 197, 210, 313n3
European (person), 58, 65, 75
Eudaimonia, 169–170
Eugenics, 42–43, 48n28, 49n33, 66, 297
Evaluation, 17, 23, 27, 42, 86, 126, 144, 147, 154–155, 181, 204–205, 209, 215, 228, 323–324, 269, 287, 313n3, 317
Evolution, 9, 27, 38, 76, 214, 217n19, 260–269, 290, 304, 306, 320
  biological, 4
  cultural, 9
Excitability, 132
Exclusion. See Disclosure, Minority, Social exclusion
Exhibitionism, 75
Existence (existentia), 11, 36, 47n20, 53, 68, 72, 79, 128, 187, 246, 298, 301, 305, 309–311, 321–322
Experiment, x, 24, 38, 88, 198, 200–206, 212, 236n1, 242
Explanation, 11–12, 29, 32, 36, 40, 43, 48n28, 49n33, 87, 113, 175, 207, 215, 224, 234, 239, 241, 247, 265, 268, 286, 300, 309, 328
Extraversion, 139–143, 290
Extreme-male-brain theory, xi, 40, 208, 238, 240–253, 255–256, 258–259, 262, 268, 277, 288, 296, 298, 301

Face, facial, 17, 23–24, 41, 58, 83, 92, 94, 118, 125, 129, 132, 141n1, 143, 205, 229, 242, 250n2, 256
  expression, 34, 39, 85, 90, 95, 118, 133, 139, 141, 223, 231–232, 290, 293
Faking, 20, 124, 145. See also Cheating; Lying; Pretending
Family, 13, 17, 33, 48n28, 58, 71, 74, 76, 79, 165–171, 174–175, 189, 194, 225–226,246, 261, 280

Father, 71, 81, 83, 122, 170, 254, 261, 268, 280. See also Patriarchy
Fear, 31, 33, 65, 75, 90, 125n1, 155, 175, 176n4, 183, 205, 223, 226–228, 250, 270, 309–311, 320
Feedback, 87–96, 148, 224, 226, 301
Feeling, 2–3, 22–23, 27, 29–33, 38, 45, 55–56, 60, 78, 82, 94–95, 126, 154–157, 162, 173, 176n4, 207–208, 226–228, 232, 248, 260, 273–276, 287, 289, 298, 311, 318, 320, 324–325
  gut, 222–223, 259
Female choice, 260, 270
Feminalism, 20, 261, 314n6
Femininity, feminization, 11, 58, 72, 189, 272, 275–276
Feminism, feminist, x, 2, 20, 29, 69, 70–71, 79–80, 156, 163, 261, 285, 298, 314n6. See also Technofeminist
  science, 16, 40–44, 76, 86, 193–195, 216n1, 253, 255
Fertility, 73
Fetish, fetishism, 13, 76, 211, 247
Field, 10, 21, 25, 29, 31, 34, 36–41, 46n2, 154, 157, 161–162, 164, 176n2, 186–187
  cultural, 160
  emotional, 160
Film, 193, 227, 229–233, 236n2, 237–238, 244, 259, 267, 272, 275, 277–279, 291
Flooding (emotional), 274–275
Flow, 87, 158–159, 239, 241, 243
Fragile-X syndrome, 264
Frame, framework, 267
Framing, 294
Friendship, friend, 33, 82–83, 146–147, 168–171, 244, 246, 278
Frontal cortex, 222
Frontal lobe, 137
Fronto-insular cortex (FI), 203
Frustration, 186
FTM (female-to-male transsexual), 78

Function, 2–11, 19–22, 25 (color plate 5), 28–29, 33–39, 45, 58, 65, 67, 72–79, 103–115, 122, 131–134, 144, 158, 162, 165, 167, 174–175, 182, 194–195, 199, 205, 207, 216n12, 221–224, 227–228, 230, 234–235, 239–244, 249, 251, 257–262, 266–267, 273, 277, 279, 282, 290, 300–301, 310, 317–319, 326. *See also* fMRI; HFA
    executive, 250, 289, 302, 313n1
    Functional Elite Theory, 17
    of pop science, 294–295, 301, 303
Functionality, 30, 38, 44, 207, 215, 224, 226, 244, 293, 299, 310
Functional magnetic resonance imaging (fMRI), 5, 22, 25–29, 37, 46n2, 104–105, 111, 113, 195, 200–203, 247–250, 283, 292. *See also* Magnetic resonance imaging (MRI)

GAIA (hypothesis), 304–306
Game theory, 194, 199–200, 217n13. *See also* Ultimate game
Gamete, 76
Gatherer, 288, 326
Gay, 18, 38, 240–241, 254–255, 277, 282–283, 303. *See also* Homosexual(lity); Inversion; Same-sex sexual(ity)
Gender equality, 197
Gender equity, 19, 70
Gender mainstreaming, 11, 70, 197
Gender medicine, 44
Gender order, 74, 76
Gender pay gap, 16–17
Gender role, 1, 10–13, 18, 43, 75, 171, 197, 206, 267, 276, 298–303
Gene, 35, 238, 242, 247, 279, 284–285
Genetic, 11, 48n29, 76–77, 110–112, 121, 241–245, 252–253, 279–285, 290–293, 297, 302–303
    testing, 110, 238, 284–285
Genital, 8, 282–283
Genitalia, 73–74, 78–79
Genius, vii, x, 21, 48n28, 53, 135, 238, 253, 255, 261, 266, 272, 275–278, 281, 285–300

Genome, 246, 279–280
Genomic imprinting, 280–281
Genotype, 243, 246, 253, 292
Genus, 58
Gesture, 85, 95, 230
Girl, 61, 170, 275, 299
Girlfriend, 277. *See also* Lover
Glass ceiling, 190
Global, 16, 28, 41, 165–167, 183, 249, 264–265, 280, 298
Globalization, 164–167, 180
God, goddess, 73, 286
Gonadal, 8, 29, 76–77, 243, 261, 279–283
Gonads, 76, 252, 282–283
Graph, 188, 263–266
Gray matter, 249
Greenlander, color plate 6
Group, 23, 38, 40, 43, 53, 61, 73, 107, 112, 121, 136, 182, 184, 197, 202, 207, 222, 253, 256, 270, 298, 303, 325
    occupational, 137
    social, 24, 160, 165–167, 262, 305, 326
    status, 162
    watchdog, 70
Growth, 74, 76, 136, 153, 181, 224, 242–243
    personal, xii
Guilt, 10, 25–26, 31, 39, 152, 276, 289, 321
GWSIT (George Washington social intelligence test), x, 118

Habit, 151
Habitual, 32, 122, 158
Habitus, viii, xi, 19–20, 160–171, 177n11, 303
Happiness, 29, 39, 124–125, 153, 169, 184, 212, 228, 250, 289, 303
Harmony, 95, 180, 256, 305
Harvard University, 53, 68n1, 72, 264, 272, 306
Health, 44, 78, 112–114, 122, 124, 144, 151, 160–161, 171, 183–189, 200–201, 256, 278, 281, 303, 314n3, 327
    care, 44, 256, 278, 281, 327
Heart, 34, 41, 44, 72, 83, 97, 151, 167, 186–187, 201, 226, 296, 301

Hemisphere (brain), 26, 222, 261, 283, 300, 304

Heredity, hereditary, 40–41, 253, 264, 279–280

Hermaphrodite, 36, 76

Heterosexuality, ix–x, 3, 8, 24, 44, 78–79, 146, 205, 241, 245, 247, 273–278, 299–300

Hierarchy, 16, 34, 38, 40, 61, 71, 76, 79, 132, 143, 152, 171–172, 176, 180, 183, 189, 224, 269–270

High-functional autist (HFA), 250–254, 266–267, 286, 298, 300–302. *See also* Asperger's syndrome

Historian, 7, 36, 43, 47n22, 72, 77, 92, 96–97, 98n2, 295, 304

HIV (human immunodeficiency virus), 79

Hollywood, 193, 237, 257, 257, 267, 274, 299

Homeostasis, 320, 324

Homo duplex, 310

Homo oeconomicus, xi, 30, 192–194, 199–207, 211–214

Homo sapiens, 29

Homosexual(ity), 12, 71, 75, 241, 282, 284. *See also* Gay; Inversion, Same-sex sexual(ity)

Hormone, x, 20, 29, 46n2, 77–78, 106, 198, 213, 243, 249, 252, 259, 261, 263, 282–284, 289, 291

Hottentot woman, color plate 7

Housewife, 10

Human being, xii, 29–30, 33–34, 46n4, 55, 192, 201, 211, 246, 251, 259, 271, 297, 300–311, 314n17, 322

Human Genome Project, 279

Human relations movement, 180

Humanities, 4–5, 9, 12, 20, 32–36, 45, 69, 85, 256, 307, 317, 327–328

Humanoid, 5, 241, 277

Hunter, hunting, 261, 269, 288, 326

Husband, 17, 75–76, 166, 170, 261, 274, 276

Hybrid, 35

Hyperfemale, 251, 282–284

Hypermale, 239, 249–251, 262

Hypervigilance, 122

Hypothalamotomy, 291

Hypothesis, 8, 22, 27, 31, 39, 121, 128, 189, 243, 246, 253, 264, 278–282, 304–305

Icon, 5, 78, 247, 254, 285, 296, 308

Iconology, 12

Idea, 2, 4, 6–7, 11–12, 17–19, 24–28, 31–35, 40–44, 47n17, 49n35, 55, 66–67, 77–81, 84, 90, 97, 98n6, 118–120, 132–133, 148–157, 181, 185, 192, 196, 199, 204–214, 222, 242, 245–256, 261–165, 271–278, 281, 285–311, 314n17, 319–329, 324

Ideal, idealistic, xii, 4, 93, 177n16, 179, 181, 188, 196, 208–209, 235, 250, 275, 283, 302, 310

Idealtype, 243, 245, 251, 253, 266–267, 271–272, 298, 301

Identity, 4, 36, 46n4, 61, 78, 80, 139, 243, 254, 259, 327

corporate, 28

gender, 8, 24, 77–78, 80, 85, 170–171, 282

sexual, 73, 78, 252

social, 153, 155, 162, 175, 314n17, 326

Ideology, 43, 71, 79, 157, 284

Idiocy, 21

Idiopathic, 279

Ignorance claim (of science), 294

Illiteracy, 134, 143, 274

emotional, 134

Illusion, 229, 251, 307

Image run, 250

Imagery, 88, 90, 247, 264

Imagination, 7, 91, 142, 267–271, 325

Imitation, 323–324

Immediacy, 31, 257

Immortality, 60, 184, 286, 307. *See also* Life, eternal

Immune system, 77, 301

Impact, 22, 30, 39, 45, 91–92, 106, 109, 114–117, 121, 123, 127, 134, 137, 145, 154, 170, 214, 234, 267, 301, 306

Imperturbability (male), 274

Impotence, 80n3, 260, 291

Impulse, 81, 122, 290

Impulsive, 139

Income, 75, 112, 168, 180, 264. *See also* Wage; Payment

Incompetence, 157–160, 175, 310

Incorporation, 78, 241

Independence, 55, 84, 118–119, 123–124, 192, 257, 296

Individualism, 74, 174–175, 192–193, 257

Individualist, 192–193, 301

Individuality, 56–57, 115, 164, 175, 202, 209

Industry, 154, 161, 163, 267, 272

Inequality, 169, 175–176, 189–190, 212–213

Inferiority, 21–22, 26, 41, 60, 65–66

Information, 20, 46n8, 88–89, 97, 105–106, 109–118, 139, 143, 177, 182, 185, 192, 221, 224, 231–234, 241, 252–253, 271, 276–277, 287, 313, 319–320, 325, 327

Inhibition, 89, 152, 223

Innate (congenital), 19, 21, 37–40, 75, 129, 147, 196, 221, 224, 228–234, 235n1, 236n1, 269, 272, 285–286, 301, 306

Inner Self Helper, 248, 263

Innovation, 1, 42, 180–182, 286, 294

Institution, 53, 70, 114, 168, 207, 257, 277

Institutional, 180, 212, 294

Instrument, 24, 133, 154, 166, 197, 256, 298

Instrumentalism, 133

Intellectual, 9–10, 21–22, 41, 54, 56, 59, 118, 132, 156, 249, 254, 271, 277, 283, 291, 293, 298, 304–306, 318

Intelligence
  general (*g*), 22, 48n28, 118–123, 127–129, 130n2, 132–133
  human, 41, 132
  inferior, 21
  interpersonal, 119, 124, 134
  intrapersonal, 119, 124, 134
  multiple, 155
  social, 34, 93, 117–123, 127, 133, 322–323

Intelligence quotient (IQ), 1, 10, 37, 41–42, 117, 121, 132–139, 145, 156, 160, 171, 185, 238, 250, 254–257, 263–272, 282–283, 287–288, 293–294, 318. *See also* Type, IQ type

Intelligence test. *See* Test

Intention, 91, 146

Intentional, 27, 91–92, 96, 183, 222–223, 228, 232

Interaction, 84, 92, 115, 137, 146, 162–163, 174, 186, 205–206, 221, 226–234, 245, 281, 286, 293

Intercourse, 69, 75, 260

Interest, 26, 30–34, 41, 43, 65, 84, 109, 117, 119, 128, 155, 157, 165–170, 186, 189, 191, 193, 199, 204, 214, 226, 249, 257, 277, 291, 293, 305, 319, 321. *See also* Self-interest

Intersex, 36, 77

Interview, 120

Intimacy, 153, 167–175, 185, 225, 231, 234, 244, 287, 327

Intrauterine, 243, 245, 259, 282–283, 289

Intrinsic, 327

Introspection, 159–160, 163

Introversion, 139

Inversion (sexual), 75–76. *See also* Gay; Homosexual(ity); Same-sex sexual(ity)

Inversion (genetic), 279

Ivy League, 18–19

Jealousy, 83, 157–158, 170, 321

Jew, 61, color plate 8

Job, 37–38, 96, 109, 117, 120, 123–124, 127–128, 145, 154–155, 161–162, 180–183, 186, 189, 196, 261, 290, 302, 306. *See also* Employment; Unemployment
  obsolescence, 180
  performance, 127, 183

Journal, 3, 41, 65, 117, 139, 193, 256, 272, 283, 292, 295, 306

Journalist, 46n2, 155, 295

Judge, 79, 120, 124–125, 146, 258

Judgment, 59, 84, 94, 276, 333
Justice, 38, 41, 48, 132, 167–169, 204, 255, 258, 287, 294, 328

Kinship, 73, 169
Klinefelter's syndrome, 243
Knowledge, 12, 18, 23, 32, 43, 54–55, 65–68, 73, 93, 108, 111, 113, 140–141, 145–146, 151, 153, 158, 172, 196, 203, 211, 215, 233, 246, 255–259, 262, 271–274, 287–296, 300, 307, 325, 326–327
  cultural, 158
  manipulation of, 172
  self-, 145, 262
  stored, 158
  tacit, 158

Labeling, 157–159, 188, 193, 201, 244, 266, 297
Laboratory, lab, ix, 6, 11, 19, 22–25, 31, 36, 43–44, 89–90, 119, 144, 186, 198–202, 240, 249, 272, 300
  MIT Media Lab, 188
Language, 7, 9, 12, 20, 55, 65–73, 77, 83, 86, 89, 91, 99, 144, 163, 167–174, 184, 186, 213, 237–238, 241, 257, 274, 283, 288, 290, 293, 322, 330
Law (lawyer), vii, xii, 78, 86, 99, 109, 214, 256, 258, 317, 326–328. See also Legal
  universal, 74
Lay, laypeople, 1, 87, 13, 103, 117, 119–122, 129, 294
  press, 5
  reader, 295
Leader, 182, 208–209, 301–302, 308
Leadership, x, 6–7, 13, 17–18, 38, 127, 155, 161–164, 182, 196–197, 207–210, 215, 217n17, 262, 264, 269, 300–304
  primal, 207–208
  transactional, 209
  transformational, 208–209
Learning, 27, 35, 41, 97, 111–112, 159, 196, 200, 276, 323

Left-handedness, left-hander, 283–284
Legal, 21, 43, 60, 70, 79, 114, 322, 326–328
Leib, 32
Lesbian, 18, 197, 206, 240, 252, 255, 282–283, 300, 303
Liberal, 7, 70
Libertarian, 212, 216
Liberty, 82, 97, 100n30
Libido, 75–76, 153, 155
Lie detector, 327
Life, 11, 16, 21, 24, 30–35, 86–87, 99n14, 115–123, 128, 131, 134–136, 151–152, 156, 168–169, 173, 176, 185, 238, 246–248, 274, 285, 296, 300, 305, 311, 320–321
  biological, 16, 36, 184, 242–243, 277, 297, 305, 320, 325
  economic (work), 46n2, 73, 153, 171, 180, 226
  emotional, 2, 10, 84, 136, 145–146, 153–155, 160, 165
  eternal, 307
  form of, x, 85–92, 96–98
  mental, 60, 237, 248
  private (family), 1–2, 6, 21, 37, 48n32, 74, 110, 158, 163, 180, 184, 285, 295
  public, 1–2, 6, 204, 255, 295
  real (everyday), 19, 36, 44, 113, 133–137, 144–145, 174, 184, 193, 199, 201–203, 207, 217n15, 233, 287
  social, 6, 81, 87, 136, 153, 164, 199, 204, 317, 325
Life science, 9, 247, 268, 298, 317. See also Biology
Limbic system, 31, 318
Linguistic market, 257, 294
Lion, 58
Lobotomy, 291
Loneliness, loner, 245–248, 255
Love, 39, 74, 76, 81–85, 97, 151, 158, 167, 212, 275, 277
Lover, 157–159, 261. See also Boyfriend; Girlfriend

Low-functional autists (LFA), 254
LSD (lysergic acid diethylamide), 134
Lust, 193, 291
Lying, 276. *See also* Cheating; Faking;
    Pretending

Macho, 171. *See also* Man (idealtype)
Magazine, 134, 270
Magnetic resonance imaging (MRI), 4, 41,
    105–106, 111, 201, 249. *See also* Functional
    magnetic resonance imaging (fMRI)
Magnetoencephalography (MEG), 104, 111,
    200
Mammal, mammalian, 4, 8, 35, 73, 213, 260,
    297, 322
Mammon, 167
Man (idealtype), xii, 15, 41, 70, 80n1, 194,
    203, 238, 259. *See also* Macho
"The New Man," xi, 151, 164, 166
Management. *See also* Self-Management
    conflict, 135
    economic, 136, 142, 179–181, 183, 208
    emotion, 76, 100n29, 126, 141–142,
        145–147, 154, 160, 176n4, 179, 182,
        185–189, 303
    health, 114, 188–189
    of procreation, 73
    strategy, 122, 180
    scientific, 180
    social, 156, 208
    stress, 124
    technique, x, 38
Manager, 136, 161, 163, 165, 179–183,
    208–209
Manipulation, 113, 158–159, 172
Market, 4, 7, 9, 17–18, 37–44, 80, 105, 110,
    163–164, 167, 176, 180, 183, 193–198, 201,
    206, 212, 239, 250, 257, 262, 270, 277,
    292–309
    market participant, xi, 196
    marketplace, 112, 153
Marketing, 111, 191, 198, 200, 204–205, 261,
    278, 295, 303–306. *See also* Neuromarketing

Marriage, 71, 78–83, 87, 97, 98n1, 157–159,
    165, 169, 171–175, 274, 300–301. *See also*
    Wedding
Masculinity (virility), 11, 58, 70–77, 166,
    171–174, 189, 276, 303, 326
Masochism, 75–76
Mass, 86, 151, 201, 254, 286, 309
    media, 221, 295, 307
    society, 16, 151
Masturbation, 79, 302
Match, matching, 78, 88–89, 267, 275,
    288
Materialism, 59–60
Materialist, 56
Materiality, 79, 81, 88, 90–92, 96, 99n14,
    239–244, 261, 290
Mathematician, mathematics, 12, 59, 106,
    130n2, 132–134, 141, 254–256, 264–265,
    268, 272, 275, 277, 283
Mating, ix, 5, 29, 46n2, 175, 252
    m. intelligence, 5, 29
Mean(s), ix, xi, 30, 32, 61, 97, 183, 208, 240,
    244, 257, 301
Mean average, 263
Meaning, 5, 10–11, 21–24, 39, 46n6, 55, 72,
    77, 86, 88, 95, 99n17, 143, 151, 158,
    168–169, 210, 235, 246, 290, 297, 305–309,
    324, 328
Measure(s), 12, 23, 27, 58–60, 74–75, 84,
    104
    ability, 139
    maximum-performance, 139–140
    self-report, 145
    typical-performance, 139–140
Measurement, xi, 12, 23, 27, 104, 107, 119,
    123, 126, 131, 136, 138–144, 175, 187, 192,
    207, 209
Media, xi, 31, 242, 257. *See also* Mass media
    audiovisual, 221, 228–234
    entertainment, 227
    communication, 221, 225–226
    coverage, 137
    star, 254

Mediality, 242

Medicine, 20, 28, 44, 59, 72–79, 109, 112, 114, 195, 238, 242, 245, 247, 253, 258, 281–285, 290, 305

Meditation, 308–309

MEIS (multifactor emotional intelligence scale), 140, 143, 147

Melancholy, 226, 286

Melodrama, 95, 226–227, 234

Memory, 22, 61, 89, 91, 108, 110, 118, 145, 198, 256, 288, 291–292, 297, 324

Mendelian genetics, 280

Menopause, 261

Menschenbild, 41, 67, 239

Mental health, 144, 161, 171

Mental illness, 21, 134, 296

Mentality, 184, 245, 303

Mental retardation, 21, 254, 264, 281

Mental state, 21, 113, 187, 193, 207, 246, 250, 318–324

Mercury, 245, 263, 278–279, 313n3

Merit, 17, 215

Meritocracy, 18–20

Meta-emotion, xi, 225–227, 236n2

Metaphor, x, 7, 9, 24, 32, 39, 93, 151, 232, 240–246, 252, 268, 288, 310–311, 324

Meta-subject, 35, 326

Method, methodology, vii, x, xii, 1, 12, 18–23, 27–30, 61, 66–67, 85, 103–110, 113, 115, 125–129, 198, 204, 263–264, 282–292, 317, 327–328

Microanatomy, 66

Microscope, microscopic, 76, 249

Microstructure, 66

Middle Ages, 309–310

Milieu, 73, 166, 177n11

Mimics, 237

Mind, 3–7, 11, 17–18, 27, 32–35, 45, 55, 58, 83, 86, 91, 113, 162, 169, 193, 196, 213, 239, 241–289, 304, 308–310, 318–328

  mastermind, 45

  theory of, 4, 6, 193, 241–243, 250–251, 268, 292, 322, 324

Mindblindness, 241, 246, 251. *See also* Systemblindness

Mind reading, 6, 263, 303

Mineness, 310

Minority, 42, 79, 156, 197, 210, 278, 299

Mirror neurons, 36, 223, 231–232, 241, 252, 262, 273–274, 323–324

Misogynist, misogynous, 4, 36, 60, 285, 306

MLQ (multifactor leadership questionnaire), 209

Modality, modal, 30, 48n31, 229–230, 234, 252, 298

Mode, 235

Model, vii, ix, xii, 2, 4, 8, 30, 40, 60, 66, 72–73, 83, 91, 118–123, 128, 133, 135, 143, 152, 154, 168–171, 192–194, 207–213, 224, 239–249, 256, 259–261, 267, 269, 274, 279, 288, 294, 297–304, 320, 323–327. *See also* Self-model

  cultural, 164, 171

  emotional, x, 171, 224, 288

Modernism, 305

Modernity, 165, 171, 174, 306

Module, 241, 243, 268

Molecule, molecular, 35, 105, 280

Mongolian type, 41

Money, 17, 28, 37, 43–44, 152, 175–176, 190, 198–199, 203, 211, 216–217, 262, 269

Monitoring, 105, 108, 115, 156, 222

Monkey, 46n2, 61, 213–214, 235n1, 237, 269, 322–322. *See also* Ape

Monkey fissure (*Affenspalte*), 61

Mood, 30, 122–127, 141, 144, 225, 230, 234, 236, 291–292

Moral, 21, 55, 61, 74, 79, 97, 120–121, 133–135, 156, 169, 233–234, 258, 264, 276, 285, 287, 290, 302, 327

Morphology, 40, 59, 77, 244

Mortality, 30. *See also* Death

Mother, 71, 75, 81, 170, 172, 238, 243, 245, 251, 257, 259–260, 268, 271, 277–282, 301. *See also* Nurture

Motivation, 33, 119, 158, 208, 223, 226, 234, 236n2, 243–244, 320, 324
  extrinsic, 44, 127, 225, 326
  intrinsic, 122, 176n4, 183, 264, 319
MSCEIT (Mayer-Salovey-Caruso emotional intelligence test), x, 125–127, 129, 140–143, 146–148
Multiple personality disorder (MPD), 247, 255, 257, 263, 298
Multiple sclerosis, 105
Museum, 295
Music, musician, 48n22, 229–231, 242–243, 285, 311
Muslim, 308
Myers-Briggs type-indicator, 154
Myth, 210, 300

Narration, narrative, 118, 165, 170, 174, 227–234, 269
Nation, 28, 76, 167, 264, 314n17
National Institutes of Health, 70, 280
National intelligence, 41
Naturalization, 8, 35, 54, 167
Nature, 7, 10, 13, 16, 27, 30, 34, 39–42, 54–55, 59, 67, 79, 70–81, 86, 93–97, 125, 146, 151, 170, 193, 201, 213–214, 224, 229–230, 240–243, 248, 256, 261–262, 268–275, 285–288, 295–298, 302, 305, 308, 310, 322–326
  human, 29, 36, 54, 81, 240, 294, 297–298
Near infrared spectroscopy, 104
Needs, 174–175, 180, 183, 300
  emotional, 156, 235
  organizational, 183
  societal, 240, 246, 258
NEO-FFI (NEO-five-factor inventory), 290
Neoclassical economics, 192, 194–195
Neocortex, 318
Neoliberalism, 180, 184. See also Liberal
Nerve, 67, 298, 320
Network, 195, 268
  associative, 222, 228
  neural, 30, 36, 203, 222–223, 245, 249, 288

  random scale-free, 279
  social, 163, 165, 181
Neural, 3, 7, 22, 29, 35, 46n2, 104, 106, 202, 222–224, 249, 252, 273, 281, 288, 291, 299–300, 308, 311, 317, 319, 323–327
Neuroanatomy, 65
Neuroarchitecture, 37, 248
Neurobiologist, 37–38, 314n14
Neurobiology, xii, 1, 22, 28, 35–37, 43, 45, 185, 191, 213, 272, 282, 289–290, 320, 325, 328
Neurodiversity, 254
Neuroeconomics, viii, xi, 5, 30, 45, 47n10, 191–215
Neuroendocrinologist, 8, 299
Neuroendocrinology, 243, 279
Neuroimage, ix–x, 12–13, 22, 27–28, 38–39, 202, 238, 242, 247–248, 264–265, 288–289, 294. See also Brain image
Neuroimaging, 23, 28, 30–41, 103–116, 195, 201, 210–211, 292, 311, 319. See also Brain imaging
Neurologist, 61, 305
Neurology, 105, 137
Neuromarketing, 191–192, 195, 202, 205
Neuromythology, 35
Neuron, 35–36, 77, 89, 144, 213, 244–245, 273, 290–291. See also Mirror neuron; Spindle neuron
Neurophilosophy, 5, 36, 45, 317–318
Neuroplasticity, 8, 30, 297. See also Plasticity
Neuropsychology, 22, 107, 235
Neurosis, 152, 163
Neurosociology, xii, 5, 317, 324
Neurotheology, 5, 43, 308–309
Neuroticism, neurotic, 122, 124, 139, 290
Neurotransmitter, 2, 4, 84, 89, 213, 249, 289, 291
Neurotypic, 238, 254, 256
Newspaper, 211, 272, 277, 295, 304. See also Journal; Magazine
Nobel Prize, 194
Nonknowledge, 18, 257, 279, 294, 309

Normality, 5, 21–24, 44, 75, 108–110, 200,
    237–248, 250–254, 259–268, 275–280,
    287–289, 294–298, 319, 327
Normative, 5, 11, 22, 29, 32, 36, 39–43, 92,
    96, 100n30, 125, 171, 179, 182, 186, 215,
    222, 228, 235, 247, 289–290, 295, 298, 328
Norms, 2, 9, 13, 27–28, 73–74, 79, 82, 84, 92,
    96, 174, 184, 201–210, 221, 227, 232,
    234–235, 238, 268, 278, 287–289, 291, 295
  emotional, 82, 92, 96–98, 235
  social, 258, 268, 278, 287, 289. *See also*
  Recognition
"Nothing," 310–311
Novel, 257, 324
Nucleus accumbens (NA), 2, 15, 84, 203,
    color plates 2–3
Nurture, 10, 76–77, 193, 214, 224, 272–273.
    See also Mother
Nymphomania, 75

Object, 7, 11, 13, 40, 44, 53, 55, 74, 77, 89,
    90, 159, 201–202, 231, 238, 240–241,
    247–249, 255–256, 260–262, 274, 280, 286,
    296–298, 318, 320
  epistemic, 240, 279, 284
Objectification, 202, 217n16, 259, 296
Objectivation, 35, 259
Ontology/ontic, 5, 13, 22, 30, 34, 40, 42,
    241–242, 257, 259, 263, 289, 309–310
Open-minded, 209
Openness, 44, 123
Oppression, 7, 80, 175, 291
Optimism, 123–124, 129, 134–135, 148, 189
Orbitofrontal cortex, 2, 203
Organ, 8, 22, 31, 34, 37, 55–56, 242, 282,
    284, 292, 296
Organic, 75, 252
Organism, 4, 29, 301, 305, 320–321
Organization, 6, 153, 160–161, 164, 171,
    180–184, 189, 192, 195, 207, 209–210, 254,
    326
Organology, 55–59
Orgasm, 21, 75, 260, 275

Originality, original, 5, 27, 42, 58, 77, 89,
    112, 188, 244, 255, 257, 263, 270, 301,
    323
Othering (otherness), 239, 245, 254, 280,
    294, 297, 301. *See also* Alien
Ovary (Ovaries), 283
Oxytocin (OT), 212–213, 249, 252, 289

Pain, 2–4, 14–15, 31, 37, 39, 48n, 82–83, 91,
    97, 99n26, 111, 175, 202–207, 260, 265,
    273, 288, 298, 310–311, 320
Paradigm, paradigmatic, 89–90, 159, 168,
    172, 175, 200, 202, 215–216, 282
Parents, parenthood, 8, 48n28, 77, 82, 129,
    225–226, 285, 302
Parthenogenesis, 281
Participation, 6, 168, 197, 294
Pathologization, 21, 75, 258, 299
Pathology, 21, 28, 72, 74, 78, 105, 113–114,
    160, 253, 258, 271, 298
Patient, 46n4, 105, 112, 114–115, 157, 253,
    258, 291, 296, 316, 327
Patriarchy, 74
Pay gap, 17
Payment, 17, 256
Peacock's tail, 205
Pedophilia, 109
Penetration, 72. *See also* Intercourse
Penis, 74, 77
Perception, 15, 31–32, 40, 67, 84, 109, 112,
    125–128, 144, 185, 198, 202, 229, 231, 239,
    259, 284, 292
Perfection, 184
Performance, 221, 227, 229–230, 234, 237
  job, 127, 183
  maximum, 139–140
  performative action, 300
  typical, 139–140
  work, 154, 174, 182
Performativity, 19, 98n7, 237
Performer
  star, 16, 181–182, 189, 301
  top, 161, 301

Person (human), 4, 29, 44, 71, 240, 246, 261, 318, 324–325. *See also* Personhood
Personality, 1, 5, 9, 18, 29, 33, 115, 122–131, 134–147, 153–154, 163, 176, 209, 236n3, 237, 247, 252, 257, 262–263, 277–279, 285–292, 301, 309, 323–326
traits, 124, 140, 290–291
Personhood, 29, 224, 258, 273, 326
Pervasive developmental disorder (PDD), 254, 292, 313n1
Perversion, 75–76
Pessimistic, 41
Pharmacogenetics, 4, 279, 292
Phenomenology, xii, 31–32, 133, 246, 252, 258, 305, 311
Phenotype, 8, 11, 238, 245–248, 253, 281, 284, 292, 294
Philosopher, 8, 42–43, 60, 86–87, 90, 98n5, 99n16, 133, 217n19, 241, 245–246, 253, 255, 273, 304, 306–307, 311, 314n17, 317, 324
Philosophy, xii, 23, 36, 40, 72, 85, 87, 133, 239, 241, 274, 276, 314n17, 319
cultural, ix, 6, 39
of science, 6, 40, 43, 244, 279, 284, 291
Photograph, 23–24, 28, 39, 103, 105, 125, 141, 205, 242–250, 287–288. *See also* Picture
Physical, 3, 5, 11, 29, 32–38, 48n31, 53, 70–74, 104–105, 115, 141, 174, 186, 204, 229–234, 240, 244–245, 286, 311, 318, 321
Physiognomy, 58–61
Picture, 59, 107, 120, 122, 156, 230, 296, 321–322, 324. *See also* Brain image; Neuroimage; Photograph
Placenta, 243
Plant soul (*anima vegetativa*), 242
Plasticity, 8, 30, 67–68, 107, 115, 224, 297. *See also* Neuroplasticity
Pleasure, 20–21, 75, 151, 211, 233, 235, 260, 320
Pluralism, 45, 157, 193, 257, 314
Plurality, 171

Poet, 57, 241
Poetry, 94
Policy, ix, 16, 39, 197, 200, 212, 253, 279, 306
Political correctness (PC), 27, 41, 53, 69, 71–72
Politician, 12, 46n6, 185, 241, 247,
Political scientist, 121
Politics, 16, 18, 27, 33, 40–45, 46n6, 53–55, 60, 66, 69–79, 85, 92, 96–97, 121, 153, 155, 168–169, 180–189, 197, 211–215, 253, 257, 259, 264, 287–296, 300, 306–309, 314n17, 317
biopolitics, 13, 285, 292
life, 169
memoro-politics, 287–288, 292
Polygamy, 261, 275, 302
Poor, 151, 167, 200
Pop Science, vii–viii, xi, 1, 3, 6–7, 12, 19, 43–46, 208, 211, 238–239, 245, 260–267, 281, 294–311
Pornography, 79
Pose, 54–55, 84–86
"the cool pose," 175
Position, 17, 19, 66–67, 114, 132–133, 152, 158, 162, 170, 176, 205, 209, 215, 273, 309
Positron emission tomography (PET), 104–105, 112, 292
Possibility, 43–44, 45, 86, 126, 175, 205, 241, 252, 257, 285
Poststructuralism, 85–86, 97–98
Potentiality, 242–243
Potentials, 3, 30, 243–244, 258, 285, 291, 299
Power, 16–18, 28, 56, 67, 91, 113, 133, 159, 176, 182, 192, 195, 205, 209–210, 215, 240, 243, 251, 255, 257, 270, 272, 277, 292, 296, 298, 300
Practice, 18–19, 36, 72, 76, 85–87, 91, 96–98, 115, 144, 154, 160, 164, 182, 186, 225, 258
Predator type (*Raubtiertypus*), 61

Prefrontal cortex, 26, 109, 222–223

Prefrontal lobe, 318

Prenatal, 77, 106, 259, 265, 282–289

Prestige, 81, 152, 176

Pretending, 38, 88, 276. *See also* Cheating; Faking; Lying

Primitive, 3, 35, 37, 58, 61. *See also* Savage; Tribal

Prisoner's dilemma game (PDG), 202–203

Private. *See* Life, private

Probability, 199, 260, 281

Processing, 2, 7, 12, 19, 29, 84, 88–91, 99, 105, 115, 133, 138–139, 143, 145, 156, 158, 201, 229–230, 241, 256, 269, 319–320, 325

Procreation, 73–75, 189

Productivity, 10, 134, 144, 160–161, 179–190, 212

Profession, professional, 37, 39, 48n33, 61, 65–66, 95, 114, 154, 158–161, 164–170, 179, 184, 196, 203, 226, 326

Profile, 42, 110, 137, 166, 233

Profit, 137, 161, 184, 191, 247, 302, 304

Projection, 229–230

Property right, 42

Prospect theory, 216

Prostitution, 79

Prototype, prototypical, 122, 222, 228–232, 277, 310

Provocation, 109, 251, 273, 303–304

Pseudoscience, xi, 303

Psychiatrist, 238, 249, 254, 281

Psychoanalysis, 36, 143, 151, 154, 169–170, 328

Psychological persuasion, 153, 157–158, 170

Psychological test, 112, 136, 249. *See also* Test

Psychologist, 6, 8–9, 34, 36, 39, 41, 48n33, 84, 87- 91, 107, 114, 117, 119, 121–122, 132–134, 144, 154–155, 157–161, 163, 165–171, 176n2, 179, 213, 238, 242, 244, 258, 272, 281–282, 300, 314n14, 322

Psychology, ix, xi, 4–5, 7, 27–28, 34–37, 39–41, 48n31, 56, 66, 87, 90, 99, 103, 112, 117–120, 122–123, 133, 136, 139, 144, 164,

176, 184–185, 191, 208, 213, 217, 221, 238–242, 248, 255–259, 279, 287–288, 299–301

applied, 131, 258

clinical, 155, 157

cognitive, 106–107, 121, 159, 241, 289

differential, 138

evolutionary, 263, 269, 290, 328

Psychopathology, 145, 247, 282, 289

Psychotherapy, 288

Public, 123, 229, 272, 300

Publicity, 295

Punishment, 3, 37–38, 48n31, 100n30, 204

Purification, 43, 74

Purity, 79, 152, 184, 275

Qualia-problem, 47n19, 207

Quality, 8, 109, 115, 127, 135, 137, 146, 151, 207, 211, 215, 224

Queer, 12

Questionnaire, 7, 42, 65–66, 121, 321. *See also* MLQ; Trait Emotional Intelligence Questionnaire

Race, 7, 23–25, 40–42, 48n28, 56, 61, 65–66, 109, 121, 197, 210, 256, 321. *See also* Blackness; Ethnicity; Whiteness

Racism, 61, 68, 264, 327

Rat, 77, 269

Rationality, 5, 28, 32–33, 44, 47n18, 182, 184, 188–192, 196, 199, 202, 213, 298, 300, 314n17, 317–318, 326

Reaction, 38, 84, 89, 117, 125, 191, 194, 201–202, 205, 207, 231, 293

Realism, 193, 255

Reality, 39, 43, 77, 87, 123, 185–186, 190, 196, 209, 229, 303–308, 314n6. *See also* Augmented reality

The Reality Club, 304–307

Reason, 6, 19, 21, 28, 34, 40, 56, 65, 67, 71, 84, 86, 91–96, 113, 119, 136, 138, 168, 212, 229, 242, 244, 254, 265, 278, 298, 323–326

Recognition (philosophical), xii, 88–92, 176, 188, 245, 277

Recognition (sociological), 168, 287

Recognition (psychological), 117, 135, 145, action, 274

face, 118, 141, 223, 250

race, 141

speech, 41, 90–92, 118

visual, 89, 118, 256

word, 41, 91

Recruitment, 17–18, 28, 161, 181

Regulation, 30, 38, 48n32, 80, 135, 145, 182–183, 187, 200, 222, 231, 290, 320–321

Relationship, 5, 8, 54, 68, 123, 130n2, 139–142, 146, 152–153, 158, 170–174, 184, 201, 205, 208, 238, 278, 290, 317

Religion, 13, 25–26, 33, 43, 55, 72–73, 131, 286, 307–308, 328, *See also* Neurotheology

Representation, 5, 7, 12, 31–33, 56, 61, 221–222, 227–234, 247–248, 263–265, 286, 311, 320, 323–325

Reproduction, 5, 29–30, 42, 73–74, 76, 78–79, 106, 113, 214, 247, 251, 253, 268, 275, 281, 284, 302–303, 306, 310

social, 156, 168

symbolic, 168

Resource(s), 73, 88, 153, 157, 167–168, 171, 174, 181, 189, 194, 213, 257

economic, 53

emotional, 37, 152

symbolic, 252

Response, 15, 35, 79, 97, 105, 107, 109, 139, 186, 245, 320, 324

Emotional, 26, 33, 39, 41, 90, 100n30, 107, 158–159, 175, 201, 206, 222, 224

Social, 26

Responsibility, 10, 28, 54, 184, 190, 194, 211, 296

Revenge, 15, 38, 203–207, 288–289

Reward, 17, 20, 35, 37, 79, 152, 199–207, 212, 289, 291

reward center (of the brain), 20, 199, 205, 212

Risk, 109, 114, 116, 155, 157, 199, 216n12, 268, 279, 284, 311, 321–327

Ritual, 74, 94, 162, 294, 238

Robot, robotics, 5, 7, 19, 30, 239–242, 246, 252, 277, 319

Role congruity theory, 210

Romance, 76, 234

Romantic, 56–58, 74, 81

Rule, 53, 59, 81, 86–87, 141, 158–165, 171, 174, 179, 197, 203, 221, 226, 230–234, 257, 269, 272

Sad Film Scale, 227

Sadism, 75

Sadness, 29, 125, 176n4, 225, 227–228, 250

Same-sex sexual(ity), 12, 24, 74–75, 79, 251, 253, 302–303. *See also* Gay; Homosexual(ity); Inversion

Satisfaction, 38, 127–128, 134, 146, 169, 180, 209

Satyriasis, 75

Savage, 238, 268–269. *See also* Primitive; Tribal

Savant, 134, 254

Scenario, 66, 187–188

Schizophrenia, 110, 239, 253, 258–259, 262, 267, 292–293

School, 17–18, 42, 79, 109, 133, 165, 258

Scientific citizenship, 294

Scientific community, 78, 103, 117, 194, 215, 250, 253, 264, 295, 302, 306

Science writer, 44, 46n3, 303–307

Scientist, 1, 5, 8, 11–12, 20–24, 29, 35, 42–44, 58, 60–61, 69–76, 86, 103, 111, 114–119, 121–123, 131–132, 185–186, 199–203, 212–215, 238–244, 250, 253–260, 268–273, 280, 284, 295, 303–308

Scoring, 124, 126–128, 132, 136, 139–142, 146, 255, 264–268, 277, 299, 301, 306

consensus, 125–126, 141

expert, 125–126, 141

target, 125, 141

Screening, 109, 113, 154, 253

Seduction, 261

Selection, 41, 76, 114, 123, 145, 161, 214, 255, 262, 269, 304, 326

Self, xii, 3–6, 9, 13–17, 28–44, 72, 82–87, 91, 94, 96, 120, 155–159, 167, 170, 177n10, 179, 183, 188, 192, 194, 196, 222, 234, 239–263, 268, 277, 290, 296, 307–310, 314n17, 315n17, 317, 319, 320–327. *See also* Technology of the Self

 no-self, 308

 second, 247–248, 263, 288

Self-abnegation, 251, 284

Self-assessment, 135

Self-assertion, 165

Self-awareness, 135, 160–161, 170, 176, 208, 222–223, 252, 322. *See also* Awareness

Self-care, 184, 187. *See also* Care

Self-confidence, 135, 162, 189, 226

Self-consciousness, 94, 139, 158, 167, 177n16, 321, 324

Self-control, 33, 122, 134, 135, 176n4, 182, 224, 251, 252, 257

Self-dignity, 175

Self-discipline, 121, 123

Self-distance, 309

Self-enhancement, 13, 124, 209, 214, 227

Self-esteem, 252, 325

Self-fashioning, 303

Self-government, 181

Self-healing, 296, 309

Self-help, 170–171, 275

Selfhood, 163–171, 177n16, 310

Self-image, 28, 44, 116, 129

Self-insight, 145

Self-interest, 155, 193. *See also* Interest

Selfishness, 33. *See also* Egocentrism

Self-judgment, 276

Self-maintenance, 305

Self-management, 135, 163, 165, 180, 184, 187, 208

Self-model, 320, 324, 327. *See also* Model

Self-motivation, 183, 319

Self-observation, 163

Self-occupancy, 193, 246. *See also* Egocentrism

Self-organization, 252, 304

Self-preservation, 325

Self-rating, 145

Self-regard, 124, 129

Self-report, 123–124, 129, 139, 142, 145–147, 303

Self-representation, xi, 320, 324

Self-responsibility, 186, 190

Self-transcendence, 307

Self-transformation, 179, 185

Self-understanding, 191, 310

Semantic, 39, 88, 99

Sensation, 31, 141, 202, 206, 260

Senses, 10, 22, 31, 40, 163, 186, 229, 275, 293, 327

Sensibilité, 47, 95

Sensitivity, 14, 22, 39, 47, 59, 89–90, 93–97, 104, 108, 110, 114–116, 120, 128–131, 135, 176, 185–186, 189, 206, 215, 270, 275, 291, 293

Sensorimotor, 111, 224, 228, 232, 234, 287, 289

Sensors, 186–188

Sentiment, 30, 167

Sentimental, 82

Sentimentalist, 97

Sexism, 41, 61, 68

Sexist, 59, 204

Sex object, 77

Sexual abuse, 255, 289, 299

Sexual arousal, 20–21, 46n2, 47n15, 103, 110, 250, 260–261, 298

Sexuality, 2, 9–12, 20, 44, 47n21, 48n27, 72–80, 251, 261, 283, 303

Sexualization, x, 8, 273, 286

Sexual identity, 24, 73

Sexual life, 78, 174

Sexual offender, 302

Sexual orientation, 108, 210

Shame, 33, 93, 155, 320–321

Signal, 13, 35, 69, 72, 91, 104, 160, 201, 205, 212, 248, 321–322

Simulation, 212, 228, 273

Single photon emission computed tomography (SPECT), 104

Skills, 38, 90, 96, 118–122, 129–130, 135–136, 140, 147–148, 155–156, 160, 163, 165, 170–176, 182–183, 193, 208, 221–228, 234–236, 248, 251, 255, 258, 262, 265, 267, 275, 278, 281, 287–290, 302

Skin, 31, 61, 179, 185, 186, 201, 244
   enhanced second skin, viii, xi, 179, 185

Skull, x, 56–57, 61, color plate 6

Smart clothes, 185

Sociability, 122, 162–163, 278, 319

Social cognitive science, 24, 40, 239, 268, 292

Social dominance, 205, 322

Social mobility, 16, 152–156, 287

Social neuroscience, 4, 13, 22–23, 25–27, 34, 37, 240, 250, 253, 259, 288–290, 298, 319, 328, color plates 3–5

Social system, 13, 252, 269, 326–327

Sociality, 193, 212–213, 240, 273–274, 321

Socialization, 128–129, 156, 165, 226–227, 315n17

Sociology, xii, 6, 13, 16, 22–23, 36, 43, 48n25, 151–156, 167–168, 174, 176, 193, 197, 208, 258, 319, 321, 328

Sociologist, 16, 34, 43, 78, 98n5, 156, 158, 160, 165, 167, 174–175, 208, 294, 304

Sociophobe, 237

Soul, 4–5, 32, 60, 241–247, 256, 259, 287, 292, 322, 327

Spatial, 9, 12, 16, 30, 37, 104–108, 145, 231–240, 243–244, 271, 283, 308, 322

Species, 4, 29–30, 76, 217, 255, 273, 310, 322–323

Sperm, 76, 260–261

Spindle neurons, 35, 244. *See also* Neuron

Spinster, 152

Spontaneity, 10, 153, 164–165, 181, 222, 277, 293

Stability, 67, 110, 139, 151, 197, 242, 290

Standardization, 115, 202, 209

Star, stardom, 16, 181–182, 189, 287, 299

Startle reflex, 27

Statistics, 12, 22, 59, 118, 121, 207, 247, 263, 279, 283, 287

Status, 17, 28, 34–35, 40, 46n6, 53, 59, 78, 81, 103–106, 121, 131, 136, 158, 162–169, 197, 205–207, 239, 243, 259, 263–264, 269–270, 298, 303

Stereotype, 2, 8, 10–13, 18–19, 23–24, 37, 39, 42, 53–54, 58, 116, 129, 136, 147, 166, 197, 204, 206, 209–210, 214, 230, 256, 267, 270, 276, 294, 306

Sterile, 72, 76

Stigma, 1, 22–25, 27, 41, 47n17, 115, 278

Stigmatization, 23–25, 61, 238, 278, 290

Stimulus, 24, 37, 89, 107, 109, 134, 143, 203, 205, 213, 216, 222–229, 231–235, 323

Stoic, Stoicism, 82, 94, 274

Stone Age, 38–39, 268

Strategy, 126, 197, 262, 269, 273, 285, 295, 301–308, 314n10

Stratification (social), xii, 153, 156, 176, 287

Stress, xi, 10, 21, 39–41, 108, 109, 114, 122, 124, 129, 139, 182, 187–189, 259, 285, 290
   See also Coping, stress

Structural magnetic resonance imaging (sMRI), 104

Structure, 5, 8, 12, 16, 24, 33–34, 40, 42, 50, 56–66, 71, 74, 79, 91, 96, 104–108, 151, 153, 163–169, 181, 204–205, 231–232, 237, 243, 245, 252, 257–258, 261, 267, 272, 277, 279, 298, 303, 36

Style, 22, 59, 72, 85, 96, 100n30, 122, 129, 131–132, 163, 166–167, 208–209, 266, 269, 277

Subculture, 7

Subject, 4, 6, 22, 30, 55, 60, 84, 86, 89–90, 95, 114–115, 123, 157, 163, 174, 179–184, 189–190, 197, 200–202, 214, 224, 246, 248, 261, 283, 287, 290, 297, 317–318

Subjectification, 184

Subjectivation, 35, 259, 302

Subjectivity, 4, 6, 30, 33, 36, 71, 86, 217, 326–327

Subordination, 70

Success, 2, 19, 43, 46n5, 85, 96–97, 108, 117, 121, 123, 132–136, 144, 153–154, 160, 179–185, 189, 210, 290, 296, 301–304, 321, 328

Suffering, 31, 82, 97, 157, 174, 238, 278, 290

Superiority, 112, 115, 144–145, 234, 254

Surgery, x, 28, 46, 78, 109–111, 296

Surprise, 10, 78, 125, 241, 276, 288, 307

Survival, 1, 4, 8, 29, 73, 205, 214, 206, 268–269, 289, 308, 320–325

Susceptibility (of genes), 290

Symbol, x, 79, 182, 276, 286

Symmetry, 2

Sympathy, 10, 21, 69, 129, 142, 201, 209, 226–227, 232, 235, 238, 259, 263, 266, 273–274, 290, 320–322

Systemblindness, 251, 303. *See also* Mindblindness

Systemizer, 208, 251, 265, 270, 288. *See also* Type, S-type

Systemizing (cognitive style), 2, 208, 256–267, 270–271, 277, 286, 300, 302, 305, 310

Systemizing quotient (SQ), 265–266, 276–277, 287, 303

Systems biology, 247, 251, 288

Talk show, 176n5, 314n10, 314n14

Tax, 211–212

Taylorism, 180

Team, teamwork, 127–128, 136, 147, 249

Technical, 7, 69, 148, 161, 181, 186, 188, 242, 244, 249, 308

Technique, x, 2, 5, 9, 12, 28–32, 38, 76–77, 104–105, 110, 116, 131, 137, 180–184, 189, 197, 201, 205, 233, 249, 258, 270, 284, 290, 292, 300, 319

Technofeminist, 19

Technofuturism, 4, 307–308

Technology, 19–20, 28, 104, 111, 179, 183, 188–189, 240, 249, 253, 262, 272, 276–277, 280, 284, 294, 303

Technology Assessment, x, 103

Technology of the self, xi, 179, 183–184, 188–189

Technomorphous, 297

Technophobia, 283

Temper, 36, 93

Temperament, 34, 140

Temporal, 37, 105–108, 199, 223, 250, 308, 310, 324

Test, x, 18, 37, 40, 42, 48n28, 49n35, 106, 110–111, 118–148, 156, 161, 197, 209, 249–250, 263–266, 272, 275–276, 287, 301, 306. *See also* GWSIT; MSCEIT; NEO-FFI; Questionnaire

autism spectrum quotient (AQ), 314n7

Binet's, 21–22, 42

finger ratio, 282–283

genetic, 110, 112, 284–285

language, 283, 290

maximum performance, 138–142

paper-and-pencil, 119

performance, 124–127, 129, 139, 141

personality, 124, 153–154, 176n2, 290–291

prenatal, 282, 284–285

psychiatric, 115

reading-the-mind-in-the-eyes, 274, 287

scholastic, 154

Social Insight, 118

Verbal Scholastic Aptitude, 146

Testing culture, 27, 37, 42–43, 196, 293

Test person, 37–38, 105, 107, 109, 200–209, 323, 327

Test situation, 113

Testis, testicle(s), 283

Testosterone, 8, 29, 76, 78, 243, 249–252, 259, 262, 265, 282–283, 289, 299

Therapeutic culture, 7, 1, 58, 190, 238

Therapeutic language, 150, 170–171

Therapy, xi, 28, 43–44, 78, 109, 111, 164, 167–170, 238, 253, 291, 301

Therapist, 160

Thiomersal (also thimerosal), 244, 287, 313n3

Tissue, 89, 105

Tolerance, 121, 278
  stress, 127, 129

Tool, 6, 96, 105–106, 109, 111, 124, 156, 170,
  268–269, 282

Topos, 257

Tradition, 9, 25–26, 40, 75, 91, 94, 118, 140,
  144–145, 152, 162, 176, 185, 189, 192–199,
  202, 206, 267, 279, 292, 305, 326

Training, 5–6, 16–17, 33, 46n9, 94, 111, 114,
  121, 129, 137, 154–155, 164, 179–189,
  217n18, 226, 290, 297–301, 305

Trait, 122, 139
  Trait Emotional Intelligence Questionnaire
  (TEIQue), 140

Transcranial magnetic stimulation (TMS), 292

Transgender, 79, 272, 283, 311

Transhumanism, 304, 307–308

Transsexuality, x, xv, 23–26, 36, 77–79, 109

Tribal (society), 305, 321, 326. *See also*
  Primitive; Savage

Trieb, 242. See also Drive

Trust, 83, 170–175, 199–200, 203, 212, 268.
  See also Distrust

Truth, 1, 21, 27, 32, 83, 86, 126, 138, 262,
  270, 327

Type, 4–5, 22–27, 36–44, 61, 85, 108, 110,
  114, 127–138, 166–168, 205–209, 217,
  237–244, 258, 268–293, 300–302, 320 *See
  also* Genotype; Idealtype; Mongolian type;
  Phenotype; Predator type; Stereotype
  Clint Eastwood type, 274
  E-type, 265, 271
  pure EQ type, 10, 39, 308
  pure IQ type, 10
  S-type, 265

Ultimate game, 198, 200, 217n14. *See also*
  Game theory

Ultrasound, 284

Underacting, 228

Unemployment, 180, 184. *See also*
  Employment; Job; Work

Universe, 10–11, 272, 304–307

Uterus, 243, 249, 284. *See also* Intrauterine;
  Womb

Utility, 92, 192, 194, 198–199, 214, 216

Utopia, 38, 243, 271

Vaccination, 244

Vaccine, 263, 313, 313n3

Vagina, 72, 74

Validation, 23, 110, 115, 235

Value, 9–10, 31, 37, 40, 43, 55, 79, 91,
  99n14, 124, 144, 147, 156, 169, 171, 182,
  204, 215, 296, 303, 321

Variability, 9, 13, 71, 76–77, 92, 187

Variation, 84, 92, 241, 326

Vegetative nervous system, 32, 242, 244, 281

Viagra, 78, 80n3

Victimization, 302

Victorian, 376

Video(tape), 306

Vineland Social Maturity Scale, 118

Virgin, virginity, 81, 301

Virtue(s), 45, 73, 168, 314n17

Visibility, 249

Visualization, 12, 249, 262, 284

Vocal expression, 223

Volition, 317

Wage, 16, 38, 197. *See also* Income; Payment

Wealth, 163, 168, 200, 205, 211–212, 223

Weapon, 269

Wedding, 92. *See also* Marriage

Welfare state, 181, 184, 190

Well-being, 127–128, 146, 167–169, 175, 235,
  294, 308, 320–324

Weltoffenheit, 310

Whale, 35, 275

White matter, 55

Whiteness (as cultural category), 12, 24, 39,
  56, 65, 121, 175, 197, 294, 304

WHO (World Health Organization), 314n4

Wife, 17, 66, 76, 93, 97, 151, 155, 157, 166,
 172, 173, 274–276
Wikipedia, 255
Williams-Beuren syndrome, 245
Wisdom, 136–137, 184, 189, 221, 325
Wolf, 58, 322
Woman (idealtype), 12, 17, 20, 23–24, 29, 37,
 41, 43, 54, 56, 71, 74–75, 82, 128, 145,
 171, 176, 205, 210, 255, 259, 275–276, 281,
 301, 326
 "women's film," 234
Womb, 243, 247–250, 265, 284. *See also*
 Uterus
Work, 1, 17, 21, 37, 39, 58, 75, 114, 127,
 134, 146, 152, 158, 169, 171–172, 196–198,
 209, 249, 256, 260
 experience, 179
 performance, 154, 174, 182
 satisfaction, 127, 180 (*see also* Satisfaction)
Worker, 179, 181, 183, 189, color plate 8
Workplace, ix, 21, 37, 136, 146, 160, 167,
 170, 174, 179–190, 196, 209
Workshop, 164–165
World, 16, 31, 67, 88, 96, 155, 167, 232, 234,
 238, 248, 259, 263, 275, 277, 285, 295,
 297, 300, 303–305, 309–311
 life (real), 6–7, 10, 24, 32, 36, 133, 145,
 237–238, 240, 246, 262, 274, 288, 290, 298,
 300, 307
 industrialized (economic), 78, 196
 social, 22, 24, 144, 244, 249, 252, 272, 286,
 292, 324
 unseen, 86
Wunderkind, 299

X chromosome, 280–281
XX-type (chromosomal), 72, 244
XY-type (chromosomal), 72, 243

Yanomamo people, 268
Yin and Yang, 74

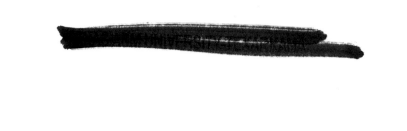